W9-ATP-803

Age Erasers

for Women

The revolutionary new plan to strip away
10 years *or more*!

BY THE EDITORS OF WOMEN'S HEALTH®

RODALE®

Mention of specific companies, organizations, or authorities in this book does not imply endorsement by the author or publisher, nor does mention of specific companies, organizations, or authorities imply that they endorse this book, its author, or the publisher.

Internet addresses and telephone numbers given in this book were accurate at the time it went to press.

© 2009 by Rodale Inc.

All rights reserved. No part of this publication may be reproduced or transmitted in any form or by any means, electronic or mechanical, including photocopying, recording, or any other information storage and retrieval system, without the written permission of the publisher.

Rodale books may be purchased for business or promotional use for special sales. For information, please write to:
Special Markets Department, Rodale Inc., 733 Third Avenue, New York, NY 10017

Women's Health is a registered trademark of Rodale Inc.

Printed in the United States of America
Rodale Inc. makes every effort to use acid-free ⊗, recycled paper ♻.

Book design by Davia Smith with Bess Yoham; contributing designer Holland Utley
Adapted from *Age Erasers for Men* designed by John Seeger Gilman
with George Karabotsos, Design Director, *Men's Health* Books

Photo Editing by Marianne Butler

Library of Congress Cataloging-in-Publication Data

Age erasers for women : the revolutionary new plan to strip away 10 years or more! / By the editors of Women's Health.
    p.   cm.
  ISBN-13: 978–1–60529–482–7   direct mail hardcover
  ISBN-10: 1–60529–482–9   direct mail hardcover
  ISBN-13: 978–1–60529–467–4   trade hardcover
  ISBN-10: 1–60529–467–5   trade hardcover
  1. Women—Health and hygiene.   I. Women's Health (Rodale Press)   II. Title.
RA778.W2268 2009
613'.04244--dc22   2009024744

Distributed to the trade by Macmillan

2 4 6 8 10 9 7 5 3 1   direct mail hardcover
  2 4 6 8 10 9 7 5 3 1   trade hardcover

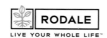

LIVE YOUR WHOLE LIFE™

We inspire and enable people to improve their lives and the world around them
For more of our products visit **rodalestore.com** or call 800-848-4735

Age Erasers

Age Erasers

Contents

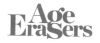

Introduction

Why Some Women Stay Young

(and How You Can, Too)

*I*f you were a Hollywood actress who reached "a certain age"—about 35—a few decades ago, your career took a noticeable turn. As new starlets appeared on the scene, studios relegated yesterday's stars to roles such as plain-as-dirt spinsters, kindly apron-wearing moms, matronly socialites, bland better halves, and no-nonsense secretaries. That transition wasn't necessarily the kiss of death (Bette Davis, for one, earned an Oscar at 42 for *All about Eve*), but they weren't especially glamorous roles (she played an aging actress being replaced by a young upstart). As for sexy, mature female icons, there simply weren't many: Coo, coo, ca-choo, Mrs. Robinson!

But today you've no doubt noticed a new breed of post-40 women. They're everywhere—magazines, advertisements, movies, television shows—and, so long as they haven't had too much work, they look *good*. Take, for instance, Kim Cattrall of *Sex and the City*, whose audacious alter ego, the 50-plus sex bomb Samantha Jones, treats men as mere notches on her Dolce & Gabbana belt. Or what about the ridiculously buff 51-year-old Madonna, who could crush Hannah Montana's microphone with a single bare hand? Or *Law & Order's* 45-year-old Mariska Hargitay—casing crime scenes, busting the perps, and making handcuffs look . . . well, actually kind of kinky.

Christy Turlington, Diane Lane, Michelle Pfeiffer, Sheryl Crow, Cate Blanchett, Salma Hayek—all 40 or older and looking as good as ever.

So how is it possible that some women can hold their own against the younger crowd? It's simple, really: They know the secrets of Age Erasers.

Sooner or later, every woman has a light-bulb moment when she realizes that her fresh looks are no longer something she can just take for granted. (Look at this photo of Marilyn—even she took precautions!) Throughout our twenties, we'll inhale a pint of Ben & Jerry's, spend Saturdays sprawled on the sofa watching *Lifetime* marathons, and even forgo our daily SPF—all the while knowing that our bodies will bounce back. But when we reach our thirties, the story begins to change. Skip a workout and your body feels softer. Our favorite expensive jeans start feeling a little too tight. Climb a few flights of stairs, and you're as winded as if you'd just finished a 5-K. Skip the moisturizer and eye cream in a rush to get out the door for work, and you're (literally) looking at a day of dry skin. Worst of all, sex by candlelight is no longer a mood-enhancer, but rather a crafty "let's hide the wrinkles" necessity.

In fact, youthful looks can slip away faster than dollars at a white sale. But know this: Smooth and glowing skin, healthy and lustrous hair, and a toned body are not something you have to kiss buh-bye as you get older. Beauty isn't the domain of just one decade—nor is it about the number of candles on your birthday cake. Youth is something you can hold on to in your forties, fifties, and beyond. All it takes is a bit of strategizing, some wisdom, and a little hard work.

That's where this book comes in. Consider it your ultimate guide to staying younger longer. We'll show you how to defy the decades so that you can feel as toned, athletic, vital, and sexy as you deserve to be. What's age got to do with it? Not a whole heck of a lot. Just ask Tina Turner—she's entering her eighth decade! Today, the ideal age is the one you're at right now.

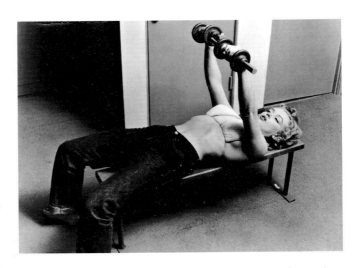

What You'll Gain from This Book

For the past five 5 years, *Women's Health*, the world's fastest-growing women's magazine, has been dispatching some of the country's best journalists to interview top doctors, dermatologists, personal trainers, nutritionists, and more—all with one goal in mind: to help you better understand your own body now and through the years. Now, everything we've learned is right at your fingertips, in this truly cutting-edge book. As you pore through these pages, you'll learn to transform not only your body—but also your life. Just think:

• **You'll get gorgeous skin and sexy hair!** We reveal the sneaky tricks the country's top stylists use to make celebrities and top models look their best—including the latest, most cutting-edge anti-aging tips. Follow their insider advice every single day to turn heads by looking 5, 10, even 15 years younger!

• **You'll learn how to achieve success—without stress!** These easy time-management skills will actually seem to lengthen your days and help you get more done in less time, and you'll discover how simple activities that you already love, such as dancing, can actually help you boost your brainpower.

• **You'll get flat abs, a firm butt, and a gravity-proof bust!** Specially designed workouts created

You can hold on to your youth, but it takes is some strategy, some craft, and some wisdom— and that's what this book has to offer you.

by more than a dozen of the country's top personal trainers help you turn the gym from a dreaded destination into your most important ally. Your dream body awaits!

• **You'll rev up your sex life and learn the secret to being irresistible to men.** Discover the secrets to a better relationship with our red-hot sex boosters—like workouts that do wonders for your sex life, food that'll get him in the mood, and naughty games guaranteed to bolster the action between the sheets.

• **You'll end aches and pains—and feel younger than ever.** The exclusive Age Erasers program is designed to firm and strengthen your entire body, putting an end to back pain, sagging energy, and annoying aches and pains.

• **You'll spend less time in the doctor's office— and add years to your life.** Heart disease is the leading cause of death for American women. How to protect yourself from such a silent, lethal killer? Follow our eight foolproof tips for keeping your ticker in top shape.

• **You'll lose weight—while you eat! With our exclusive, fat-burning eating and exercise plan, you'll see dramatic changes in your body in just weeks.** And you won't be eating rabbit food or rice cakes. We're talking delicious food your belly will crave!

• **You'll learn the smartest styles for your shape!** Top designers and fashion stylists to the stars share their sneakiest tips, like how to fake a fabulous body by choosing the right clothes, and how to conceal your biggest figure flaws—from a less-than-toned tummy to a flat butt. It's chock-full of get-chic advice for each decade!

Test Your Age—And Change It!

How old are you, really? Don't look at your driver's license, or the calendar on your BlackBerry, or the candles on your birthday cake. Chronology and your true age are two very different things, as our list of leading ladies shows.

In this book, we'll give you the tools to test your true age: Your Age Erasers Score, the definitive breakdown of just where you fall on the youth/age continuum. And then, we'll give you the tools to improve that score, to actually turn back the clock, to get younger even as the world gets older. We'll give you the tools to accurately assess your physique, your sexual performance, your brain function, your risk of disease, and more, and you'll begin to understand exactly where you fit in on the great bell curve of life. More important, you'll be able to assess your position on that bell curve, and begin to change it—to make the little changes that will slowly move your age backward, even as the clock moves forward. Throughout this book, we'll take you through the principles of the Age Erasers program and show you exactly how and why you can take total control of your life's direction.

Ready to dive in?

Turn the page, take our quiz to determine Your Age Erasers Score, and get ready to change your life, starting today!

Chapter One

What's Your True Age?

TAKE THE AGE ERASER HEAD-TO-TOE
DIAGNOSTIC AND FIND OUT HOW YOUR SCORE
COMPARES TO THE AVERAGE WOMAN

Introduction

Men, it's been said, dress up to impress women. And women dress to impress . . . other women.

Comparison is part of every woman's DNA. From tussles in the sandbox, to the mean-girl moments of junior high, to the struggles to find the perfect job, the perfect mate, and the perfect home, a woman is always testing herself against others. We understand how well we are living our lives only if we can compare them to those of our fellow citizens. That's the allure of celebrity gossip—seeing that the rich and famous are subject to conflict, romantic setbacks, and body issues means that we're not so unusual ourselves.

Well, in this chapter, we're going to find out how you're doing. We're going to give you a measurement tool that will truly mark your spot on the map—not by measuring your income or romantic conquests, or which school your children will attend. This is a measure of the most irreplaceable qualities of all: youth and vitality. We call this measurement Your Age Erasers Score.

When it comes to this score, we all start at the same basic place. Youth and vitality can't really be inherited—Mom and Dad may give you the basic building blocks, but how you manage them is entirely up to you. You certainly can't steal youth, no matter what Snow White's stepmother thought. And as for luck? Sure, it plays a small part, but when it comes to staying young, we each make our own luck—the lifestyle decisions we make every day are the biggest determining factor in how we're going to look and feel year in and year out.

And here's the great thing: Your Age Erasers Score—the definitive measure of your youth and vitality—isn't an unchangeable number. It can be improved, by making smart lifestyle choices and by following the advice in this book. Once you've keyed in on the problem areas that are hurting your overall score, you can begin to attack them, and suddenly, you'll begin to look and feel younger, stronger, healthier than you have in years.

Are you ready to take the challenge? Then let's get started!

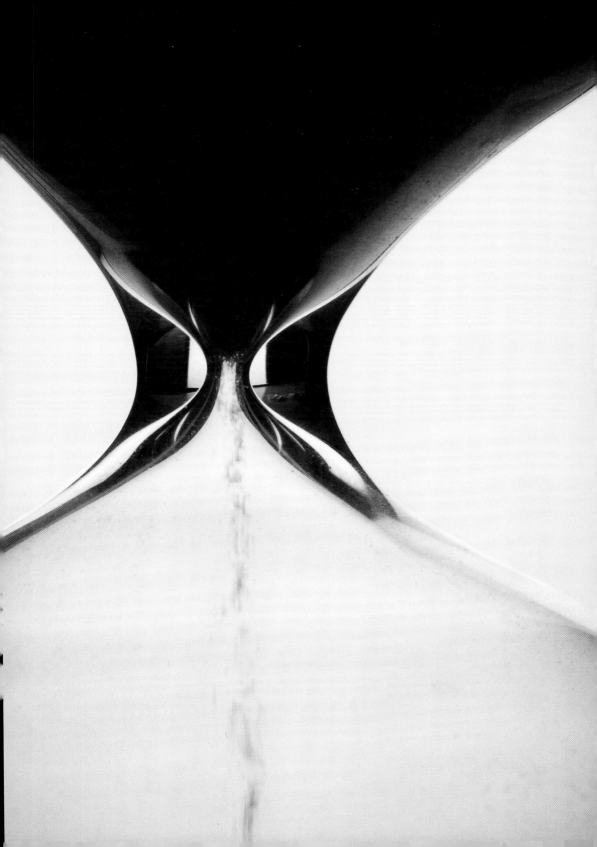

1. How Fit Are You?

1. Lower-Body Strength: Wall Sit

How long you can literally hold your own weight is the ultimate measure of your muscular endurance—the amount of time your muscles can keep going full force. That's key for everything, from being wobble-free in your favorite Ashtanga class to hauling your new flea market finds upstairs.

Instructions: Stand with your back to a wall, your feet hip-width apart. Press your head, shoulders, back, and hips against the wall, then lower your hips until your thighs are parallel to the floor. Hold for as long as possible.

		Points
Aspiring	30–59 seconds	**5**
Solid	1 minute to 1:29	**3**
Strong	1:30 or more	**1**

2. Core Strength: Hover

This move hits your transverse abdominus, one of the muscles that stabilize your core. When your core is weak, your entire body is less stable, putting you at a higher risk for sprains and strains. Beyond that, a strong middle gives you the power to sprint like a track star or serve like a Wimbledon regular.

Instructions: Get in the plank position. (This looks very similar to the starting position of a pushup, except that your forearms should lay flat on the floor with your elbows directly below your shoulders.) Contract your abdominals, glutes, and hamstrings. Hold your body perfectly straight—don't let your back arch or drop—for as long as possible.

		Points
Aspiring	Less than 45 seconds	**5**
Solid	45–59 seconds	**3**
Strong	1 minute or more	**1**

3. Upper-Body Strength: Balance Pushup

According to a 2007 study published in the journal *Applied Physiology, Nutrition, and Metabolism,* placing your hands on a Swiss ball to do pushups makes your arms work 30 percent harder than when you have them on the floor.

Instructions: Mastery of regular pushups is recommended before attempting this exercise. Get in the bottom of a pushup position with your hands on a Swiss ball. Keeping your legs and body straight and your feet hip-width apart, balance on your toes. Extend your arms and contract all your torso muscles to lift off the ball until your arms are nearly straight. Return to the starting position and repeat as many times as possible with good form.

		Points
Aspiring	1–4 pushups	**5**
Solid	5–7 pushups	**3**
Strong	8 or more pushups	**1**

4. Balance and Flexibility: Standing Bow Pose

Talk flexibility and everyone wants to know if you can touch your toes. But it's really the muscles that make up the front of your body—especially your hip flexors and quads—that are the most likely to be as stiff as frozen taffy.

Instructions: Stand tall with your feet together and your arms at your sides. Lift your left knee and balance on your right foot. Then reach back and grasp your left foot with your left hand. Raise your right arm in front of you for balance. Keeping your hips square, slowly tilt your upper body forward as one long unit while you lift your left leg even higher behind you.

		Points
Aspiring	Torso vertical to 45 degrees toward floor	**5**
Solid	Torso 46–90 degrees toward floor	**3**
Strong	Torso 91 degrees or more toward floor	**1**

5. Endurance: 5-minute Run

Running is the hallmark of cardio fitness.

Instructions: Warm up with a brisk walk for 3–5 minutes. Then up the pace and run as far as you can in 5 minutes. For the easiest scoring, do this on a treadmill.

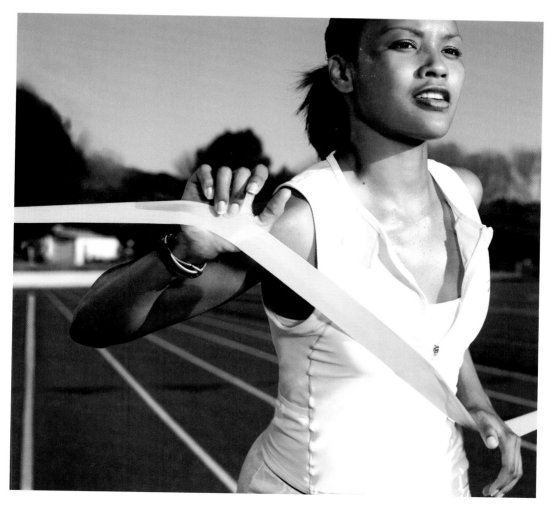

		Points
Aspiring	10-minute-mile pace or slower $^1\!/_2$ mile or less	**5**
Solid	8- to 10-minute-mile pace more than $^1\!/_2$ mile to $^2\!/_3$ mile	**3**
Strong	8-minute-mile pace or faster more than $^2\!/_3$ mile	**1**

Your Fitness Age

Add your points and compare with the following chart:

Your Points	Your Fitness Age
If you failed a test	**50**
21–25	**45**
16–20	**40**
11–15	**35**
5–10	**30**

Add your points to determine Your Fitness Age: ___

Note: The ideal scores for optimal fitness are based on reference ranges for 20- to 29-year-old women. Get a physical exam before you take these tests if you're over 40 or have two or more of these risk factors for heart disease: you're overweight, you're sedentary, you smoke, or you have high blood pressure or high cholesterol.

Reviewed by Carol Espel, MS, exercise physiologist and national director of group fitness at Equinox Fitness Clubs

2. How Old Is Your Skin?

Instructions: This test is the only one that begins with your actual age. After you answer a question, add or subtract the corresponding value from your age. Keep track of your total as you take the test.

1. Your mom's appearance can give you a clue about how genetics will affect your skin over time. How does your mom look for her age?

Pick the Best Answer   Points
a. Pretty damn amazing—she still gets looks from men half her age!.. -2
b. Not bad—she actually looks slightly younger than her age. .... -1
c. Basically, she looks her age. 0
d. She looks older than her age. .... +1

2. The pigment in naturally darker skin offers some ultraviolet UV ray protection that can slow the aging process. Describe your natural skin color.

    Points
a. Paler than nonfat milk .... +1
b. Somewhere between vanilla and café au lait 0
c. A shade of mocha .... -1
d. Rich and dark, like espresso .... -3

3. Weight changes stress your skin, but you also need some fat to keep your face looking full and young. How has your weight changed since high school?

    Points
a. I can still get into my prom dress. 0
b. I've gained a few pounds from my senior-year size. .... +1
c. Okay, I've gained more than a few pounds, but my weight stays mostly consistent. 0
d. Like hemlines, my weight goes up and down over the seasons. .... +2

4. It's no coincidence that Arizona, the sunniest state in the United States, has the country's highest rate of skin cancer. Where in the country have you lived longest?

    Points
a. Northwest.. -1
b. Southwest .... +2
c. Northeast and Midwest... 0
d. Southeast.. +1

5. Exercise improves circulation, reduces stress, and lowers blood pressure—all of which help preserve your skin's health. But too much activity can counteract all the good you're doing. Describe your level of activity:

    Points
a. I feel ashamed! I do not exercise with any regularity and know that I could be in better shape .... +2
b. I work out at least once a week, but I'm not a fanatic about it. My workouts typically last about 30 minutes, and cardio tends to play a larger role than resistance or weight training. I'm not in terrible shape . . . but I'm not in great shape, either. 0
c. I exercise three or four times a week for about an hour a session, and I regularly challenge myself with cardio as well as resistance or weight training. I feel like exercise is a priority in my life and that I'm in very good shape. .... -1
d. I'm one of the fittest people I know. I can count my rest days over the past month on one hand, and I often have marathon workouts that last multiple hours. Weights, cardio— doesn't matter. I excel at both. .... +1

6. Pinch the fleshy part of your hand between your thumb and index finger. The faster the rebound, the stronger your skin's collagen and elastin, both firming proteins. (It's best to do this test in the morning or before bed, when your body is hydrated.) How many seconds does it take for the skin to bounce back?

    Points
a. Less than a second.. -1
b. 2–3 seconds 0
c. 4–5 seconds .... +1
d. More than 5 second.. +2

7. Damage from UV rays is the biggest threat to your skin. (Wear sunscreen!) The more unprotected exposure you've had, the older you're likely to look. Which of the following statements more or less describes your sunning habits?

Points

a. I've been religious about protecting myself from the sun for years. I've almost never been burned, and having a tan isn't really a priority of mine. SPF 45 is about as low as I go, and I'll even wear sunscreen during the winter. .... **-2**

b. I've had a few bad sunburns over the years, but I usually apply plenty of sunscreen. The moisturizer I use every morning is SPF 15. I opt for SPF 30 or 45 if I'll be in the sun all day, and I reapply every few hours. .... **-1**

c. I tan throughout the summer and whenever I'm on vacation. I often apply sunscreen after I've already been in the sun for an hour. I'll use SPF 30, but 15 is more my style because I like a good tan. I'm not very good about reapplying sunscreen, though, so I tend to get a little too red. And I know I shouldn't let it happen but I get sunburned about once a summer. .... **+1**

d. Sunscreen is an afterthought. I frequently spend a few hours in the sun without protection, I get sunburned multiple times a year, and I don't have reservations about using a tanning bed. .... **+2**

8. Oily skin is rich in natural moisturizers believed to keep skin supple. Dryness and other sources of irritation cause damage below the surface that adds up over time. Which best describes your skin type?

Points

a. Oily .... **-1**
b. Normal or combination **0**
c. Dry .... **+1**
d. Dry, sensitive, and flushes easily .... **+2**

9. Check off each product below that is part of your regular skin-care routine:

○ Moisturizer
○ Sunscreen or moisturizer with sunscreen
○ Antioxidant cream or cleanser with exfoliants
○ Retinoid cream (prescription or over-the-counter)

Directions

Subtract 2 points for each check mark; using each of these products has proven antiaging, skin-preserving benefits.

10. We all have them, so fess up. What are your bad habits? Check off all that apply.

○ If I sit back and think about the food I consume, most weeks I eat almost as much junk—fast food, sweets, potato chips, processed foods, etc.—as fresh fruits and vegetables, if not more.

○ I've smoked more than a single pack of cigarettes in my life. (If you've quit, congratulations! But you still need to check the circle. If you haven't quit or are still stealing drags off your friends' cancer sticks, kick the habit. Nothing compounds the effects of aging as much as smoking.)

○ I probably drink more alcohol than I should. (In other words, you'll often finish more than three drinks at a sitting, drink on multiple weeknights, and/or overindulge on weekends.)

○ I'm inconsistent about all those little "healthy" habits I know I need to do daily, such as flossing my teeth and applying sunscreen.

○ I have erratic sleep patterns and often get less than 6 uninterrupted hours a night.

Directions

Add a point for each check mark. Smoking and drinking expose healthy cells to damaging toxins. And without enough sleep and nutrients, your skin can't repair the damage.

Your Skin Age

Add up your points and compare with the chart below:

Your Points	Your Skin Age
26 or more	**85**
24 or 25	**75**
21 to 23	**65**
17 to 20	**55**
13 to 16	**45**
9 to 12	**35**
6 to 8	**30**
4 or 5	**25**
0–3	**15**

Enter Your Skin Age here: ___

Reviewed by Francesca J. Fusco, MD , assistant clinical professor of dermatology at Mount Sinai School of Medicine in New York City.

3. How Strong Is Your Heart?

1. Heart disease tends to run in families. My:
a. mother and/or father has/had heart disease **10**
b. biological aunt or uncle has/had heart disease at some point..**5**
c. family has been blessed with healthy hearts. There's no history of heart disease in my family..**0**

2. When it comes to smoking cigarettes, I:
a. have never touched them **0**
b. have finally kicked the habit, still sneak a few a week, or am exposed to second-hand smoke..**3**
c. can't imagine anything coming between me and my nicotine...**5**

3. The last time I saw my doctor, he or she told me that my cholesterol levels were:
a. within a healthy range **0**
b. a little higher than they should be, but nothing to be too alarmed about...**3**
c. off the charts and that I needed to make changes to get them under control **5**

4. I'm in good physical condition and exercise for at least 30 minutes on most days.
a. True, I exercise regularly **0**
b. Well, sort of—I squeeze in some activity when I can find the time, but I'm not consistent..............**5**
c. False, I don't exercise at all.......................................**10**

5. In the past, my doctor has told me that my blood pressure is:
a. within normal range..**0**
b. off the charts...**5**

6. The stress level in my life is:
a. very manageable. My life is fairly stress-free.........**0**
b. high at moments, but I don't feel like it's running my life **3**
c. really high. I'm pretty wired most of the time **5**

7. My weight is:
a. my ideal body weight...**0**

b. higher than I'd like it to be; I have about 10 pounds to lose.....................................**3**
c. too high. I need to drop 20 pounds or more............**5**

8. I have diabetes or take medicine to control my blood sugar.
a. True **10**
b. False **0**

9. My age is:
a. 50 or older..**5**
b. 40–49...**3**
c. 39 or younger **0**

10. My alcohol consumption is generally:
a. Nonexistent. I don't drink at all **0**
b. No more than about a drink per day **3**
c. I have many drinks several times a week................**5**

11. My doctor has told me that I have angina.
a. True..**5**
b. False **0**

12. I have had a heart attack.
a. True **10**
b. False **0**

Your Heart Age
Add up your points and compare with the chart below:

Your Points	Your Heart Age
60–80	**60**
45–59	**50**
35–44	**45**
30–34	**40**
0–29	**30**

Enter Your Heart Age here: _____

Note: This is not a diagnostic tool. This is a quiz to provide you with a general appraisal of your risk level. If your score raises concerns, make an appointment with your doctor to discuss the test and your results.

Test courtesy of Arthur Agatston, MD, author of The South Beach Diet Supercharged

4. How Sharp Is Your Memory?

Remember these words:
Apple, television, lamb

Remember this name and address:
Jane Doe, 2745 Broad Street, Philadelphia, PA

1. Think about what you've done in recent weeks. Is it difficult to remember specifics?
○ Yes   ○ No

2. Has it been harder for you to remember lists?
○ Yes   ○ No

3. Have you noticed a decline in your ability to make calculations, such as for tips?
○ Yes   ○ No

4. Have you been forgetting to pay bills?
○ Yes   ○ No

5. Have you had trouble remembering names?
○ Yes   ○ No

6. Have you had trouble recognizing people?
○ Yes   ○ No

7. Is it ever difficult to find the right word?
○ Yes   ○ No

8. Do you ever forget how to do simple tasks?
○ Yes   ○ No

9. Do memory lapses interfere with your functioning at work?
○ Yes   ○ No

10. What about at home and around friends?
○ Yes   ○ No

11. Name the last three mayors of your town.

12. The past five presidents:

13. What was for dinner the last two nights?

14. Name the last two movies you've seen.

15. Write the three words you had to remember.

16. Also write down that name and address.

Directions
For the first 10 questions, score 1 point for each "no."
For the rest, score 1 point for each correct answer.

Your Mental Age
Add up your points and compare with the chart below:

Your Points	Your Mental Age
27–28	20
25–26	25
23–24	30
21–22	35
18–20	40
16–17	45
0–15	50

Enter Your Mental Age here: _____

Test courtesy of Richard C. Mohs, PhD

Determine Your Age Erasers Score

Complete the following equation:

Your Fitness Age
+ Your Skin Age
+ Your Heart Age
+ Your Mental Age
÷ 4

= Your Age Erasers Score! ___

Head-to-Toe Tune-Up

JUST LIKE YOUR CAR, YOUR BODY NEEDS ROUTINE MAINTENANCE. HERE'S AN EASY SCHEDULE FOR WHAT TO DO WHEN YOU'RE IN YOUR TWENTIES, THIRTIES, AND FORTIES.

Daily

Insert floss Decay-causing bacteria between teeth can lead to gum disease, which raises the risk of heart disease, stroke, and even preterm deliveries.

Step on the scale Studies show that people who weigh themselves are more likely to maintain a healthy weight.

Take a multivitamin It'll provide a boost of iron and folic acid (good in your twenties and absolutely essential before and during pregnancy), and the calcium and vitamin D will help keep your skeleton strong (important in your thirties and forties).

Weekly

Knock the boots Research has shown that having sex boosts production of immunoglobulin A, an antibody that fights viruses and bacteria, by 30 percent.

Semi-annually

Say "ahh" After your dentist has cleaned your teeth and checked for cavities, ask for an oral cancer inspection. The disease spreads quickly, so early detection is crucial.

Screen for STIs Get tested for sexually transmitted infections whenever you have a new partner. Putting it off could compromise your fertility and your health. The big three to check for are chlamydia, gonorrhea, and HIV.

Yearly

Show your dermatologist some skin The incidence of melanoma—the deadliest form of skin cancer—is on the rise in women, and 25 percent of those cases occur before age 40. And always keep an eye out for moles that are asymmetrical, have irregular borders, or have changed color.

See an ob-gyn Show up for the routine poking and prodding, i.e., breast and pelvic exams and a Pap test. (It's safe to reduce the frequency of your Paps if you've had two or more consecutive normal tests and no new sexual partners.) If you're at high risk for cervical cancer, ask your doctor for a human papillomavirus (HPV) test, too: Research shows that it's nearly 40 percent better than the Pap at detecting precancerous lesions.

Have your eyes examined Get tested for glaucoma, macular degeneration, and cataracts starting at age 35.

Get a mammogram Do it yearly starting at age 40. If you have a family history of breast cancer, get checked at least 5 years before the earliest age that cancer was diagnosed in your family.

Every 2 to 3 Years

Have a physical Heart disease, the top killer of women, can't be detected during an ob-gyn visit. You'll want an old-fashioned checkup to determine if you're at risk for that (or anything else for that matter). At the very least, ask your doc to examine your heartbeat, blood pressure, and weight.

Check for diabetes Get your blood glucose levels checked once you hit 45. Go earlier if you're overweight, have a family history of diabetes, or are trying to get pregnant.

Every 5 Years

Order a full lipid profile Beginning at age 20, have your LDL, HDL, total cholesterol, and triglyceride levels checked. If your LDL, total cholesterol, and triglyceride levels are high and your HDL is low, you may need to be screened more frequently.

Get a thyroid check More than 8 of 10 thyroid disease patients are women, and you may not even realize you have a problem because the symptoms often sound like common complaints. Begin having your thyroid hormone levels screened when you're 35.

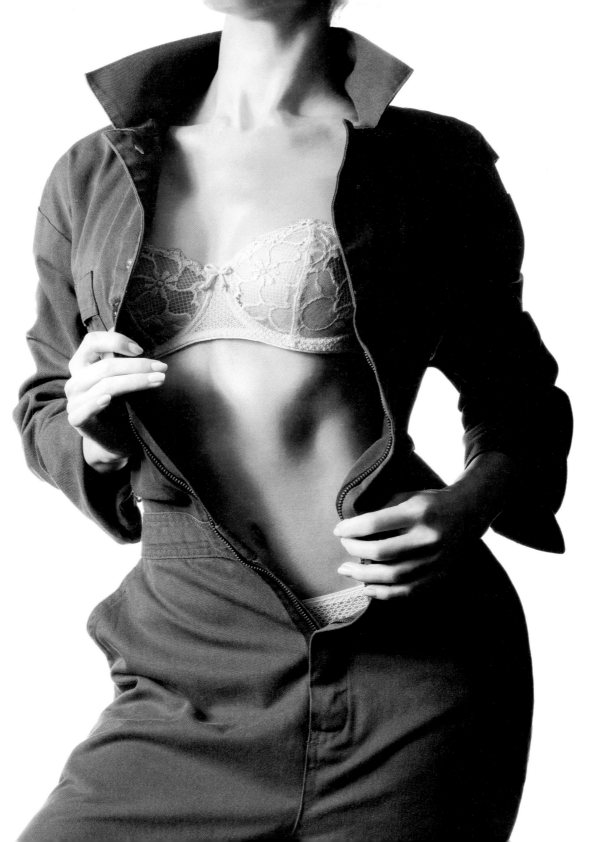

Chapter Two

The Age Eraser Food Plan

WHAT TO EAT IN YOUR TWENTIES, THIRTIES, FORTIES, AND BEYOND TO IMPROVE YOUR AGE ERASER SCORE

INVESTMENT: 4 WEEKS
AGE ERASED: 2 YEARS

Introduction

Part One:
Perfect Nutrition, Day After Day
- 25 Foods Every Woman Should Eat
- The Real Power of Antioxidants

Part Two:
Superfoods for Each Decade
- Nutrition at 20+: Stress-Relieving Snack Strategies
- Nutrition at 30+: Fat-Melting Diet Upgrades
- Nutrition at 40+: Protect and Reenergize

Part Three:
Eat Well, Live Better
- 7 Rules for Longevity
- The Antiaging Meal Plan

Introduction

*I*n a world where you can inhale half your daily allotment of calories as you turn left out of the drive-thru, often the only thing standing between you and a few extra chins is willpower—that oh-so-elusive ability to halt the urge to indulge. If your powers of resistance are lacking, you'll be psyched to hear this: Research shows that willpower is a kind of mental muscle, and like any muscle, it can get stronger. "We now know that the capacity for self-control can be increased," says Roy Baumeister, PhD, a professor of psychology at Florida State University in Tallahassee who studies the subject.

Sadly, American women have been sold a bill of goods: that happiness resides in some magical combination of the rich, sweet, and creamy, and billions are spent every year in reinforcing that message. And it works. The evidence of that unfortunate success is everywhere. Wander through the streets, shopping malls, and office buildings of today's America and you'll surely notice something: People are fat. Not just a little fat, but a lot fat. If there's any aspect of our lives that we should exert more personal power over, it's eating.

The perks of eating healthy aren't exactly news. We all know how important it is to eat our five to seven servings of fruits and vegetables every day. Yet one-third of our daily vegetable intake comes from just two sources: iceberg lettuce and potatoes. When you consider that most potatoes are polished off in the form of French fries or potato chips, American women are barely eating any vegetables at all. Even with fruit, we rarely venture out of our comfort zone: Half of the typical consumer's daily servings come from just six sources, including—surprise—apples, oranges, and bananas. Any way you slice it, we're failing to eat the wide variety of produce recommended by the USDA.

What's more, as the researchers, scientists, doctors, and nutritionists in this chapter will tell you, our bodies change with age and require different foods to function at their finest. When you apply the simple lessons from their latest science, you'll upgrade your diet immediately and harness the age-erasing power of healthful foods!

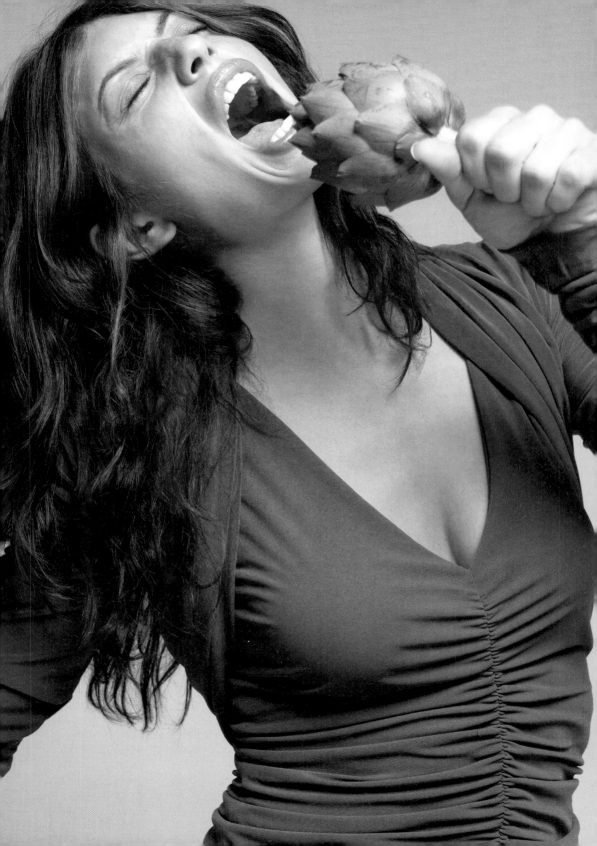

Perfect Nutrition, Day After Day

25 Foods Every Woman Should Eat

KEEP YOUR IMMUNE SYSTEM STRONG, YOUR SKIN SOFT,
AND YOUR ENERGY LEVEL SKYROCKETING.

By Matthew G. Kadey, MS, RD

T he most powerful weapon against aging isn't a plastic surgeon's scalpel—it's the food you put into your body. Outsmart fate by filling your shopping cart with foods that will fight for your right to look and feel amazing. From your brain to your breasts to your bones, researchers agree that these edibles have healing powers that can help keep you in top shape inside and out—for life.

Your Hair
Low-Fat Cottage Cheese
Hair is almost all protein, so attaining a strong, vibrant mane starts with eating enough of the stuff. Reduced-fat cottage cheese is a protein heavyweight, with 14 grams in half a cup.

Pumpkin Seeds
Add a tablespoon of these zinc-heavy seeds to cereal to reduce shedding, says Francesca Fusco, MD, assistant clinical professor of dermatology at New York's Mount Sinai Medical Center.

Your Girl Parts
Blueberries
From vision-protecting vitamin C to appetite-quelling fiber, there are plenty of reasons to be sweet on these antioxidant powerhouses. And scientists now believe that, like cranberries, blueberries battle urinary tract infections, says Elizabeth Somer, RD, author of *Age-Proof Your Body*. Opt for wild blueberries whenever possible as they contain 26 percent more antioxidants than cultivated blueberries.

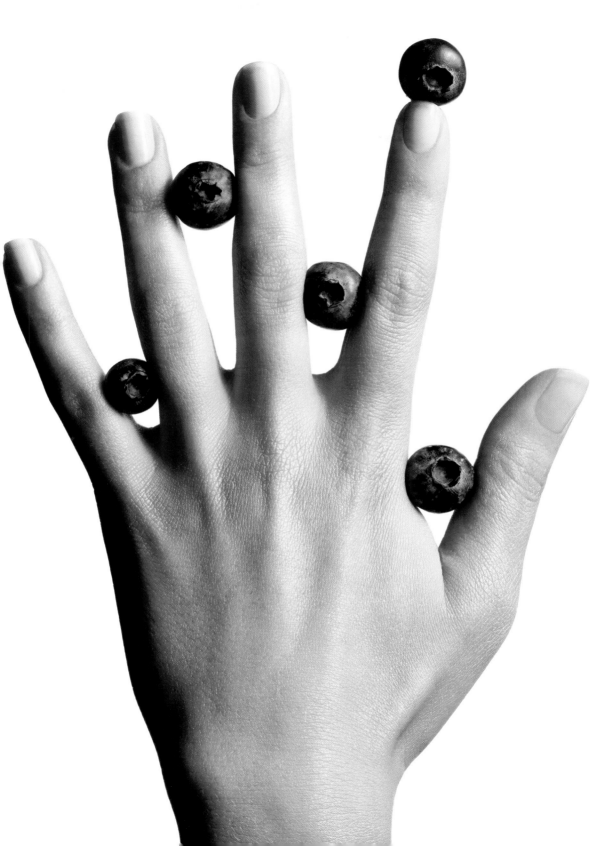

Kefir

Yeast infections put a serious damper on bed play. "Having lots of fermented milk products, including kefir, is a good way to reduce infections," says Anne VanBeber, RD, PhD, a nutrition professor at Texas Christian University in Fort Worth. These products may add beneficial bacteria to the vagina, keeping infectious bacteria in line, early research indicates. Blend ½ cup low-fat plain kefir (Lifeway is a delicious, easy-to-find brand.) with 1 cup fat-free or low-fat milk, a handful of berries, and 1 tablespoon almond butter for a creamy smoothie.

Your Brain
Arctic Char

This cold-water fish is a great source of the omega-3 fats docosahexaenoic acid (DHA) and eicosapentaenoic acid (EPA), which can improve brain function and ward off the blues, says Somer. Omega-3s help squelch inflammation in the brain and regulate feel-good neurotransmitters. Sprinkle fillets with sea salt, ground black pepper, and fresh lemon juice, then pan-fry on medium-high until one side is slightly brown. Flip and cook until the inside is slightly pink (6 to 8 minutes total).

Kale

Feed the 100 billion neurons in your noggin with nutritious kale. A study in the journal *Neurology* found that getting two-plus servings per day of veggies—especially leafy green ones like kale—slows cognitive decline by 40 percent. Temper kale's bitter flavor by cutting a single bunch into inch-wide ribbons and sautéing it with 1 teaspoon lemon juice, a chopped garlic clove, 2 tablespoons pine nuts, and a pinch of salt.

Your Nose
Sunflower Seeds

Hay fever affects more than 40 million Americans, according to the National Institutes of Health. Halt the drip with vitamin E. Researchers suspect

40
Percentage you can slow cognitive decline by eating vegetables

it calms the parts of your immune system involved in allergies. An ounce of these seeds contains 49 percent of your daily vitamin E needs.

Your Eyes
Whole Eggs

Add a yolk to that egg-white omelet. The yolks are an all-star source of two antioxidants—lutein and zeaxanthin, carotenoids that fight cataracts as well as macular degeneration, the leading cause of blindness. (The hands-down best source of these antioxidants, though, is kale.) Don't worry about your cholesterol levels. University of Massachusetts researchers have concluded that eating an average of one egg yolk a day will not raise them.

Orange Cauliflower

Food scientists at Cornell University in Ithaca, New York, reworked the standard white variety to provide 25 times as much beta-carotene, which maintains the protective covering of the cornea. As with any low-calorie vegetable, you can enjoy peachy cauliflower with reckless abandon, provided you don't drown it in salt and butter. Try steaming it or roasting it with curry powder and paprika instead.

Your Skin
Tomatoes

As if you needed a reason to cozy up to your nearest Italian eatery, this ubiquitous red fruit is especially beneficial when cooked—more of the carotenoid lycopene makes it into the skin, where it can limit ultraviolet (UV) damage to lower skin cancer risk and hold off wrinkles.

Hemp

The omega-3 fatty acids in hemp help your skin retain moisture so you don't look like a cast member from *Twilight*. Toss a tablespoon each of lemon juice, pine nuts, and shelled hemp seeds into a blender with 1 cup hemp seed oil, a chopped garlic clove, a pinch of salt, and ½ cup fresh basil. Whirl to create a delicious and healthy pesto.

The Real Power of Antioxidants

SEVEN MAGNIFICENT NUTRIENTS THAT WILL PROTECT YOU FROM AGING AND DISEASE.

Selenium: This overachieving trace mineral does double duty—it acts as an antioxidant itself and speeds up your body's natural antioxidant-making process. In a study at Cornell University and the University of Arizona of 1,312 patients with skin cancer, those who got 200 micrograms of selenium daily for 10 years reduced their risk of dying from any cancer—not just skin cancer—by 18 percent, compared with those who took a placebo.
Shoot for: The dietary reference intake (DRI) of 55 micrograms a day
Best food sources: Brazil nuts, snapper, and shrimp

Vitamin E: This antioxidant fights heart disease, boosts immunity, and helps stop cell damage that leads to skin cancer. What's more, it also keeps the ravages of time from showing up on our faces. In a Korean study, mice exposed to UV sunlight were less likely to wrinkle when they consumed vitamin E (along with a host of other antioxidants).
Shoot for: The DRI of 55 micrograms a day
Best food sources: Sunflower seeds, hazelnuts, and peanut butter

Vitamin C: It's not just for colds anymore. Now we know it protects your DNA and helps your body use vitamin E more efficiently. Research has shown that C has a talent for protecting blood vessels and reducing the risk of heart disease and stroke. In a 6-year study of 5,197 people at the Erasmus Medical Center in Rotterdam, the Netherlands, those who consumed the highest amounts of vitamin C had the lowest risk of stroke.
Shoot for: At least the DRI of 75 milligrams a day
Best food sources: Papaya, bell peppers, and broccoli

Carotenoids: These pigments help protect your eyes and skin from sun damage. In a study of 5,836 people in the Netherlands, consumption of beta-carotene—one of the many carotenoids—reduced the risk of macular degeneration, the leading cause of blindness.

Shoot for: Scientists have no standard goal for carotenoid intake other than the dietary reference intake of 2,310 IU for vitamin A
Best food sources: Carrots and butternut squash

Isothiocyanates: These antioxidants put cancer-causing enzymes in a headlock. In a study of more than 1,400 people at the University of Texas MD Anderson Cancer Center in Houston, researchers found that people who ate more isothiocyanate-rich foods reduced their risk of bladder cancer by 29 percent.
Shoot for: Scientists have no standard goal for isothiocyanate intake.
Best food sources: Broccoli, Brussels sprouts, and cauliflower

Polyphenols: Raise a glass of pinot noir to polyphenols—they've turned our favorite vice into a virtue. Researchers at Columbia University in New York City studied 980 people and found that those who drank up to three glasses per day of wine—rich in flavonoids, a polyphenol—were less likely to develop memory-loss problems such as dementia or Alzheimer's disease. In a test-tube study at the Leeds Dental Institute in the United Kingdom, the polyphenols in cocoa reduced the growth of two types of bacteria that can trigger gum disease.
Shoot for: Scientists have no standard goal for polyphenol intake.
Best food sources: Dark chocolate (the higher the cocoa content, the better), red wine, tea, and coffee

Coenzyme Q10: Its nickname—CoQ10—sounds like R2-D2's cousin, and this is a cell-protecting machine. It's also been linked with the prevention of migraines, which it may accomplish by guarding brain cells. In a study of 42 migraine patients in Zurich, those who took CoQ10 had half as many headaches over 3 months as those who took a dummy pill. The enzyme may also help lower blood pressure.
Shoot for: Scientists have no standard goal for CoQ10 intake.
Best food sources: Lean beef, chicken breast, and fish (all types)

A study of 74,000 women found that those who got more fiber were 49 percent less likely to experience weight gain.

Your Lips
Walnuts

To get moist, beautiful, chap-free lips, your body needs to constantly replace old skin cells with new ones. "Omega-3 fats help regulate this turnover so that it happens all the time," Dr. Fusco says. And unlike much-lauded almonds, walnuts have tons of these fats. So do your lips a favor and pucker up to an ounce (about 14 shelled halves) a day; eat them plain or add them to oatmeal, trail mix, or your favorite muffin recipe.

Your Nails
Beef

Of all the sources of highly absorbable iron in your supermarket, beef is among the best. Low iron levels, which are common in women, not only zap your zip, but, Dr. Fusco says, they can also cause brittle nails. With the least fat of the common cuts, top round (and other round cuts) deserves high billing on your broiler pan. Opt for grass-fed beef whenever possible, as its ratio of detrimental omega-6 fatty acids to beneficial omega-3 fatty acids is about half that of corn-fed beef, says Susan Bowerman, MS, RD, assistant director of UCLA's Center for Human Nutrition.

Your Breasts
Broccoli Sprouts

Sulforaphane, which is found in baby broccoli, fires up enzymes that may stop breast cancer cells from growing. Researchers at Johns Hopkins University in Baltimore discovered that broccosprouts have up to 20 times more of this compound than full-grown plants (scientists there also developed them). Boost your sandwiches and salads with 1/2 cup; a 1-ounce serving contains 73 milligrams of the naturally occurring precursor of sulforaphane.

Your Heart
Asparagus

Italian researchers have found that the B vitamin folate reduces homocysteine, an amino acid believed to promote inflammation, which can up your risk of heart disease. Eight steamed asparagus spears deliver 20 percent of your daily folate requirement, as well as other heart-chummy nutrients like potassium.

Purple Grape Juice

Pull over, OJ! According to researchers at the University of Glasgow, purple grape juice is high in phenolics, "a group of powerful antioxidants that swallow up heart-damaging free radicals," says Dr. VanBeber. To cut calories while guarding your arteries, mix equal parts grape juice and seltzer.

Your Belly
Prunes

These high-fiber fruits help keep your gastric system working like a finely tuned machine. They may shrink your stomach, too. A study published in the *American Journal of Clinical Nutrition* found that of the 74,000 women surveyed, those who ate more fiber were 49 percent less likely to experience weight gain. Make your own trail mix with a handful of chopped, pitted prunes plus walnuts, pumpkin seeds, dried blueberries, and hemp seeds.

Tempeh

Made from whole soybeans that are then fermented, tempeh pads our guts with beneficial bacteria. After taking up residence, Dr. VanBeber says, these live microorganisms improve digestion, reduce gas production, and kill bacteria that cause ulcers. Like tofu, tempeh soaks up the flavors around it, so crumble a block and toss it into chili, soup, or pasta sauce.

Your Bones

Chocolate

Chocolate is rich in magnesium, vital to bone health. "It forms the crystal lattice that gives bone its structure," Dr. VanBeber says. That may be why University of Tennessee scientists linked a higher magnesium intake with greater bone mineral density. Nibble an ounce, or about half a bar, of the dark stuff each day.

Canned Salmon

Research suggests that omega-3s in these fatty swimmers can boost bone density. Canned salmon in water is inexpensive and typically lower in heavy metals like mercury than many other fish. "Canned salmon [with bones] is also a good source of calcium—another bone must," Somer says. For a better burger, make patties starting with 1 can of salmon, an egg, $\frac{1}{4}$ cup bread crumbs, $\frac{1}{4}$ cup chopped onion, and $\frac{1}{2}$ tablespoon cumin powder.

Your Teeth

Mango and Kiwifruit

Together, these fruits deliver more of the proven gum protector vitamin C than an orange. Researchers in Italy have also found that each fruit portion you down daily—even a single kiwifruit—reduces your risk for oral cancer by nearly 50 percent.

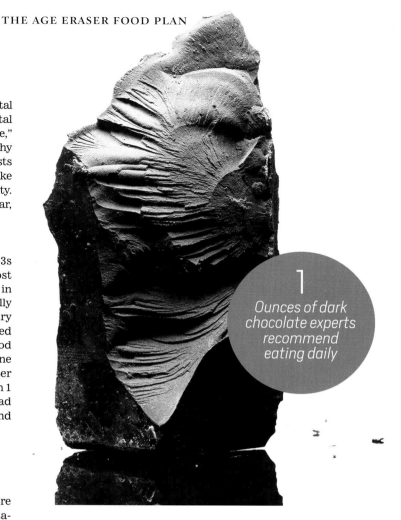

1
Ounces of dark chocolate experts recommend eating daily

Shrimp

Research has shown that vitamin D can put the smackdown on cytokines, proteins that stimulate inflammation. Three ounces of shrimp provides 65 percent of the dietary reference intake of vitamin D, so cast them into a wok with vegetables.

Your Muscles & Joints

Ricotta Cheese

Loaded with all of the amino acids muscles need to grow and mend, whey protein is a virtuoso when it comes to helping you build a buff bod. While milk curd is used to make most cheeses, ricotta is produced from the whey that's left behind in the cheese-making process. Mix low-fat ricotta with scrambled eggs, salsa, and broccoli sprouts for a killer breakfast.

Extra-Virgin Olive Oil

Ditch fat-free dressings. Olive oil contains oleocanthal, an anti-inflammatory that may work like ibuprofen, report scientists in the journal *Nature*, and it's known to lower bad cholesterol levels while raising the good. Start drizzling 2 teaspoons of extra-virgin olive oil onto your veggies before grilling or sautéing them.

Part Two:
Superfoods for Each Decade

Nutrition at 20+: Stress-Relieving Snack Strategies

FIGHT BACK TODAY—WITH YOUR MOUTH.

By Phillip Rhodes and Elizabeth Callahan

Thanks to a smorgasbord of stressors—the kind that come with 60-hour workweeks, copious dating, and late nights on the cocktail circuit—the first episodes of depression often hit women in their twenties. And it's not just your mind that pays the price. A busy, high-stress lifestyle often leads to a diet of convenience—one that lacks vitamins and minerals and is overloaded with sugar, fat, and calories. The result is a body that can never realize its full potential. A poor diet not only inhibits your ability to do that, but also increases your risk of disease, weight gain, and mental breakdown, now and in the decades ahead.

Sports Injuries

Whether it's because you're bombing down black diamonds or entering too many charity 5-Ks, you are seven times more likely to tear an anterior cruciate ligament as a man in the same age group.

The Fix: Beef. It's the perfect muscle food because it's packed with protein and creatine—both build muscle, which acts like bubble wrap around tendons and joints. Try this ligament-loving Tex-Mex salad recipe: Brown $1/4$ pound extra-lean ground beef over medium heat. As it cooks, sprinkle it with ground black pepper, 2 teaspoons chile powder, and a dash of hot sauce. Place the beef,

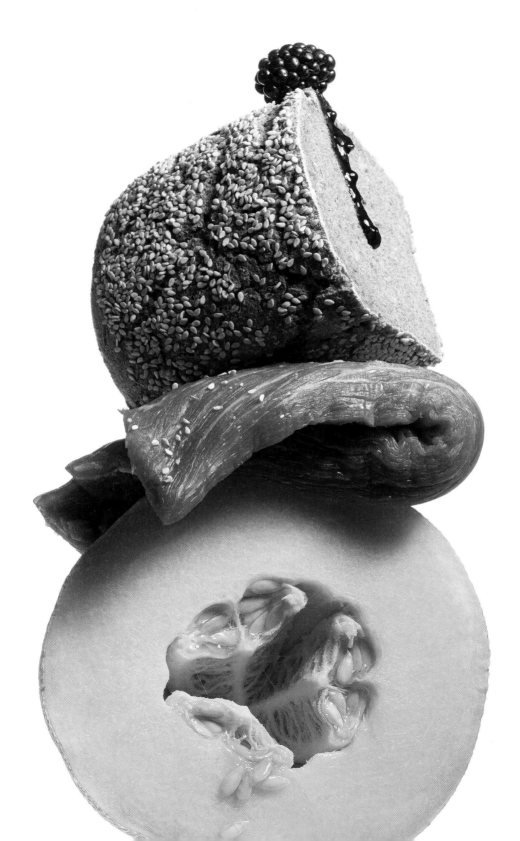

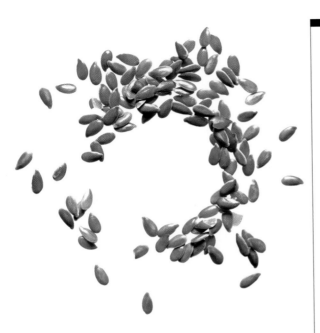

one chopped tomato, and 2 tablespoons low-fat cheese over a bed of lettuce and top with salsa.

The Bone-Building Clock Is Ticking

This is your last chance to strengthen your skeleton. When you hit 30, you're pretty much stuck with what you've got.

The Fix: Drink two 8-ounce glasses of vitamin D–fortified low-fat milk every day. You'll get 581 milligrams of calcium and 5 micrograms of vitamin D, the perfect nutrient combo to develop break-resistant bones. Broccoli also deserves a place on your menu. It contains a respectable 43 milligrams of calcium per cup and is also home to magnesium, vitamin K, and phosphorus, all of which, research shows, play a major role in keeping you upright from here to Social Security. Find naked broccoli unbearably boring? Top it with a nearly decadent layer of melted low-fat Cheddar cheese for the ultimate bone-friendly side dish, says ADA spokesperson Kerry Neville, RD.

3 Quick and Healthy Dishes to Serve Tonight

Pasta Primavera
Total Time: 40 MINUTES *Serves:* 4

Ingredients
⅔ cup reduced-fat ricotta cheese
1 cup vegetable broth
1 tablespoon extra-virgin olive oil
1 shallot, finely chopped
¼ pound white button mushrooms, sliced
½ pound plum tomatoes, chopped
2 large cloves garlic, minced
¼ teaspoon salt
¼ teaspoon ground black pepper
½ pound multigrain spaghetti
3 cups small broccoli florets
1 medium carrot, julienned
¼ pound asparagus, cut into 1" chunks
¾ cup frozen shelled edamame (green soybeans), thawed
½ cup fresh basil, thinly sliced
⅓ cup grated Parmesan cheese

Directions
1. In a food processor, combine the ricotta and broth. Process until smooth. Set aside. Bring a large pot of water to a boil.
2. Heat the oil in a large, nonstick skillet over medium-high heat. Add the shallot and mushrooms. Cook, stirring frequently, for 3 minutes, or until the mushrooms begin to brown. Reduce the heat to medium. Stir in the tomatoes, garlic, salt, and pepper. Cook for 2 minutes, or until the tomatoes begin to soften. Reduce the heat to very low and cover to keep warm.
3. Cook the pasta. Two minutes before it's al dente, add the broccoli, carrot, asparagus, and soybeans to the pot. Drain when finished cooking.
4. Return the hot pasta and vegetables to the pot. Add the basil, the mushroom mixture, and the ricotta mixture. Toss and sprinkle with the cheese.

Nutritional Facts per Serving
· Calories 401 · Fat 9 g · Saturated fat 3 g
· Cholesterol 16 mg · Sodium 423 mg · Carbohydrates 62 g
· Total sugars 9 g · Dietary fiber 12 g · Protein 21 g

(continued on page 27)

A busy, high-stress lifestyle often leads to a diet of convenience—and one severely lacking in vitamins and minerals.

Keep Your Spirits High—And Your Weight Low

The next time you're powering through spin class, take a look at the 30 other women sweating around you. Five of them either currently take antidepressants or have taken them at some point in the past year. But even if you're not using antidepressants to treat those pesky rain clouds, you can still improve your long-term outlook with a little-known powerfood.

The Fix: Eat 1 tablespoon of ground flaxseed every day. It's the best source of alpha-linolenic acid, a fatty acid that researchers say improves the operation of the cerebral cortex. That's the area of the brain that processes sensory information, including pleasure signals. Bonus: Unlike whole flaxseed, "flaxseed meal is easily digested and rich in lignans, prebiotic compounds that nourish bacterial cultures in the gut," says Susan Kleiner, PhD, author of *The Good Mood Diet*. In fact, flax has the most lignans of any food. These estrogenlike compounds are also found in sesame seeds, hummus, and dried fruits—and women who eat the most lignans have the lowest Body Mass Index (BMI). In animal studies, estrogen reduces appetite and shrinks fat cells, and phytoestrogens may have a similar effect in people, says

Anne-Sophie Morisset, RD, of Laval University in Quebec. To meet your quota, sprinkle ground flaxseed on salads, vegetables, and cereal, mix it into a smoothie or a shake, and look for the ingredient in multigrain bread. If your grocery store doesn't carry it, you can make it yourself with a coffee grinder.

No Time to Eat Right

Between jobs, boyfriends, seeing your parents, and trying to keep some measure of a social life, who has time to eat, let alone eat healthfully?

The Fix: Choose microwave-friendly meals that have the perfect balance of protein, carbs, and veggies in one package, such as Kashi's Sweet and Sour Chicken. In general, look for these qualifications when choosing a frozen feast: 450 milligrams or less of sodium and no more than 3 grams of total fat and 1 gram of saturated fat per 100 calories, says Constance Brown-Riggs, RD, spokesperson for the ADA. MorningStar Farms' Spicy Black Bean Burger and Lean Cuisine's Grilled Chicken Primavera (though the recipe for a home-cooked alternative is on page 24) are two other meals that take the guesswork out of grocery shopping. Bonus: Harvard scientists found that every one-serving increase in daily vegetable intake decreases your risk of heart disease by 4 percent. So sauté your favorite greens with some olive oil and garlic while you nuke your entreé.

25

Nutrition at 30+: Fat-Melting Diet Upgrades

WHAT TO NOSH IN THE PRIME OF YOUR LIFE.

By Phillip Rhodes and Elizabeth Callahan

The metabolism that once let you go out for dinner and drinks and then hit the fridge after midnight is now dropping slowly but surely. And even if the number on your scale isn't rising, the number on the tag of your little black dress probably is. In a study published in the *American Journal of Clinical Nutrition*, people who managed to maintain their weight swapped lean body mass for blubber each decade. Sagging body parts aren't your only hazard. Starting at 30, your systolic blood pressure rises 4 points per decade and your joints can start acting up. The good news is that your thirties is the decade when you can stiff-arm health ailments that previous generations just accepted as part of getting older.

Corroding Joints

Arthritis doesn't usually set in until later in life, but the damage that causes it is happening now.

The Fix: Eat three 6-ounce servings of cold-water fish per week. A serving of salmon, mackerel, trout, halibut, or white tuna—each packs more than 1,000 milligrams of DHA and EPA omega-3 fatty acids. A small UK study found that getting this amount of fish oil daily appeared to reduce cartilage-eating enzymes in a majority of patients facing joint-replacement surgery. Fish oil slows down cartilage degeneration and reduces factors that cause inflammation, says Bruce Caterson, PhD, of Cardiff University in Wales, a lead researcher in the study.

Cracks in the Facade

You're cool with getting older—you're smarter, wiser, and having fun. What's not cool are the tiny lines starting to show up on your face.

The Fix: Stroll down the bean aisle. An Australian study of 453 elderly people found that those who ate the most legumes and vegetables had fewer wrinkles and less sun-related skin damage. Beans are rich in antioxidants that help the body deal with free radicals. Keep hummus on hand as a sandwich spread and carrot dip, toss black beans into soups or lentils into pasta sauce, or serve canned beans as a convenient side. Mix them up

Seared Wild Salmon with Mango Salsa

Total Time: 20 MINUTES *Serves:* 6

Ingredients

Salsa:
1 ripe mango, peeled and cut into small cubes
½ cup chopped red bell pepper
½ cup chopped red onion
3 tablespoons freshly squeezed lime juice
2 tablespoons chopped fresh mint
1 tablespoon finely chopped jalapeño chile pepper

Salmon:
Juice of 1 lemon (about ¼ cup)
½ teaspoon paprika
2 wild salmon fillets (1 pound each, about 1 inch thick)
1 tablespoon olive oil

Directions

1. Prepare salsa: Toss together mango, bell pepper, onion, lime juice, mint, and jalapeño chile pepper in small bowl. Season with salt and ground black pepper to taste. Cover and chill at least 1 hour.
2. Prepare salmon: Combine lemon juice and paprika in large, shallow baking dish. Season with salt and ground black pepper. Place salmon in dish and flip to cover both sides. Marinate, covered, for 20 to 60 minutes in refrigerator.
3. Remove fillets from marinade. Discard marinade. Heat oil in large nonstick skillet over medium-high heat. Sear fillets 15 minutes, turning once, or until just opaque. Serve with salsa.

Nutritional Facts per Serving
· Calories 276 · Fat 12 g · Saturated fat 2 g
· Cholesterol 83 mg · Sodium 69 mg · Carbohydrates 11 g
· Total sugars 8 g · Dietary fiber 2 g · Protein 31 g

(continued on page 30)

with face-saving, antioxidant-rich veggies, like asparagus, broccoli, celery, eggplant, onion, and spinach—all of which were also found in the study to be the skin's fountains of youth.

Yaaaaawn!

You're climbing the company ladder, having kids, dealing with your finances . . . you're stretched and stressed to your limits. Oh yeah, and your sex life is about as revved up as a rusty tractor.

The Fix: Go nuts. Peanuts, hazelnuts, and walnuts are loaded with vitamin E, an antioxidant that bolsters the immune system. They're also chock-full of B vitamins, which prepare your body for physical ramifications of stress like high blood pressure and off-kilter hormones. Nuts are also a great food source of arginine, an amino acid that improves bloodflow—to help you get from dead tired to orgasmic. Eat a handful (unsalted and raw) per day.

A Pokey Metabolism

Your skinny jeans fit as if they just came out of the dryer—even though you haven't washed them in weeks and you work out like Olympic-great Dara Torres. It's a bitch to stay thin when you're doing all the right things but your metabolism is conspiring to add flab.

The Fix: Low-sugar, high-protein snacks will keep your metabolic furnace stoked and leave you less likely to binge. Have a slice (1 ½ ounces) of cheese—like Cheddar, Swiss, or provolone—once a day. Cheese has up to 11 grams of protein per serving and almost no sugar, which keeps your blood sugar in check. Other options: Greek yogurt, beef jerky, or almonds.

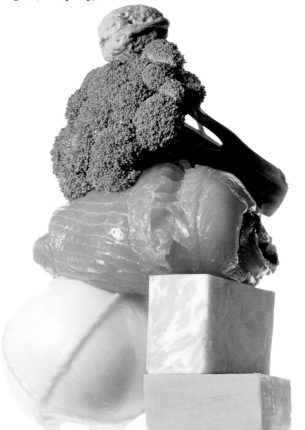

Nutrition at 40+: Protect and Reenergize

LAUNCH A PREEMPTIVE ATTACK ON YOUR BODY'S NATURAL ENEMIES.

By Phillip Rhodes and Elizabeth Callahan

U ntil your forties, you were more likely to be killed in the street by a falling piano than anything else. But now the big words—heart disease and cancer—start showing up as the leading health problems in women. As you reach your fifties, there's also an elevated risk of nonfatal but still nasty diseases, such as macular degeneration, the leading cause of blindness. And even if you managed to sidestep weight gain in your thirties, keeping your waistline in check becomes even harder now as your metabolism begins to slow and your hard-earned muscle gives way to fat. The solution: a preemptive attack on your body's natural enemies. Your weapons, as usual, are a knife and fork.

Cancer-Prone Skin

After all those years you spent soaking up the sun covered by nothing but a string bikini and a thin coating of SPF 2, it's payback time.

The Fix: Melanoma is scary, but food can help. National Cancer Institute researchers found that the skin cancer risk of people with the highest intakes of carotenoids (pigments that occur naturally in plants) was significantly lower than in those who ate the least. "Beta-carotene is an internal sun protector," says Regina Goralczyk, PhD, of DSM Nutritional Products. "The plant pigment is transported in the bloodstream to the skin, where it is enriched and helps fight the

28

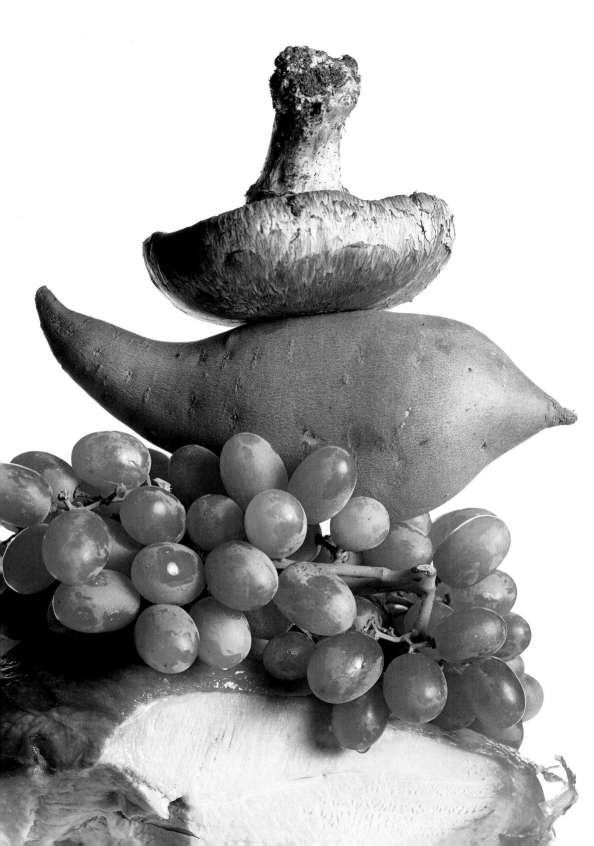

damaging effects of sunlight." As a preventive tool, eat two sweet potatoes every week. They'll give you plenty of beta-carotene. Other great sources: carrots and cantaloupe.

Narrowing Arteries

Heart disease scores as a top-three killer of women in this age group.

The Fix: Grab a handful of red grapes every day. Antioxidants in their skins have been linked to lower LDL cholesterol and a lowered risk of clogged arteries. A glass of red wine is beneficial too. In a Spanish study, scientists found that red wine significantly reduced markers of arterial inflammation. The booze also helps prevent clots, just as a daily aspirin does.

Shrinking Muscles

You've gone soft—in the arms, legs, and booty—because your muscle mass continues to decline as you age.

The Fix: Tuna. Ounce for ounce, it's one of the best sources of protein. Grill your way to a better body with this muscle-building recipe: Brush a 4-ounce tuna steak with olive oil, lightly season it with ground black pepper, and place it on a preheated grill. Cook until medium-rare to medium, for 4 to 5 minutes per side. Meanwhile, mix 3 tablespoons peanut butter, 1 tablespoon lemon juice, 1 tablespoon balsamic vinegar, 1 teaspoon brown sugar, and 2 tablespoons water in a bowl and microwave for 30 seconds. Drizzle over tuna.

Weakening Vision

Even if your peepers are still 20/20, two eye conditions that can lead to vision loss—cataracts and macular degeneration—can start developing during this time. (And for reasons scientists have yet to put their finger on, women are at higher risk for macular degeneration than men.)

The Fix: You might be sick of hearing that it's time to go green, but when it comes

Roast Pork with Sweet Potatoes and Apples

Total Time: 2 hours 30 minutes
Serves: 10

Ingredients:
1 boneless pork roast (4 pounds), trimmed of fat
⅓ cup honey
¼ cup orange juice
¼ cup frozen apple juice concentrate, thawed
1 tablespoon ground black pepper
1 tablespoon packed brown sugar
3 large sweet potatoes, halved
3 large apples, cored and quartered

Directions
1. Preheat the oven to 375°F.
2. Coat a large Dutch oven with cooking spray and place over medium-high heat until hot. Add the pork. Cook for 2 minutes, or until brown. Turn and cook for 2 minutes, or until brown. Remove from the heat.
3. In a medium bowl, combine the honey, orange juice, apple juice concentrate, pepper, and brown sugar. Spoon over the pork. Place the sweet potatoes around the pork. Cover and bake for 2 hours, or until the pork has an internal temperature of 150°F.
4. Place the apples around the pork. Bake uncovered, basting frequently, for 20 minutes, or until the apples are just tender. Let the pork stand for 10 minutes before slicing. Serve with the sweet potatoes and apples.

Nutritional facts per serving
· Calories 276 · Fat 12 g · Saturated Fat 2 g
· Cholesterol 83 mg · Sodium 69 mg · Carbohydrates 11 g
· Total sugars 8g · Dietary Fiber 2 g · Protein 31 g

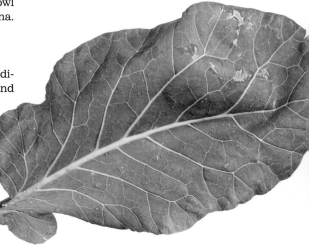

Studies have found that consuming about 6 milligrams of lutein and zeaxanthin daily should protect our vision. We average 2.

to your eyes, you don't have a choice. Kale, collard greens, spinach, and turnip greens all contain lutein and zeaxanthin, two antioxidants that act like chemical sunglasses—they help protect your eyes from the UV rays that can lead to these two conditions, says Judith Delgado, director of the Macular Degeneration Partnership. In a 15-week study, people who ate a diet high in lutein and zeaxanthin had a higher density of macular pigments, a factor that has been shown to safeguard against macular degeneration. Studies have found that about 6 milligrams of each daily should protect your vision; most Americans average about 2 total. That's where the greens come in: A cup of chopped kale has 26.5 milligrams of total lutein and zeaxanthin. Make sure you drizzle your spinach salad or sauté your greens with olive oil—healthy fats help your body absorb the antioxidants more effectively.

The DHA-fortified milk (Horizon Organic offers a couple varieties) gets you a nice dose of the omega-3 fatty acid that's been shown to decrease the risk of dementia. Each of these ingredients protects gray matter on its own, too, so use all of them freely.

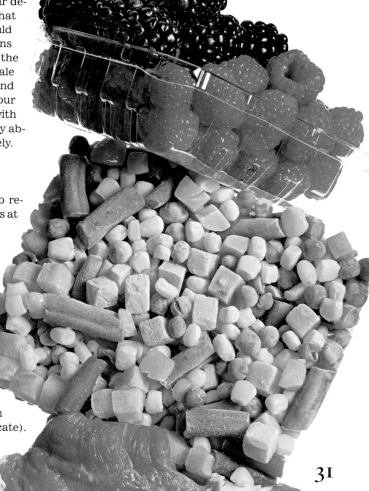

Brain Freeze

It's taking you just a little longer to remember your co-workers' kids' names at the company picnic.

The Fix: Dust off the blender and mix up this concoction for your noodle—$1/2$ cup DHA-fortified low-fat milk, 1 cup blueberries or blackberries, 1 cup cherry juice (look for CherryPharm all-natural tart cherry juice), and a handful of crushed ice. Berries and cherries are rich in anthocyanins, which have been linked to better memory (researchers think they help your brain improve the way neurons communicate).

7 Rules for Longevity

WHAT (AND HOW) TO EAT SO YOU'LL STAY
STRONG AND SEXY FOR DECADES.

By Matt McMillen

*T*he fountain of youth has yet to be found, bottled, and sold for $3.99 at Whole Foods. But that doesn't mean the secret to living a long, healthy life can't be bought at the supermarket. Use these seven no-fail food rules to give yourself the best possible chance of staying lean, sexy, and glowing for longer than you ever imagined you could.

1. Go for Color

The biggest antiaging breakthrough in recent history comes from new discoveries about the power of antioxidants, which you can learn even more about on page 19. For those who have heard the word but are fuzzy on the details, here's a crash course. As the cells in our bodies metabolize oxygen, unstable molecules called free radicals form. These cause cell damage that has been linked to age-related illnesses like Alzheimer's and heart disease. Many scientists think that all symptoms of aging are the direct result of free radicals attacking our cells. Antioxidants (cue the superhero music) neutralize free radicals, preventing them from doing any damage and thereby slowing the aging process. "Antioxidants can even reverse damage to our cells," says Bonnie Taub-Dix, RD, a spokesperson for the American Dietetic Association (ADA). While there's ongoing debate about how many of

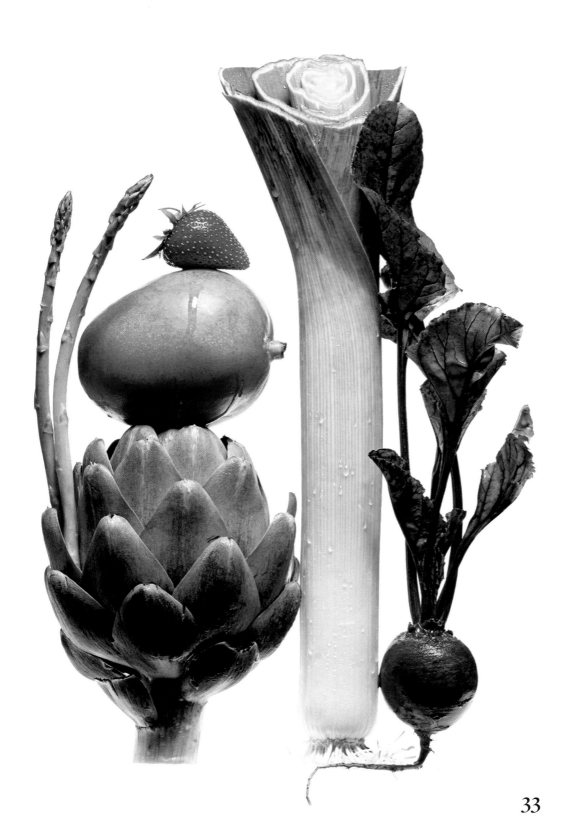

33

Your body typically digests whole foods more slowly than processed foods, and that can help you stay thin.

the large variety of food-derived antioxidants our bodies can actually use and how efficiently we can use them, a convincing pile of research points to a strong connection between foods loaded with antioxidants and a longer, healthier life. Luckily, spotting foods high in the amazing stuff is easy, thanks to a handy trick of nature: They're the ones bursting with color. Berries have tons of antioxidants, and according to James Joseph, PhD,

a neuroscientist at the USDA Human Nutrition Research Center on Aging at Boston's Tufts University, they help maintain cognitive and motor functioning as we age. Pomegranates have been found to reduce the risk of heart attack and stroke. And results published in the *British Journal of Cancer* show that broccoli and Brussels sprouts contain compounds that can help prevent breast cancer.

The Perfect Shopping List

TAKE THIS TO THE GROCERY STORE AND STOCK UP ON THE MOST POTENT ANTIAGING FOODS.

- ❑ Dry Goods
- ❑ Almonds
- ❑ Chickpeas
- ❑ Green tea
- ❑ Oatmeal
- ❑ Extra-virgin olive oil
- ❑ Pecans
- ❑ Walnuts
- ❑ Whole-grain pasta
- ❑ Whole wheat bread
- ❑ Fish
- ❑ Albacore tuna
  (in water, if canned)
- ❑ Salmon
  (wild, if possible; in
  water, if canned)
- ❑ Trout
- ❑ Produce
- ❑ Avocados
- ❑ Beets
- ❑ Blackberries

- ❑ Blueberries
- ❑ Broccoli
- ❑ Brussels sprouts
- ❑ Cherries
- ❑ Eggplants
- ❑ Onions
- ❑ Oranges
- ❑ Pink grapefruits
- ❑ Plums
- ❑ Pomegranates
- ❑ Prunes
- ❑ Raspberries
- ❑ Red bell peppers
- ❑ Red grapes
- ❑ Spinach
- ❑ Strawberries
- ❑ Sweet potatoes
- ❑ Tomatoes
- ❑ Red wine

2. Rely On Real Foods, Not Supplements

Given all the hype about antioxidants, your local health food store is probably already shilling an antioxidant pill with a label covered in promises. Well, stroll past it. Supplements have nothing on fresh, whole foods. Case in point: the massive Iowa Women's Health Study. Researchers found that among the 34,492 women participating in the study, those who ate foods rich in vitamin E, such as nuts, lessened their chances of suffering a stroke. Vitamin E supplements, on the other hand, provided no protection. Natural foods—those that have been minimally processed, if at all—contain "thousands of compounds that interact in complex ways, and if you take one out, there's no predicting how it will function on its own," says Frank Hu, PhD, associate professor of nutrition and epidemiology at the Harvard School of Public Health. He adds that large-scale trials of individual antioxidant supplements have been largely disappointing.

3. Avoid Processed Foods

Processed foods—those full of preservatives, chemicals, and added colors—simply aren't as nutritious as whole foods. And every time you eat a highly processed food, you're bypassing another food that actually can help delay the effects of aging. The classic example is whole wheat bread versus white bread. Whole

The Antiaging Meal Plan

THREE DAILY MENUS TO HELP YOU LIVE A LONG AND HEALTHY LIFE

This balanced diet, created by Bonnie Taub-Dix, RD, is packed with some of the best antiaging foods. And because research has shown that reducing calories by 25 percent has impressive antiaging benefits, it contains about 1,700 calories a day—about a quarter fewer calories than the National Academy of Sciences' average requirement for an active 30-year-old woman. Cut the last snack to drop another 200 calories or so.

	DAY ONE	DAY TWO	DAY THREE
BREAKFAST	• *8 ounces fat-free yogurt mixed with ½ cup raspberries* • *8 ounces green tea*	• *1 slice toasted whole-grain bread spread with 2 tablespoons peanut butter (or other nut butter, like almond)* • *¾ cup strawberries*	• *¾ cup high-fiber cereal* • *1 cup fat-free milk* • *½ banana*
LUNCH	• *2 cups mixed greens, ¼ cup tomatoes, ¼ cup carrots, ¼ cup red cabbage, ⅓ cup chick-peas, ⅓ cup red beans, ⅓ cup edamame, 1 ounce slivered almonds tossed with 1 tablespoon extra-virgin olive oil and as much red-wine or balsamic vinegar as you'd like* • *1 plum* • *8 ounces sparkling water mixed with ¼ cup pomegranate juice and a twist of lime*	• *2 ounces turkey breast, 3 spinach leaves, 2 slices tomato, and 1 tablespoon mustard on 2 slices whole-grain bread* • *1 cup red grapes* • *8 ounces green tea*	• *Omelet made with 2 eggs and 2 egg whites with 5 spinach leaves, ½ cup chopped red bell pepper, and 1 slice low-fat cheese* • *1 small whole wheat pita* • *¾ cup grape tomatoes mixed with ¼ cup chopped avocado* • *¾ cup blackberries*
SNACK	• *A minisandwich: 1 slice whole-grain bread with 1 ounce low-fat cheese and 1 teaspoon mustard* • *¾ cup blueberries*	• *6 ounces or one 100-calorie pack low-fat popcorn, sprinkled with 2 tablespoons freshly grated Parmesan cheese*	• *1 tablespoon peanut butter on 2 whole-grain crackers* • *8 ounces raspberry iced tea*
DINNER	• *3 ounces grilled wild salmon (weight after cooking)* • *1 cup Brussels sprouts and ½ cup thinly sliced beets sautéed in 1 teaspoon extra-virgin olive oil* • *1 small sweet potato, baked* • *One 8-ounce glass red wine*	• *5 ounces grilled albacore tuna (weight after cooking)* • *½ cup cooked whole wheat pasta tossed with ½ cup broccoli and minced garlic to taste (about 1 clove) sauted in 1 teaspoon olive oil* • *1 cup red leaf lettuce and ¼ cup shredded fresh beets topped with 1 tablespoon chopped pecans and 1 tablespoon dried cranberries, tossed with 1 teaspoon olive oil* • *½ pink grapefruit* • *1 glass red wine*	• *1 veggie burger on a whole wheat bun* • *⅓ cup cooked brown rice* • *⅓ cup black beans* • *1 cup sautéed yellow and green squash* • *1 cup mesclun greens with ¼ cup shredded carrots, topped with 1 tablespoon chopped walnuts and ½ cup diced apple* • *1 glass red wine*
SNACK	• *½ cup high-fiber cereal* • *1 cup fat-free milk*	• *3 graham crackers, topped with 2 tablespoons low-fat whipped cream cheese and ¼ cup sliced berries of your choice*	• *½ cup low-fat frozen yogurt with ⅛ cup fresh berries of your choice*
	1,710 calories	*1,730 calories*	*1,740 calories*

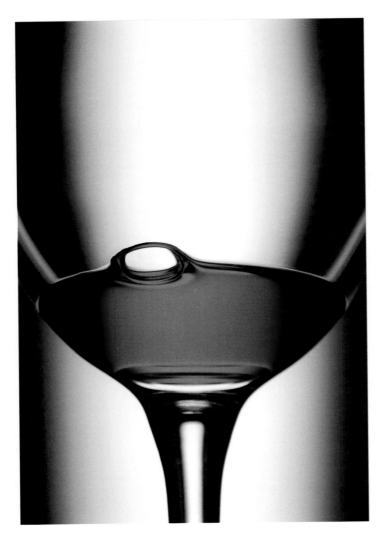

Hu says. And because whole foods pack fewer calories per gram, they can ward off weight-related illnesses like heart disease and stroke.

4. Don't Be Afraid of (Good) Fats

"Fat" is not a four-letter word. "Unsaturated fats from vegetable oils, nuts, avocados, and fish improve insulin sensitivity and reduce blood lipids," Dr. Hu says. That translates into a lower risk of heart disease, diabetes, and stroke. Healthful fats are the base of the Mediterranean-style diet—consisting mostly of vegetables, nuts, beans, olive oil, and fish—and are what make it so superior. The Harvard School of Public Health and University of Athens Medical School found that this type of diet reduces the risk of death from heart disease and cancer by 25 percent. And a Columbia University Medical Center study reported that it can lower the risk of Alzheimer's disease by 40 percent. Treating yourself two to four times a week to salmon and other fish that deliver omega-3 fatty acids, along with a small handful of nuts a day,

wheat is proven to fight heart disease, thanks to its abundance of fiber and other nutrients. White bread isn't. "Many nutrients are taken out during processing, and few are put back," says Lisa Hark, PhD, RD, director of nutrition education at the University of Pennsylvania School of Medicine in Philadelphia.

Your body also typically digests whole foods more slowly than processed foods, which keeps blood sugar and insulin levels from fluctuating rapidly (and that can help you stay thin!). "In the long term, this may help you avoid diabetes," Dr.

may reduce your risk of heart disease by 30 percent and lower your cholesterol as well, according to research from Harvard. Your skin will benefit, too. Early evidence suggests that the more omega-3s you consume, the more your rivals from high school will hate you when they see how great you look at the 30th reunion. Heh, heh.

5. Sip Red Wine

Another revelation of the Harvard/Athens study was the benefits to be had with red wine. Drinking one glass a day, four to

A diet heavy in vegetables, nuts, beans, olive oil, and fish reduces the risk of death from heart disease and cancer by 25 percent.

five times a week (preferably with a meal), has been shown to reduce the risk of heart attacks, diabetes, and other life-threatening illnesses. Part of the credit goes to the alcohol, which helps soothe inflamed arteries. But specific to red wine—especially pinot noir—are antioxidants called flavonoids, which are particularly good free-radical fighters. Consuming wine conservatively (pace yourselves, people!) will help you reap all the heart-healthy benefits, but you should go easier on the bottle as you age: Alcohol consumption has been linked to an increased risk of breast cancer in postmenopausal women. If you're drinking more than three glasses at a time multiple nights a week, cut back before a plus turns into a minus.

6. Guzzle Green Tea

Packed with powerful antioxidants— these are called catechins—green tea may be the single most life-prolonging substance you can put in your cup. A mug a day will decrease your chance of developing high blood pressure by 46 percent. Drink more and reduce your risk by 65 percent. What's the best of the best? A study in the *Journal of Food Science* found that, of all 77 US brands tested, Stash Darjeeling organic green tea delivers the greatest number of catechins: 100 per gram. (At the very least, avoid any sugar-added varieties.) If you're looking for bottled green tea, reach for Honest Tea's Organic Honey Green Tea. It contains 215 mg of catechins, the most of 14 brands tested by Chroma-Dex Laboratories on behalf of *Men's Health*.

7. Eat Less

The next time you're at a wedding, look around: The dancing ninetysomething women aren't the overweight ones. Researchers at the Harvard School of Public Health found that women who stayed closest to their weight at

18 throughout their lives had a 66 percent lower risk of developing heart disease, high blood pressure, and type 2 diabetes compared with women who put on 11 to 22 pounds by middle age. Another study found that women who gained 60 pounds after age 18 were up to three times more likely to be diagnosed with breast cancer.

Of course, as we age, extra pounds seem to materialize out of nowhere. "If you keep the physical activity the same and food the same, you will put on a pound or two a year," says Walter Willett, PhD, chairman of the Department of Nutrition at the Harvard School of Public Health and one of the lead researchers on the study. Thanks to a natural decrease in hormones that help maintain muscle mass, "those muscles shrink, you burn less energy, and you accumulate fat," he says.

The key is to cut calories without sacrificing nutrients (see "The Antiaging Meal Plan" on page 35). In 2004, researchers at Washington University School of Medicine in St. Louis reported that people who consistently ate 10 to 25 percent fewer calories than the average American, while still keeping a balanced diet, had remarkably low blood pressure and low levels of bad cholesterol and triglycerides.

The National Academy of Sciences has several theories about why eating less makes such a difference. While we often strive to boost our metabolism to stay slim, some researchers believe we need to do the opposite to living longer: A low-cal diet slows your metabolism, and a slow metabolism produces fewer free radicals. When you eat less, you also produce less glucose, which has been linked to cell damage. And low-calorie diets reduce your body's core temperature and its response to insulin, which may increase longevity in humans. Doctors aren't sure how many years leaving food behind will add to your life, but studies have shown that calorie-restricted rats live 30 percent longer than rats that eat normally.

Chapter Three

The Age Eraser Workout

PERFECT WORKOUTS FOR YOUR TWENTIES, THIRTIES, AND FORTIES TO IMPROVE YOUR AGE ERASER SCORE

> INVESTMENT: 4 WEEKS
> AGE ERASED: 3 YEARS

Introduction

Part One:
Fitness at 20+: Keep Your Back Healthy
• Save Your Spine
• Lean and Fit in 7 Minutes

Part Two:
Fitness at 30+: Protect Your Muscles and Your Bones
• Get Firm—Fast!
• The 10 Best Yoga Poses for Women

Part Three:
Fitness at 40+: Claim a Body for the Ages
• Slim Down, Power Up
• The Ultimate Cardio Burn

Introduction

U nless you're one of the lucky few to hit it big in the genetic lottery, staying fit ain't easy. And if it's this difficult now, imagine what it's going to be like in ten, twenty, thirty years. Sure, slipping back into a fitness routine after a break can be daunting, especially when you consider that even a 2-month break can cause you to lose up to 35 percent of your muscle strength and 18 percent of your aerobic endurance. "As soon as you stop participating in regular activity, your body starts detraining," says Lynn Millar, PhD, a professor of physical therapy at Andrews University in Berrien Springs, Michigan. But before you begin planning your future as a wobbly, overweight hunchback, understand that getting in the shape of your life for the rest of your life is anything but a burden. In fact, if you find your fitness groove now, you'll set yourself up for success in the future. Studies show that working out may lower a woman's risk of breast cancer by 47 percent, osteoporosis by 45 percent, and heart disease by 14 percent. In tapping dozens of doctors and fitness experts to find out exactly what you should do to add years to your life, we found that there is in fact a bottom line to outsmarting that wily Mother Nature—launch a fitness plan if you don't already have one, and then simply adjust your workouts throughout the years to help your muscles, bones, and heart keep up with you. Yes, some comebacks should stay packed up in the past (leg warmers come to mind). But your prime-time return to the gym isn't one of them.

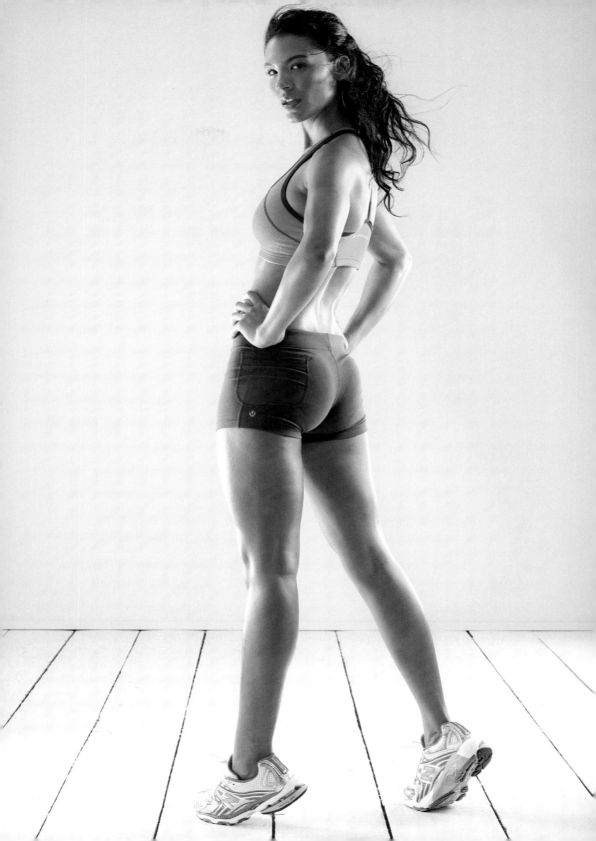

Fitness at 20+:
Keep Your Back Healthy

Save Your Spine

WOMEN BEGIN TO DEVELOP A HUNCH AS EARLY AS
THEIR TWENTIES, BUT THAT'S ONE FATE YOU CAN CHEAT.

Spending 40 or more hours a week crouched over your keyboard like a human comma probably impresses your boss, but it also compresses your spine. "That leads to slumped posture in the short term and irreversible damage to your spine over the years," says Lori Incledon, author of *Strength Training for Women*. "When your spine is held in the same posture for years, the muscles become too deconditioned to move the bones, and the bones begin to fuse together." Bone mass in your spine and hips also peaks in your mid- to late twenties, says Kara Witzke, PhD, associate professor of kinesiology at California State University in San Marcos. Building as much bone as possible now will guarantee that you have some to spare later, lowering your chances of osteoporosis. "Bones are like muscles; they get stronger at the specific region

that's stressed," says Ana Gómez, PhD, an exercise and diet researcher at the University of Connecticut in Storrs. The best bone-building moves are lower- and upper-body exercises that force you to bend at more than one joint: squats, lunges, rows, and presses. While you're at it, take a flying leap—off a 1-foot-high platform, to be exact. Do that 100 times two to three times each week and you could reduce your risk of hip fracture later in life, Dr. Witzke says. Studies show that weight-bearing impact activities minimize age-related bone loss, especially in your hips. In other words, act now and you'll be a head above the other women on your over-50 basketball team.

Instructions
Three times a week perform three sets of 10 to 12 reps, taking 1- to 2-minute rests between sets and exercises unless instructed otherwise.

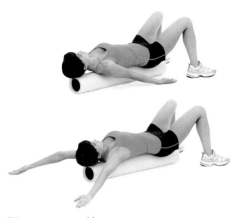

Foam Roller Snow Angel

Do this exercise every day. Lie on a 3-foot foam roller (www.power-systems.com) so that it runs the length of your spine. Bend your knees and rest your feet flat on the floor. Place your hands next to your hips, palms up, with your arms straight. Without raising your shoulders, slowly drag your hands along the floor (as if you're making a snow angel) until they're above your head. If you feel tightness in a spot, pause there for 10 to 15 seconds, then keep moving. Repeat 4 times. Note: Go slow. One rep of this exercise should take at least 45 seconds.

Front Squat

Grasp dumbbells with your palms facing each other and position your feet shoulder-width apart. Bring the weights toward your collarbone until your elbows point straight out and your upper arms are parallel to the floor. Look straight ahead, inhale, and lower your body by pushing your hips back and maintaining an arched back. Keep your heels grounded. Once your thighs are parallel to the floor (or lower), quickly rise while exhaling. Repeat.

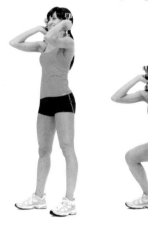
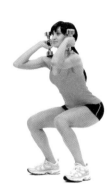

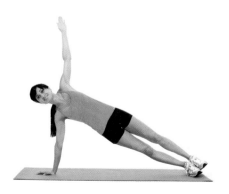

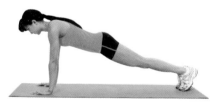

Planks and Pushups

Perform these exercises in a superset fashion: front plank, pushup, right side plank, pushup, left side plank. A front plank is the starting position for a pushup. Press back through your heels and keep your neck in line with your spine. Do not let your chest sink. Hold for 5 seconds, perform a pushup, and return to front plank.

Immediately transition to right side plank by bringing your right palm to center on the floor. Bring the outside of your right foot in line with your palm. Stack your left foot on top of your right. Press your right hand into the floor and lift your hips, making a straight line with your legs and torso. Once balanced, lift your left hand toward the ceiling so that your arms form a straight line. Contract your abs, thighs, and glutes and hold for 5 seconds. Perform a pushup, and then repeat the side plank on your left side.

Superman

Lie on your belly and draw your belly button toward your spine to tighten your abs. Keep your legs straight, your arms stretched out over your head, and your palms facing each other. Arch your back and raise your arms and legs. Hold for 5 to 10 seconds and slowly lower yourself to the floor.

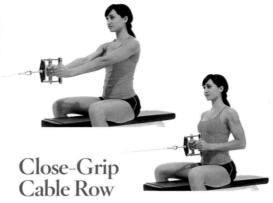

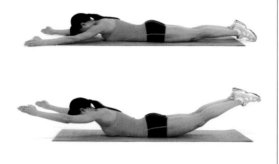

Close-Grip Cable Row

Sit with your abs tight, your lower back slightly arched, your shoulder blades squeezed together, and your torso upright. Lean forward from the hips to grasp the close-grip handles and return to the upright position. Squeeze your shoulder blades and row toward your chest, pulling the handles back as far as possible while keeping your arms close to your body. (Don't jerk your body backward to complete the movement. The rowing motion should come from your upper back, not your arms or lower back.) Slowly extend your arms to return the handles to the upright starting position.

Swiss Ball Curl

Do these exercises in a circuit with no rest to complete one set. Rest for 30 to 60 seconds between sets.

1. Bridge: Lie faceup flat on the floor with your arms extended to the sides to form a T with your body, your legs straight, and your heels on top of a Swiss ball. (The smaller the ball, the tougher the exercise.) Squeeze your glutes and lift your butt off the ground so your body forms a straight line from your shoulders to your heels. Return to the floor.

2. Leg curl: With your heels on the ball, push back up into the bridge position. Keeping your hips off the floor, bend your knees and use your heels to roll the ball toward your body. Keep your abs tight as you roll the ball out. Return to the floor.

3. Hip lift: With your heels on the ball, walk the ball toward your body. Squeeze your glutes and lift your butt until your body forms a straight line from your shoulders to your knees. Return to the floor. Rest.

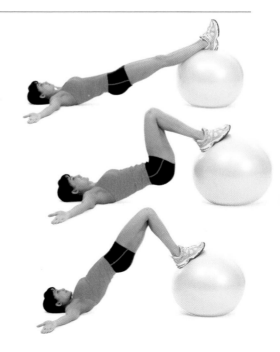

44

Straight Leg Deadlift

Stand with your feet shoulder-width apart and a dumbbell in each hand. With your arms hanging in front of your thighs, lean forward from the hips, keeping your head up, your shoulders back, and your chest out. Bend your knees slightly as you lean forward, allowing the dumbbells to lower in front of you. Push your hips backward and keep leaning forward until your torso is parallel to the floor or lower. Stop when your back starts to round. Pull your torso back to the starting position.

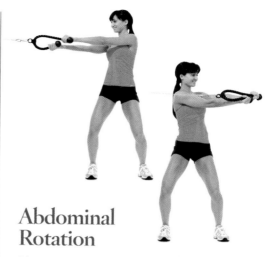

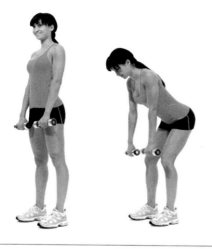

Abdominal Rotation

Stand between two pulley stacks with your arms parallel to the stacks. Position a rope attachment at chest height on the right pulley and grasp the rope with both arms extended. With your legs shoulder-width apart and your knees slightly bent, rotate your torso 180 degrees from right to left, keeping your arms completely extended. Use your abdominal muscles to work against the resistance. Repeat on the opposite side. Rest. Perform 10 to 12 reps on each side.

Prevent Weak Knees

According to the *Journal of the American Academy of Orthopaedic Surgeons*, women are most likely to sustain sports-related injuries between the ages of 15 and 25. And the knees are prime targets. That's because your hips widen slightly in your late teens. As a result, your thigh bones meet your shins at the knee joints at an increased angle, pushing your kneecaps off center, says Letha Griffin, MD, PhD, team physician for Georgia State University athletics.

To strengthen the muscles around your knees—especially your inner thighs—try lying leg circles. Lie on your left side with your head, shoulders, and hips aligned. Prop your head up with your left hand and place your right palm on the floor in front of your belly button. Bend your right knee and place your right foot on the floor in front of your left knee. Lift your left leg 8 inches (or more if you can) off the floor. With your leg straight and your toes flexed, draw 12 circles in the air with your left

heel. Lower your leg and switch sides. That's 1 rep; do 3.

Osteoarthritis, which afflicts 21 million Americans, is another source of havoc on our joints. It occurs when the joint-protecting cartilage breaks down, often from overuse or injury, causing pain and stiffness. But keep in mind that arthritis "isn't inevitable, even for marathon runners," says rheumatologist Janet Lewis, MD, assistant professor of medicine and medical director of the rheumatology clinic at the University of Virginia in Charlottesville. "Genetics has a lot to do with who gets it, and certain factors, like weight, can tip the scale in either direction." Just how important is keeping your weight in check? "Every extra pound above your ideal weight translates into 4 pounds of stress on your knees," says Patience White, MD, a professor of medicine at George Washington University and the chief public health officer for the Arthritis Foundation.

Lean and Fit in 7 Minutes

GET STRONG WITHOUT LIFTING A SINGLE DUMBBELL.

Use this get-it-done-now workout to prevent your endlessly busy life from derailing your fitness goals. Complete one circuit without stopping, rest for 60 to 90 seconds, and then bust out one or two more circuits. Aim for two to three nonconsecutive days a week. All it takes is 7 minutes—about as long as it takes to brew your morning coffee.

2. *Squat Thrusts* Targets core, legs
Stand with your feet together and your arms at your sides. Bend your knees and place your palms on the floor in front of your feet and along the outer sides of your knees. Using your arms for support, jump backward on both feet and land in the plank position. Jump forward on both feet to return to the squat. Return to standing. That's 1 rep. Do 12 to 15.

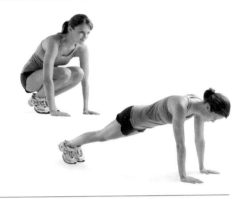

3. *Pike Walk/Pushup Combo* Targets core, upper body
Stand with your feet together and your arms at your sides. Bend over (it's okay for your knees to be slightly bent) and place your hands or fingertips on the floor in front of you. Walk your hands forward into a plank position and do 1 pushup. Keeping your hands in place, walk your feet up until they're as close to your hands as possible. That's 1 rep. Continue moving forward until you've done 5 to 6 pushups.
Trainer Tip: Keep your neck in line with your spine at all times.

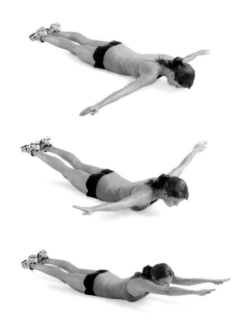

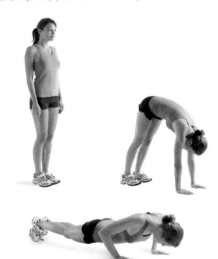

1. *Airplane/Superman Extensions* Targets core, lower back, glutes
Lie facedown and extend your arms to the sides at shoulder height, keeping your elbows slightly bent. Press your shoulder blades together and lift your arms, torso, and legs off the floor. Holding that position, bring your arms in front of you, hold for 1 count, and then move them back. Lower yourself to the floor. That's 1 rep. Do 10 to 15.

4. *Overhead Squat* Targets core, upper back, legs
Stand with your feet slightly wider than shoulder-width apart, your toes turned outward slightly. Grab a rolled-up towel with an overhand grip, holding your hands shoulder-width apart, and raise it overhead so your shoulders are roughly in line with your heels. Squat down as far as possible without letting your knees jut out past your toes. Return to standing. That's 1 rep. Do 10 to 15.
Trainer Tip: The towel helps keep your shoulders aligned. Sans towel, raise your hands overhead—but keep your shoulders and back in line with your heels.

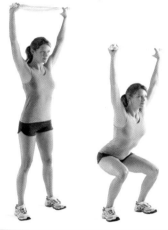

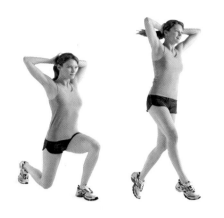

6. *Scissor Lunges* Targets lower body
Stand with your feet hip-width apart, your hands clasped behind your head. Lunge forward with your left foot and lower yourself until your right knee almost touches the floor. Explosively push up and scissor your legs in midair, landing with your right leg forward. When you land, drop down, explode up, and scissor again. That's 1 rep. Do 3 or 4.
Trainer Tip: Land as lightly and quietly as possible.

5. *Mountain Climbers* Targets core, upper body
Get in the plank position with your hands directly below your shoulders and your feet together. Bend your left knee and draw it toward your chest. Extend back to the start. Repeat with your right leg. That's 1 rep. Do 20 to 30, moving quickly.
Trainer Tip: Brace your abs and keep your back flat.

7. *Standing Bird Dog* Targets core, lower body
Stand with your arms at your sides, your right foot raised a few inches behind you. Lean forward while you extend your right leg directly backward and your left arm forward. Keep your right arm against your body. Your torso, left arm, and right leg should be parallel to the floor. Hold for 1 second, then return to the starting position. Repeat on the other side. That's 1 rep. Do 5 or 6.

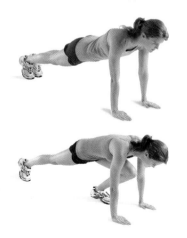

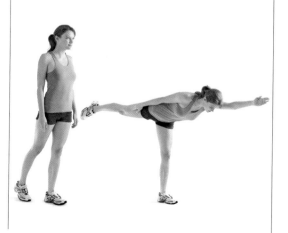

Part Two:

Fitness at 30+:
Protect Your Muscles and Your Bones

Get Firm—Fast!

TAKE THIS WORKOUT SERIOUSLY NOW AND YOU'LL OUTSMART FATE IN THE DECADES TO COME.

W hen researchers at Toronto General Hospital asked women in their thirties why they didn't exercise, 40 percent said they didn't have the time. Another 40 percent said they didn't have the willpower. Sound familiar? Even if you just strap on a pedometer and start tracking your daily steps (and take a few more of them) you'll begin to see results. University of Tennessee researchers in Knoxville found that women who took at least 10,000 steps per day had 9 percent less body fat by the time they were 50 than those who took between 6,000 and 9,999 steps. If you go for regular walks, try to add more steps in the same amount of time; you'll automatically improve your fitness level without increasing your exercise time. But to keep your muscles firm you'll also need to do a little lifting. In fact, the amount of weight-bearing exercise you do in your thirties will directly affect your bone and muscle mass in the future. Here's how to get started.

Instructions
Perform three sets of 8 reps with a 1-minute rest between sets and exercises.

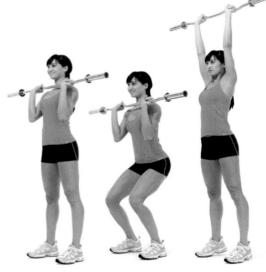

Push Press
Using an overhand grip with your hands slightly wider than your shoulders, lift a barbell to your clavicle so your elbows point down. (Hold the bar so that your knuckles point toward your body.) Squeeze your shoulder blades together and hold them there through the lift. Inhale. Bend your knees slightly, keeping your hips and back straight, and lower 3 to 4 inches into a quarter-squat. From there, exhale and drive the bar overhead until your elbows are fully extended. Slowly lower the bar to the starting position while inhaling and repeat.

48

Diagonal Dumbbell Lunge Curl

Stand with your abs tight, your shoulders back, and your arms at your sides, holding dumb- bells. Inhale. With your right leg, take a large diagonal step forward to the right. Bend your right knee to 90 degrees so that it's directly above your right foot. Keep your left knee just above the floor and your torso upright as your left heel comes up. Exhale and push off the floor with your right leg. Return to the starting position. Perform a biceps curl. Repeat, leading with your left leg.

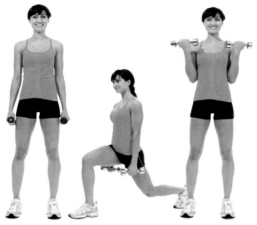

Pushup

Balance your weight on your toes and palms with your hands under your shoulders. Keeping your head aligned with your spine and your pel- vis tucked under slightly, bend your elbows and slowly lower yourself as far as possible toward the floor, then push back to start. Repeat. Note: Do not allow your lower back to sag or your hips to hike up.

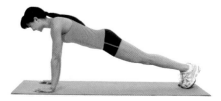

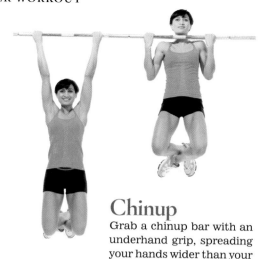

Chinup

Grab a chinup bar with an underhand grip, spreading your hands wider than your shoulders. Start from a full hanging position to work the back muscles through their full range of motion. Arch your back slightly and pull your body up. If you can, try to touch your chest to the bar. Slowly lower yourself back to hanging. Repeat.

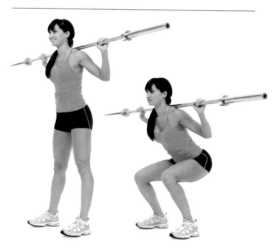

Barbell Back Squat

At a squat rack, stand with your feet shoulder- width apart. Rest the barbell on your upper back and grip it with your hands spread wide. Inhale and lower into a squat position (keep your head up, your heels grounded, and your back arched) until your legs are parallel to the floor or lower. Exhale and stand.

The 10 Best Yoga Poses for Women

WHAT TO DO WHEN YOU HIT THE MAT.

"Yoga teaches you to go to the edge of discomfort in a nonreactive way," says Alan R. Kristal, DPH, a professor of epidemiology at the University of Washington School of Public Health. In his studies Dr. Kristal found that women who practiced yoga for 10 years starting at age 45 gained 3 fewer pounds (if they were at a healthy weight) compared with those who didn't do yoga. Overweight women lost 5 pounds over the 10 years. Try practicing these 10 poses for an hour at least once a week.

Downward Facing Dog Legs, glutes, deltoids, triceps
Down-dog is a top-notch upper body strengthener.
1. Start on all fours with your feet hip-width apart. Position your hands shoulder-width apart and spread your fingers.
2. Lift your knees off the floor and straighten your legs.
3. Walk your hands forward a few inches and your feet backward a few inches to lengthen the pose. Squeeze your thighs as you press them toward the back wall. Press your heels back and down toward the floor.
4. Relax your head, neck, and shoulders. Breathe deeply. Hold for at least 1 minute.

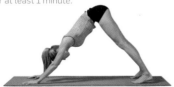

Bridge Pose Front of body, hamstrings, glutes
Bridge opens the chest and rib cage.
1. Lying on your back, bend your knees and place the soles of your feet flat on the floor about hip-width apart. Point your toes straight toward the wall in front of you. Place your arms straight along your sides, palms down.
2. Gently press into your feet as you raise your hips to the sky. Allow the front of your body to slowly expand with each breath. Hold for 5 to 10 breaths. Repeat 3 times.

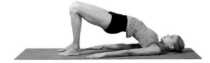

Warrior II Hips, inner thighs, chest, quads, abs, shoulders
This powerful pose will grant you long, lean, toned arms and legs as well as a firmer core.
1. Standing, step your feet to the sides until they're about 4 feet apart. Turn your right foot so the toes point toward the front of your mat. Turn your left foot inward 30 degrees.
2. Raise your arms to shoulder height so they're parallel with the floor, palms down. Bend your right knee so your right shin and thigh form a 90-degree angle.
3. Gently tuck your tailbone down as you draw in your abdomen. Hold for 5 deep breaths in and out through the nose. Straighten the right leg and repeat on the opposite side.

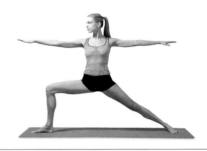

Boat Pose Core, psoas, quads
Build a bulletproof core without straining your neck.
1. Sit with your knees bent and your feet flat on the floor. Lean back slightly to balance on your sit bones. Raise your legs so your shins are parallel to the floor, knees bent.
2. Extend your arms forward, parallel with the floor and palms facing each other. Keeping your chest high and your core engaged, begin to straighten your legs. Hold for 5 to 10 breaths. Repeat 5 times.

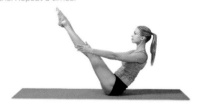

Plank Arms, back, shoulders, core, quads
The plank works all of the major muscles in your arms, back, and core and requires only your body weight.
1. Get into the starting position for a push-up with your shoulders directly over your hands.
2. Press your heels toward the wall behind you and extend the crown of your head forward to form a straight line from the top of your head to your heels. Hold for at least 1 minute.

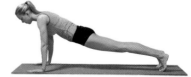

Fierce Pose Spine, quads, ankles, back

This pose strengthens your quadriceps to better support your knees, making them less prone to injury. Fierce pose also improves posture.

1. Stepping your feet to hip-width apart, spread your weight through your toes to create a stable base. As you raise your arms to the sky, palms facing each other, bend your knees and shift your buttocks backward as though you are sitting down on a chair.

2. Draw your abdomen in to eliminate any curving in your lower back. Put all of your weight into your heels and be sure your knees do not extend past your toes. Hold for 5 deep breaths. Rest for 1 minute. Repeat.

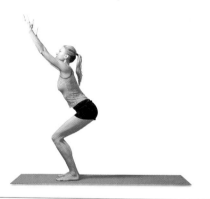

Tree Pose Hips, inner thighs, legs, spine, core

Practicing this pose will greatly improve your ability to find and maintain balance.

1. Stand with your legs and feet together and your hands on your hips. Transfer your weight to your left foot as you bend your right knee and place the sole of the right foot on the inside of your left leg (beginners, start at the ankle; more advanced yogis, raise the right foot to the inside of the left thigh). Gently press the right foot against the left leg.

2. Bring the palms of your hands together in front of your heart in prayer pose. Hold for 1 minute on each side. More advanced yogis: Raise your arms straight overhead, palms facing in.

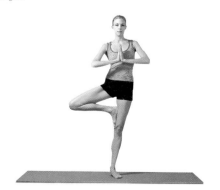

Garland Pose Low back, groin, hips, ankles

Drop into this squat to relieve tummy troubles like constipation and cramps.

1. Stand with your feet slightly wider than hip-width. Bring the palms of your hands together in front of your heart in prayer pose. Turn your toes out slightly.

2. Deeply bend your knees, squatting down between your calves. Keeping your palms together, gently press your elbows to the insides of your knees, opening up the hips. Keep the spine long and the chest open. Feel the tension in the lower back begin to melt away. Hold for at least 1 minute.

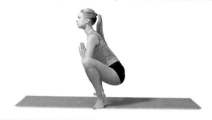

Child's Pose Hips, quads, back

This rest pose opens hips and relieves low back tightness.

1. Kneel on the floor with your big toes touching and your knees about hip-width apart. Sit on your heels.

2. Lay your torso between your thighs and bring your forehead to the mat. Extend your arms straight in front of you, palms on the floor. Close your eyes and breathe deeply. Stay here for at least 1 minute.

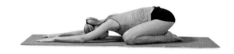

Seated Twist Outer hips, spine

You're only as young as your spine is flexible, and this move will alleviate back pain and increase your range of motion.

1. Sit with your legs outstretched in front of you. Bring the sole of your right foot to the floor outside of your left hip (so your right knee points toward the ceiling).

2. Place your right hand on the floor just behind your right hip. Lift your left arm to the ceiling.

3. Press your left elbow into your right leg, palm facing away from the knee. Inhale and rotate the shoulders and spine to the right.

4. Keeping the chin in line with the right shoulder, the neck long, look toward the wall behind you.

5. Hold for 5 to 10 deep breaths. Repeat on the opposite side.

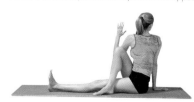

Part Three:
Fitness at 40+:
Claim a Body for the Ages

Slim Down, Power Up

FIND LEVELS OF ENERGY YOU NEVER KNEW YOU HAD.

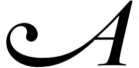fter 45, most women who don't lift weights start losing a significant amount of muscle, most of it from the lower body. Less junk in the trunk may sound like a good thing, but decreased muscle mass leads to a slower metabolism. So not only are your muscles beginning to shrink, you're also starting to feel a little chunkier. What could be worse than that? Sleep studies show that women over 40 spend more sleepless nights (and not the coed naked kind) than twentysomethings. Experts aren't sure why exactly, but one thing is clear: less sleep = less energy = half-assed everything. Here's one cure for insomnia: Exercise before work. A Northwestern University study found that sedentary women who started exercising in the morning slept better than they had before. And according to public researchers in Seattle, women who boosted their fitness levels by 10 per-

cent over a year slept better and were less likely to pop sleep meds than women who improved their fitness by only 1 percent or less. Feeling too groggy to work out? That's because it takes the brain up to 2 hours to wake up. Make yourself a bowl of instant oatmeal with ½ cup of fat-free milk before your morning workout. According to researchers at Tufts University in Boston, people who ate one packet of instant oatmeal received a shot of glucose strong enough to jolt them awake. Down that, and then do this.

Instructions
Each move has two parts and counts as 1 rep. Beginners, start with 1 to 2 reps (working up to 4) of each compound exercise, without rest. Try to do two sets of the entire circuit, pausing for 2 minutes between sets. Advance up to five sets. Start with 35 percent of the heaviest weight that you're able to lift for your weakest exercise (generally the dumbbell pullover).

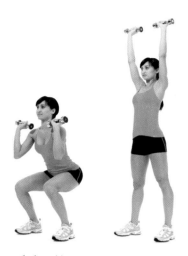

Dumbbell Back Squat to Overhead Press

Stand with your feet shoulder-width apart and your toes pointed slightly outward. Grab dumbbells with an overhand grip and bring them up to shoulder height with your palms facing outward. Inhale, bend your knees, and lower your hips into a squat. Keep your head up, your heels on the ground, and your back arched. Squat until your thighs are parallel to the floor. Then quickly return to standing and exhale. Drive both dumbbells overhead until your elbows are fully extended. Slowly lower the dumbbells to the starting position.

Dumbbell Pullover to Crunch

Lie back on a Swiss ball so it supports your lower and mid-back. Bend your knees and keep your feet flat on the floor. Raise your arms straight overhead holding a dumbbell or weight plate. Pull your arms to your chest. Crunch all the way up and slowly lower back to the starting position.

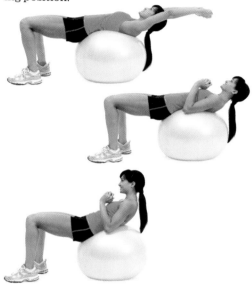

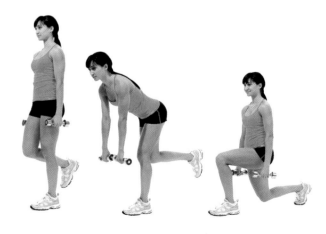

One-Leg Good Morning to Reverse Lunge

Stand on your left leg with the knee slightly bent, holding dumbbells. Keeping your abs tight, your back flat, and your knees slightly bent, slowly bend forward from your hips until your torso is parallel to the floor. Return to the starting position and lunge backward with your right leg. Forcefully push off the right leg to return to the starting position. Switch legs.

Romanian Deadlift to Row

Stand with your feet shoulder-width apart, holding a barbell (or dumbbells) in both hands with an overhand grip. Bend forward from the hips to about 90 degrees. Keep your shoulders back and your chest out. As you lean forward, lower the bar. Bend your knees slightly. Then pull the bar up toward your ribs, with your elbows pointing up. Slowly release the bar back down and lift your torso back to standing.

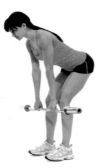

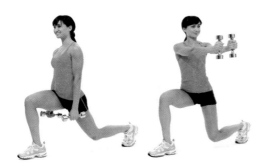

Lunge with Rotation

Stand with your abs tight, your shoulders back, and your arms at your sides holding dumbbells. Inhale. Take a large step forward with your right leg, planting your foot flat on the floor. Bend your left knee slightly. Drop your hips until your right knee is directly over your foot and at 90 degrees. Bend your left knee to 90 degrees as you roll your heel up. Keep your left knee just above the floor and your torso upright. Extend your arms straight out in front of you with your palms facing inward. Rotate your upper body to the right, center, left, and back to center. Exhale and push off the floor with your right leg. Return to the starting position and switch legs. This time rotate to the left first.

Tally Up Your Daily Burn

PICK AN ACTIVITY—OR A FEW ACTIVITIES!—TO SHED MORE CALORIES.

ACTIVITY	CALORIES PER 10 MINUTES
Yoga	30
Washing car	36
Weight training	36
Vacuuming	42
Horseback riding	48
Raking lawn	52
Gardening	54
Hiking	72
Swimming	72
Tennis	84
Circuit training with cardio	96
Cycling	96

The Spin Zone

YOU DON'T HAVE TO BE HARD CORE TO REAP THE MEGABENEFITS OF CYCLING.

You were on to something when you ditched those training wheels. Cycling fries fat and demolishes stress without pounding you into the ground. Even pedaling at an easy pace, a 130-pound woman will torch 473 calories in an hour. Up the speed to 20 mph and you'll burn 1,000 calories. You'll get sick legs, too. "Turning the pedals over 5,400 times an hour gives you serious tone in your quads and calves," says Jenni Gaertner, who coaches in Coeur d'Alene, Idaho. "In other words, the muscles you notice when you're wearing heels and a mini." To really engage those muscles, Gaertner says to make your pedal stroke a perfect circle. Push forward and then down with your quads; pull back with your hamstrings; and then use your calves and hip flexors to pull up and back. To expose the weak spots in your stroke, pedal with one leg at a time. Then concentrate on the gaps when you're back to two feet.

The Ultimate Cardio Burn

BURN 500 CALORIES DURING YOUR LUNCH BREAK.

Between their thirties and forties, lazy ladies will lose up to 6 percent of their aerobic capacity. If you want to defy their ranks, make it your goal to burn 500 calories during your lunch break. That's the gold standard—the equivalent of a gymnast achieving a perfect 10 or a director getting a thumbs-up from Ebert. "It's a great target," says Gregory Florez, a spokesman for the American Council on Exercise. "It means you've spent some serious time moving your body. Plus, seven 500-calorie workouts, added together, are really significant. That means you've exercised away a full pound." Even better, most women really can burn 500* calories in less than an hour, which means you

don't need to eagle-eye those annoying red numbers on the treadmill anymore. So put away the dog-eared copy of *Caribbean Getaways* and stop lolly-gagging it: The 42-minute cardio routine below requires undivided attention. "It gives you a great aerobic workout, hits most of the major muscle groups, and mixes it up so you're not bored and don't invite overuse injuries," Florez says. Head from one piece of equipment to the next as quickly as possible.

*Note: Calorie count is based on a 135-pound woman. If you weigh more, you'll burn more. If you weigh less . . . you get the idea.

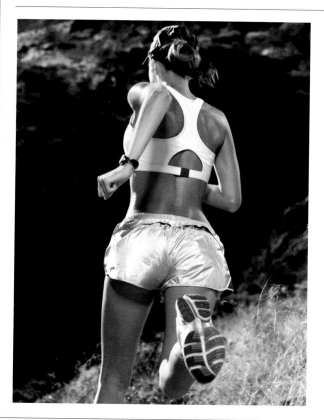

1. 15 minutes: Treadmill
To warm up, walk at 3 miles per hour (mph) for the 1st minute. For the next 4 minutes, up the speed 0.3 mph every minute. After 5 minutes, increase your speed to an easy jog (5 to 6 mph). Keep it there for 1 minute, then bring it down to $4\frac{1}{2}$ mph for a brisk walk for the next minute. Repeat this last jog-then-walk sequence 5 times.

2. 10 minutes: Elliptical Trainer
Use a full-body machine that involves arm movement. Make your arms your primary movers: Emphasize pushing and pulling them, instead of letting your legs do everything. Go hard. "You should be uncomfortable enough so that, every minute, you're checking when 10 minutes is up," Florez says. (If your gym's elliptical machines target legs only, then increase the incline on the ramp. Shoot for an incline that is about two-thirds of the maximum.)

3. 12 minutes: Tread Climber, Stairclimber, or Rowing Machine
If you have access to a tread climber—a machine that looks like a treadmill split in half—get on that. If not, a stairclimber (either with pedals or with moving stairs) or a rowing machine will do. Do 2 minutes of hard work (you should be on the verge of gasping for breath), followed by 1 minute of recovery. Get to the breathless state by increasing the incline or speed, then lower it for a minute of rest. By the end of the easier minute, you should be able to carry on a conversation.

4. 5 minutes: Stationary Bike
Pedal at a low intensity to cool down.

Chapter Four

Put Your Best Face Forward

TURN BACK THE CLOCK WITH GLOWING SKIN, LINE-FREE EYES, AND A BRIGHT SMILE

> **INVESTMENT:** 4 WEEKS
> **AGE ERASED:** 5 YEARS

Age Erasers

Introduction

Getting older may be inevitable, but looking older is optional—really! To get healthy, gorgeous skin; wide-open, beautiful eyes; and a stunning smile, you just need to think about your face (and the way you care for it) in a whole new way.

Most of us treat our skin the way we do our ovens: We count on it to function properly, then assault it with harsh chemicals and vigorous scouring when we suddenly notice what a mess it is. As early as grade school health class, we're told to scrub the grime and grease off our skin, but new science shows that our obsession with removing surface dirt and oil is like giving Steve Buscemi a haircut—it's helpful, but you still haven't fixed the problem.

Another part of maintaining a fresh look is paying attention to your eyes. On a good day, they're your best feature. On a bad one, those red rims, puffy lids, and dark circles are a road map to your worst beauty habits: the sunscreen you forgot to apply, the makeup you didn't take off, and the sleep you skipped in order to put the finishing touches on your child's model of the solar system.

Or is it your smile that's aging you? A recent Tufts University study found that 46 percent of adults over age 23 have at least one tooth with significant enamel damage. Caused by acidic foods (like soda, orange juice, and yogurt), enamel loss can leave your choppers dingy, sensitive, and more cavity prone.

Regardless of your concerns, the remedies in this chapter will help you subtract years from your appearance and give your face the bright outlook you've always wanted.

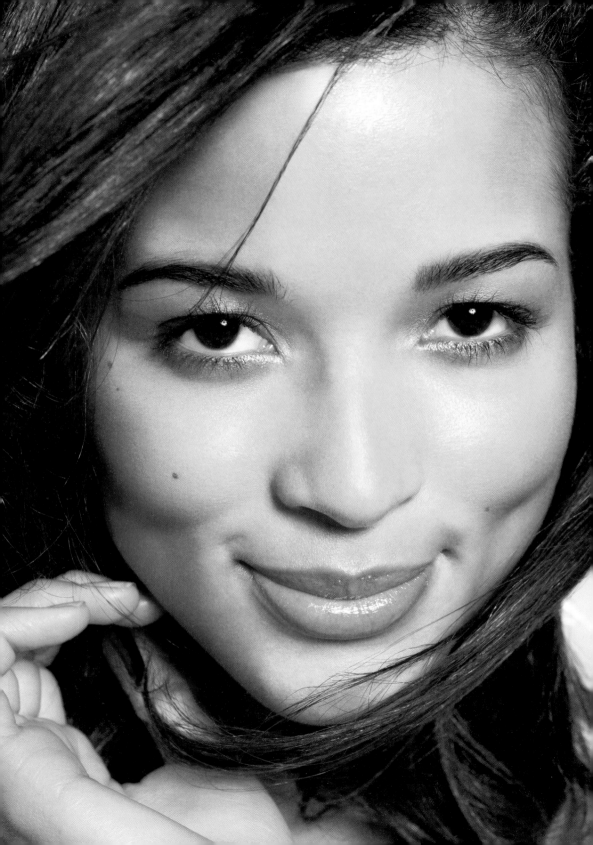

Get the Protection You Need

SHIELD YOUR FACE FROM THE DAMAGING
EFFECTS OF THE SUN'S RAYS.

*I*t's not like you need another reason to slather on the SPF, but here's one anyway: The evenness of your skin tone influences how attractive you appear, according to a study in the journal *Evolution and Human Behavior*. Researchers photographed 169 women and fitted each face onto a standard digital model using special software. They erased features like wrinkles—and nothing causes wrinkles more than too much sun—so skin tone was the only difference and then asked 198 male volunteers to rate the pictures. The men found the faces with the most even skin tones the healthiest and most attractive. "Unevenness in skin color, like veins and redness, creates contrasts [that affect] our perception of beauty," says study coauthor Paul Matts, PhD, of Procter and Gamble. The best way to protect your skin? You guessed it: sunscreen.

Still, putting on sunscreen is a lot like flossing your teeth. It's a superhealthy habit that you're totally into—in theory. But the reality is you're in a rush, and coating yourself with cream takes time. It's greasy. It makes your face shine, and you figure your pores are probably clogged enough already without that extra layer of goo.

Besides, you're only planning to be outside for a few minutes, half an hour max. Which is why it's not surprising that only a third of women lotion up before heading out the door for the day, as reported by a survey by the American Academy of Dermatology.

But skipping the slathering is a worse idea than you may realize. You don't need to bake like Donatella Versace for the sun to toy with your skin's DNA, triggering changes that can speed up the aging process and lead to skin cancer. Melanoma, the deadliest form, has increased more than 70 percent in women under 40 since 1975. That's huge. What's more, a recent study found that cases of less deadly kinds of skin cancer—basal and squamous cell carcinoma—are also rising among young women, leaving stitches and scars behind.

Unfortunately you have to be a real label hawk to know if the sunscreen in your tube is truly "broad spectrum," meaning that it protects you from both ultraviolet A (UVA) and ultraviolet B (UVB) rays. Any sunscreen with an SPF of 15 will block 94 percent of UVB rays, which penetrate the skin superficially, causing sunburn and skin

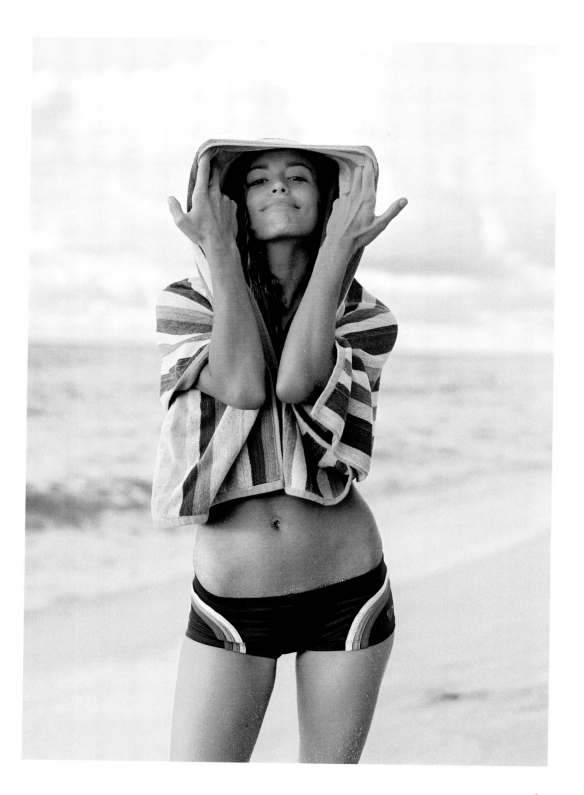

Skin Cancer Prevention

THE COMPLETE INSTRUCTIONS

More than a million cases of skin cancer occur each year in the United States, including 60,000 cases of deadly malignant melanoma. "Every photon of light can lead to a wrinkle, brown spot, or cancer," says William Heimer, MD, a board-certified dermatologist in San Diego. "Protecting your skin should be an everyday thing, like brushing your teeth." Save your hide with these tips.

Watch the Clock

Just five moderate sunburns in your lifetime doubles your melanoma risk. Wear sun protection between 10:00 a.m. and 4:00 p.m., says Adnan Nasir, MD, a clinical professor of dermatology at the University of North Carolina in Chapel Hill.

Double Your Protection

"When applying sunblock, imagine you're painting a wall," says Dr. Nasir. "You need two coats, and you want to make sure every inch is covered." Apply it 20 minutes before you go out and again every 2 hours, or each time you sweat or towel off after a swim. La Roche-Posay Anthelios SPF 40 sunscreen (www.laroche-posay.us) provides complete protection from UVA and UVB rays and contains Mexoryl SX, a compound that won't degrade as quickly in sunlight.

Dress Defensively

"A regular T-shirt has an SPF of about 5," says Dr. Heimer. "That means a lot of UV light is filtering through." If you're planning to be outside for, say, a round of golf, wear clothing with built-in SPF (www.sundayafternoons.com). Or sprinkle a laundry aid like SunGuard (www.sunguardsunprotection.com) into your wash. It increases clothing's SPF to 30.

Run on Dunkin'

A 2007 Rutgers University study found that a combination of caffeine and exercise lowered the risk of UVB-induced non-melanoma skin cancer in mice. "It enhanced their bodies' ability to kill off cells damaged by UVB, so they were eliminating precancerous cells from the skin before they caused harm," says Allan H. Conney, PhD, a study author.

Save Your Face

"Wear at least an SPF 15 sunblock on your face every day," advises Dr. Nasir. That includes cloudy days. "UVA rays easily penetrate clouds, glass, and most windows," he says. And although these rays won't leave you crispy the way UVB light can, they penetrate the skin more deeply. "Many years of UVA damage is equivalent to a few years of UVB damage," he says.

Stay Out of the Tanning Booth

A visit to the fake 'n' bake nearly triples the risk of squamous cell carcinoma and almost doubles your risk of basal cell carcinoma. "Sunlight has a mix of rays, but tanning beds contain mostly UVA rays," says Dr. Nasir. "Fifteen minutes is like 4 hours in the July sun."

cancer. UVA rays, on the other hand, cause up to 80 percent of sun-related wrinkles and age spots, and also increase your risk of skin cancer. UVA rays are trickier to fight because they penetrate the atmosphere even on cloudy days, and only four ingredients provide solid protection against them. Two of those ingredients are chemical sunblocks—avobenzone and Mexoryl SX—which work by absorbing and neutralizing UV radiation after it hits your skin, but before it can damage cells. The other two—zinc oxide and titanium dioxide—are physical sunblocks, which form a shield and actually reflect and disperse the radiation before it hits your skin.

"Stay away from any sunscreen that has an SPF of less than 15 or doesn't contain one of these four ingredients," says Coyle Connolly, DO, a board-certified dermatologist in Linwood, New Jersey. Which sunscreen you should grab depends on your needs. Physical sunblocks are effective as soon as you apply them and, because they are made from natural ingredients, can be less irritating. Chemical sunblocks are generally more waterproof, but they take 30 minutes to absorb. Mexoryl SX has been available in Europe for years, but it was only recently approved by the Food and Drug Administration (FDA). It provides excellent protection against both short and long UVA rays; the others primarily protect against long UVA rays.

Once you've picked a sunscreen, work it into your morning routine. For best absorption, rub it on clean skin. (While you're at it, swipe on some SPF lip balm.) Then add moisturizer and makeup. And make sure you put enough on. Many of us use far less than we need to get the protection promised on the tube. Apply a half teaspoon for each arm and for your face and neck, and a full teaspoon for each leg, your chest, and your back, depending on what skin will be exposed.

No matter which sunscreen you use, David J. Leffell, MD, professor of dermatology at the Yale University School of Medicine, recommends reapplying it every couple of hours. "Ignore any claims about the longevity of sunscreen," he warns. Even potions labeled "all day" wear off before 8 hours, he says, especially if you're swimming or sweating. Your goal for a weekend at the beach: finish an 8-ounce bottle of sunscreen.

Look Younger Longer

THESE 6 SIMPLE STEPS WILL KEEP YOUR COMPLEXION
SOFT, SUPPLE, AND CREASE-FREE FOR DECADES TO COME.

By Sarah Mahoney

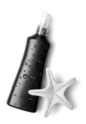

Skin care is a lot like your 401(k): There's a lot of advice out there on the best moves to make, and it'll be years before you see any return. But with this easy routine, you can start preventing the signs of aging now—and that's something you can bank on.

Step 1: Cleanser

Starting with clean skin makes the rest of your skin-care arsenal more effective. Try a gentle cleanser that leaves protective oils and moisture behind (try Dove Beauty Bar and Neutrogena Facial Cleansing Bar). "For an extra boost, use a product made with alpha hydroxy acids, or AHAs," says Francesca J. Fusco, MD, assistant clinical professor of dermatology at Mount Sinai School of Medicine and a member of *Women's*

Health's advisory board. "They exfoliate the dead cells, help plump up your skin, and give a healthy glow." AHAs make the outermost layer of skin stronger and more resistant to irritation.

Step 2: Antiaging Serum

These potent formulas pack concentrated power in small doses. The best contain antioxidants (look for vitamins C and E and green tea) or peptides (amino acid chains believed to bolster the skin's collagen production), according to Diane Berson, MD, an assistant professor of dermatology at Weill Cornell Medical College in New York City. Blend a few drops onto freshly cleansed skin—it absorbs better when pores are wide open.

Step 3: Moisturizer

When skin cells become dehydrated, they shrivel

up, making skin look older, dull in tone and texture, and even wrinkled. What's more, says Yohini Appa, PhD, a researcher at Neutrogena, "free radicals can penetrate more easily through dry skin to attack the layers of collagen and elastin." (Translation: You get saggy skin.) Look for a lightweight formula that has an SPF of at least 25 and contains petrolatum or glycerin, the gold standards for moisture retention.

Step 4: Sunscreen

Reread the previous section if you're still not convinced you need to use this every day! "Even if you've applied a moisturizer or foundation with SPF, be sure to use a sunscreen if you'll be out for more than an hour or so," says Ellen Marmur, MD, chief of dermatologic and cosmetic surgery at Mount Sinai Medical Center in New York City. Mexoryl SX is the best ingredient to look for.

Step 5: Retinoid

Antiaging ingredients aren't immediate people-pleasers; they need time to do their good deeds. Take, for example, retinoids. These vitamin A derivatives—in prescription strength, they're sold as Retin-A and Renova; in the similar but less powerful over-the-counter version, they're found in retinol—smooth away fine lines and wrinkles, help even out skin tone, and may even reverse the effects of UV exposure. However, they can make skin more sensitive to UV light, so doctors recommend applying the cream before bed. That way, it can do its thing while you doze.

Step 6: Sleep

Getting plenty of shut-eye is as good for your complexion as it is for your body. When medical researchers at New York City's Cornell University deprived 11 women of sleep for just 1 night, it was enough to deplete their skin's defenses. To make the most of your z's, try to get 7 to 8 hours of sleep a night, and use a humidifier to keep your skin moist and help your nighttime treatment sink into your pores. (Learn more about the importance of sleep—and its role in the fight against age—on page 176.)

Age-Proof Your Skin

FOLLOW THESE TIPS TO SMOOTH, MOISTURIZE, AND FIGHT WRINKLES.

Use Soap Selectively
To keep skin soft, use soap or body wash only on select areas—your face, underarms, feet, groin, and buttocks. "Rinsing with water is enough to get other spots clean and prevent you from unnecessarily stripping skin of its natural oils," says New York City dermatologist Amy Wechsler, MD, an assistant clinical professor of dermatology at the State University of New York Downstate Medical Center in Brooklyn.

Moisturize While You Wash
Amp up the antiaging benefits of your body wash by applying it with a wet mesh puff. "Pumping air into the product helps it foam more, allowing you to use less detergents, which keeps skin from becoming overly dry," says Zoe D. Draelos, MD, a clinical associate professor of dermatology at Wake Forest University School of Medicine in Winston-Salem, North Carolina.

Clean a Wet Face
Use cleanser—especially foaming or gel types—on damp skin. If applied to dry skin, they are more likely to be irritating, says Mary Lupo, MD, a clinical professor of dermatology at Tulane University in New Orleans, Louisiana.

Wash for 60 Seconds
Massage cleanser on your face for about 1 minute to break down dirt and makeup before rinsing off. "It's important to wipe away pollutants, dirt, bacteria, and product residue, which can cause dullness and clogged pores," says New York City–based dermatologist Jeanette Graf, MD, author of *Stop Aging, Start Living*.

Give Makeup a Firm Base
Splash your face with cold water before applying makeup; the coolness helps temporarily shrink pores. "It's a trick movie stars used in the '30s to tighten skin and help makeup glide on seamlessly," says Valerie Sarnelle, makeup artist and founder of the cosmetics line Valerie Beverly Hills.

Mist Up Midday
Refresh parched skin with a spritz of a facial mist on your bare skin—just be sure to apply moisturizer after to seal in the added hydration. "The dewier your skin, the less noticeable wrinkles will be," says New York City–based celebrity makeup artist Maria Verel.

Adjust Your Visor
"The left side of women's faces tends to look older because it incurs more sun damage from driving," explains Cambridge, Massachusetts–based dermatologist Ranella Hirsch, MD, past president of the American Society of Cosmetic Dermatology and Aesthetic Surgery. This one is a no-brainer. Simply move the visor in your car to your left side to block UV rays while you're driving. If you have children, consider purchasing car shades that attach to your rear windows with suction cups.

A Clear Plan

GRADUATE TO GLOWING, GROWN-UP SKIN WITH THE LATEST ACNE TREATMENTS.

Breakouts, like corsages and detention, should disappear after high school. But since we've got more stress than Jon and Kate's nanny, women still battle blemishes in their twenties, thirties, and beyond. But recent scientific advances in treating and preventing acne can help.

Stop scrubbing. New research shows that moisture is key to faster healing for acne-prone complexions, and too much washing dehydrates your skin. "Washing your face more often will not prevent or improve acne, and washing too little will not cause it," says Dr. Fusco. Hydrate with a moisturizer labeled noncomedogenic at least once a day and cleanse with a soap-free wash instead.

Think three. Combat acne with a three-pronged treatment, says Macrene Alexiades-Armenakas, MD, PhD, assistant clinical professor of dermatology at Yale University School of Medicine. Kill the bacteria that so blithely colonize our skin with an antimicrobial agent like benzoyl peroxide. Next, unclog pores with salicylic or glycolic acid. Then reduce redness with zinc or sulfur.

Follow doctor's orders. Ask your dermatologist about Solodyn (minocycline), an extended-release antibiotic that you take just once a day, which kills bacteria. Ziana Gel combines an antimicrobial agent with a retinoid that aids skin-cell turnover. And there's a version of the topical gel Differin (adapalene) that's stronger than the original.

See the light. "The biggest advance in treating acne has been light therapy," says Neil Sadick, MD, clinical professor of dermatology at Weill Cornell Medical College in New York City. Recent research from Yale shows that photodynamic therapy (in which clinicians apply a chemical called Levulan to the skin and then expose it to a light source) kills bacteria and shrinks oil glands. The treatment can clear up chronic acne in 1 to 12 sessions ($150 to $600 each). However, insurance almost never covers them.

Damage Control

DESPITE YOUR BEST INTENTIONS, SUN-CARE SLIPS HAPPEN. HERE'S HOW TO MITIGATE THE CONSEQUENCES.

Damage: A lobster-red sunburn
Rx: That tightness you feel is your skin swelling: "Take 400 milligrams of aspirin or ibuprofen every 4 hours for the first day to offset pain and inflammation," says Jeannette Graf, MD, of the Mount Sinai School of Medicine in New York City. Dab on aloe or a hydrocortisone lotion to hydrate skin until the burn subsides. Too much sun also destabilizes the skin's oxygen molecules, releasing free radicals that lead to wrinkles and sagging. Combat this effect by using a moisturizer with an SPF 30 and vitamins A, C, and E.

Damage: Swollen, sun-baked lids
Rx: Twice a day, soak green-tea bags in cold water and place them over your eyes for 3 to 5 minutes. "It feels soothing, and the polyphenols in green tea reduce inflammation," says Santa Monica, California, dermatologist Karyn Grossman, MD. Apply a layer of aloe gel around the eyes, and avoid irritating antiaging eye creams for 10 days.

Damage: Fried hair
Rx: Once a week, after shampooing, follow up with a protein-rich deep conditioner. Smooth it onto damp hair, leave it for 20 to 30 minutes, and then rinse well. For very dry, stripped hair, Dr. Graf recommends treatments that contain olive oil, ceramides, neem oil, and cholesterol.

Unveil a Wrinkle-Free Face

LINES? WHAT LINES? FROM BOTOX AND FILLERS TO LASERS AND PEELS, HERE'S HOW TO DEFY YOUR AGE—AND ERASE EVERY CREASE.

By Karyn Repinski

*M*any things improve with age, but sadly, your skin isn't one of them. Over the years (and after a lifetime of sun exposure), skin often loses its elasticity and resiliency, giving way to wrinkles. But it's never been easier to eradicate the lines and wrinkles that make you look (and feel) older than you actually are.

Here's the real scoop on the wrinkle fixers, their newfangled cousins and why some old standbys are still worth your while. We've talked to top dermatologists and plastic surgeons, who gave us loads of insider tips and expert advice to help you determine the right way to reclaim your skin.

Botox

Fixes: Crow's-feet, forehead furrows, and lip lines. Results last for up to 4 months with little to no downtime. About $400 per treated area.

Botox injections interrupt nerve impulses to the muscles used to squint, frown, and purse the lips. When these muscles relax, fine lines and wrinkles smooth out. According to a recent review of studies, patients who received Botox felt they looked about 5 years younger. It may take 2 weeks for Botox to kick in the first time. The smoothing effect lasts for up to 4 months. Repeat shots tend to take effect sooner (in as little as 2 days) and last longer. "After being in a relaxed state for so long, your muscles retrain themselves to stay that way," says David Bank, MD, a dermatologist in Mount Kisco, New York. If used early enough (ideally, in the late thirties and early forties), Botox prevents deep wrinkles from setting in.

Ouch factor: Mild stinging. "The needle is only slightly thicker than a hair, and it takes less than 10 minutes to completely treat any of these areas," says Dr. Bank. There's no downtime; you can get 'toxed during lunch and no one will be the wiser.

Risks: The low dosage levels used in a standard cosmetic injection—25 to 75 units—aren't toxic. (A lethal dose for humans is approximately 3,000 units.) Recent reports that link Botox to serious adverse reactions stem from high dosages used to treat serious medical conditions. As of May 1, 2009, however, the FDA will require the manufacturers of Botox and the recently approved anti-wrinkle drug Dysport, both of which contain the paralytic agent botulinum toxin, to carry "black-box" labels warning that the drug has the potential to spread from the injection site and affect swallowing and breathing. Still, the risk of life-threatening damage remains exceedingly rare. The most common—but still rare—side effects of

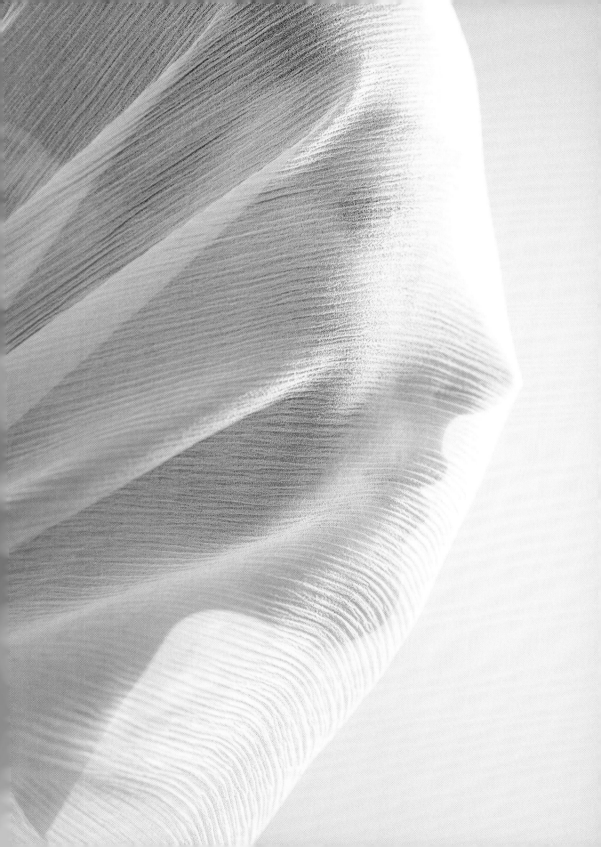

Botox when used cosmetically are slight bruising that lasts for a few days, a headache, or a strange feeling of heaviness. You may temporarily end up with an uneven brow or a droopy lid if the wrong muscle is targeted or equal amounts aren't used on each side of the face.

Maximize results: Activate the injected muscles for 30 to 60 minutes after treatment—so, for example, squint your eyes as much as you can after having your frown lines treated. "That way, more of the toxin will be taken up into the nerve that supplies the muscles," says Jean Carruthers, MD, a clinical professor of ophthalmology at the University of British Columbia in Vancouver. But don't massage the area for 24 hours or the Botox may migrate into unintended neighboring muscles.

Fillers

Fixes: "Smile" lines, marionette lines (vertical lines below the mouth), lip lines, and also deeper lines that Botox doesn't uncrinkle. Results last for up to 6 months; causes bruising for up to 10 days. Costs about $600 per treatment area.

Hyaluronic acid fillers such as Restylane and Juvéderm are smooth gels that instantly fill up wrinkles; hyaluronic acid's ability to attract up to 1,000 times its weight in water helps keep skin plumped. Repeated treatment with Restylane means longer-lasting effects because injections stimulate new collagen that "lifts" skin. "After a couple of years, patients often don't need further injections or need less filler to achieve the desired effect," says Dr. Bank.

Ouch factor: Mild to moderate. Despite the use of ultrafine needles, "some patients find it uncomfortable, especially around the mouth," says Kenneth Beer, MD, an assistant professor of dermatology at the University of Miami. Ice, topical anesthesia, and nerve blocks reduce the pain. The treatment takes less than 30 minutes but often causes bruising and swelling—so schedule treatments ahead of important events. Avoid vitamin E, St. John's wort, ibuprofen, aspirin, and other anti-inflammatories for a week prior to reduce side effects.

Risks: A lumpy feeling or asymmetry occasionally occur if the material clumps in one place instead of diffusing evenly. Massage or injection of an enzyme that dissolves hyaluronic acid usually corrects the problem.

Maximize results: Hyaluronic acid fillers are malleable, so avoid rubbing treated areas for 24 hours. Minimizing facial movements in injected areas for several hours also keeps the material in place.

Laser Resurfacing

Fixes: Fine lines and blotchiness. Skin looks badly sunburned for 2 days. Five monthly treatments are needed, at about $1,130 each.

Fractionated lasers emit very thin beams of infrared light that make microscopic wounds over only 20 percent of your skin, triggering the body's natural healing process and accelerating the production of collagen and new, healthy skin cells. A recently published study reported a 25 to 50 percent improvement in lines around the eyes and mouth following three monthly treatments with Fraxel, one type of fractionated laser. Where these lasers really excel, though, say some experts, is at wiping out freckles and blotchiness—pigment-producing cells are injured during treatment, so they pump out less melanin. It takes 3 to 6 months from your last treatment to see the final results, which last at least 2 years. But noticeable wrinkle smoothing and improvement in discoloration are possible after several sessions. "That doesn't mean every line will be erased," says Elizabeth Tanzi, MD, a dermatologist in Washington, DC, and a clinical instructor at the Johns Hopkins School of Medicine in Baltimore. "Sometimes you have to use the laser in combination with other treatments like Botox and fillers."

The best candidates for this treatment have mild to moderate sun damage.

Ouch factor: The newer Affirm and ActiveFX fractionated lasers are mildly painful, if at all, so an anesthetic is optional; a fan also cools skin to minimize discomfort. Fraxel penetrates the deepest and can

2.5
Millions of people who used botox in 2008

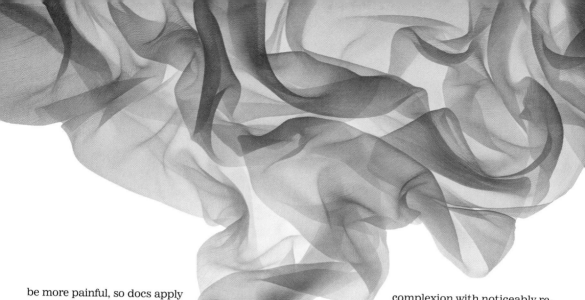

be more painful, so docs apply a numbing agent. Downtime is minimal: "You can usually be treated on Friday and be back in commission, with makeup, on Monday," says Dr. Tanzi.

Risks: Complications are extremely rare when an experienced physician performs the procedure.

Maximize results: Use a retinoid and antioxidant for 2 weeks before treatment to speed healing, says Robert Weiss, MD, president of the American Society for Dermatologic Surgery and associate professor of dermatology at the Johns Hopkins School of Medicine. "When skin is softer, you can go deeper with the same amount of energy to deliver a better outcome."

Peels

Fixes: Dramatically improves fine lines, deep wrinkles, and brown splotches. Treatment is painful, requires a week to recover. Costs $700.

During a chemical peel, doctors paint a 25 to 35 percent trichloroacetic acid (TCA) on the face like a mask to create a controlled exfoliation. Because TCA delves fairly deeply into the skin to remove the layers of damaged tissue and to stimulate collagen production, you'll need to hide out for about a week while you heal. But it's worth it: "Within 7 to 10 days, you'll have a youthful, glowing

complexion with noticeably reduced signs of sun damage," says Yael Halaas, MD, a facial plastic surgeon in New York City. "Decades of studies have shown that you'll see a 50 percent improvement in all but the deepest lines around the mouth," says Dr. Bank. The rejuvenating effect lasts for several years.

Ouch factor: Fairly high—at least briefly. For the 2 minutes it takes the acid to neutralize, you'll experience a terrible burning pain, says Mary Lupo, MD, a clinical professor of dermatology at Tulane University School of Medicine. To minimize discomfort during the 45-minute procedure, docs peel the face in sections and cool it with a fan. There's no pain post-peel, but the skin feels like it's been badly sunburned. It takes a solid week to recover—and you'll be self-conscious in public. By day 7, most of the skin has peeled off and you can cover the residual pinkness with makeup. You can also consider having a series of lower-strength TCA peels, which produce 3 days of fine flaking. Three 15 percent peels achieve nearly the same results as one higher-strength peel, says Dr. Bank.

Risks: The darker your skin's color, the higher your risk of complications such as skin discoloration and scarring.

Maximize results: Use a retinoid and a sunscreen daily to see sustained improvement.

So Long, Fine Lines

EYE CREAMS ARE YOUR SECRET WEAPONS FOR WRINKLES, BAGS, SHADOWS, AND MORE.

By Laurel Naverson Geraghty

A bag of frozen peas and some sliced cucumbers once did almost as much good as eye creams when it came to treating fine lines, puffiness, and dark circles. "Past formulations contained mainly moisturizing ingredients, so they did no more for you than a basic cream—but at quadruple the cost," says Patricia Farris, MD, a dermatologist in Metairie, Louisiana and a clinical assistant professor at Tulane University School of Medicine. But that's changing. The latest buzz: new, just-as-pricey products with a slew of much more promising ingredients. Whether you want to repair or prevent signs of aging around your eyes, here's what you need to know.

Crow's-Feet

To repair: Researchers have found that amino acids called hexapeptides can block the nerve signals that cause muscles to contract. "They work on the same principle as Botox," says Susan Weinkle, MD, a dermatologist in Bradenton, Florida. The idea: When applied, the ingredients subtly inhibit muscle movements to soften wrinkles and prevent new ones from forming. In a University of Valencia, Spain, study researchers found that the depth of participants' eye wrinkles decreased by 30 percent after 1 month.
Try: Freeze 24-7 Anti-Aging Eye Serum (www.freeze247.com) or Dermadoctor Immobile Lines (www.dermadoctor.com)

To prevent: Idebenone, a smaller version of coenzyme Q10, has emerged as one of skin care's most powerful antioxidants, gobbling up cell-damaging free radicals to keep wrinkles from forming. In a study in the *Journal of Cosmetic Dermatology*, idebenone outperformed five other antioxidants. "It helps prevent future wrinkling," says Leslie Baumann, MD, a professor of dermatology at the University of Miami and author of *The Skin Type Solution*.
Try: BeingTrue Anti-Aging I-Lift Eye Contour Concentrate (www.dermadoctor.com) or Prevage Eye Anti-Aging Moisturizing Treatment (www.amazon.com)

Puffiness

To repair: Proteins like Eyeseryl tetrapeptide are promising: "Peptides stimulate collagen production," says Diane Berson, MD, at Weill Cornell Medical College. Researchers think this boost in skin firmness forces fluids out from under eyes.
Try: Kinerase Under Eye Rescue (www.sephora.com)
To prevent: In a study of 41 women conducted by

the skin-care brand Vichy, a cream containing escinine (a botanical with anti-inflammatory properties) and manganese (a cirmineral that increases circulation) reduced the appearance of under-eye bags by 25 percent.

Try: Vichy Oligo 25 Eyes Anti-Fatigue Cooling Effect Stick (www.vichyusa.com)

Dark Circles

To repair: Scientists are targeting raccoon eyes with high-tech toning and tightening ingredients like Haloxyl and NouriCel-MD. They appear to work in a new way: by preventing stray blood cells from leaking out of under-eye vessels, potentially causing that bruised look.

Try: SkinMedica TNS Illuminating Eye Cream, with NouriCel-MD (www.skinmedica.com)

To prevent: Retinol, the vitamin A derivative mentioned earlier, can mask circles by "thickening the thin skin under the eyes, making it look less transparent," says Dr. Farris. Some products contain retinol combined with vitamin K, which helps bruises heal faster.

Try: Jan Marini Factor-A Eyes for Dark Circles (www.janmarini.com)

Arch Enemy

KEEP YOUR FACIAL FEATURES FROM PLOTTING AGAINST YOU

Sick of people saying you need more shut-eye? Your eyebrow shape and eyelid position may affect how people react to you, a study in the journal *Plastic and Reconstructive Surgery* reports. People can have a hard time projecting the image they'd like to when their facial characteristics make them look tired or sad, says study coauthor John Persing, MD, of the Yale University School of Medicine. Use these step-by-step tips from celebrity makeup artists Ramy Gafni and Emily Warren to make angry arches and lazy lids things of the past.

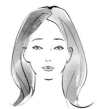 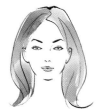 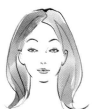 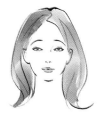

You look: *Tired*	You look: *Angry*	You look: *Surprised*	You look: *Sad*
Because: You have a pronounced space between your eyebrows and eyelids	Because: Your brows have a high, curved arch	Because: You have sparse, wide-set eyebrows with exaggerated arches	Because: Your outer brows slant straight downward
The fix:	The fix:	The fix:	The fix:
1. Lift your lids: Line the bottom of the brows with shimmery white eye shadow.	1. Thin the brows: Trim long brow hairs with scissors.	1. Thicken the brows: Fill in with a pencil that matches your brow color.	1. Ease the slope: Tweeze under each eyebrow near the bridge of your nose.
2. Widen your eyes: Shade a half-circle above each eyelid crease with light brown or gray shadow.	2. Flatten the arches: Tweeze the underside of the inner and outer corners of each brow.	2. Add width: Using the same pencil, shade just under the brows, following their natural line.	2. Create arch: Starting above the pupils, tweeze outward, removing progressively fewer hairs.
	3. Create space: Tweeze between the eyebrows.		3. Emphasize: Use a white shadow under the brow arches.

Looking Sharp

THE MUST–KNOW TREATMENTS THAT CAN ENHANCE YOUR VISION.

By Lambeth Hochwald

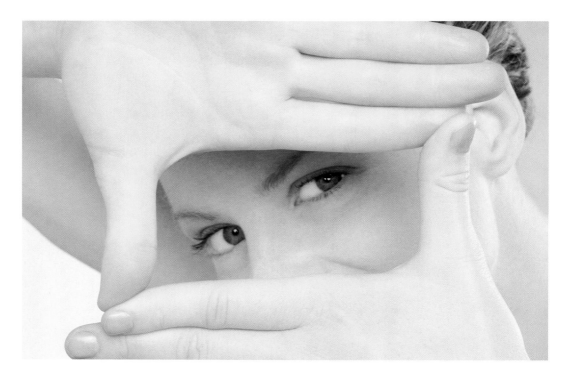

ome 1.5 million Americans—many of them women in their twenties and thirties—get surgery to fix their vision every year. But 36 million still wear glasses or contacts, some because they were told they weren't good candidates for surgery and others because of those horror stories you hear at dinner parties. Laser surgery still isn't perfect for everyone, but there have been enough recent improvements that you might take another look.

1. The Surgery Is Better at Fixing Vision

LASIK (laser-assisted in situ keratomileusis)—in which a laser beam reshapes your cornea—is the most popular kind of vision correction surgery. Now there's a better way of doing it. It incorporates a new procedure called wavefront analysis, which "allows a surgeon to see all the small irregularities in the eye and smooth these out during the procedure," says Brian S. Boxer Wachler, MD, director of the Boxer Wachler Vision Institute in Beverly Hills, California. That means much better vision in the end, especially at night and under glare conditions, adds Alan N. Carlson, MD, chief of the corneal and refractive surgery service at Duke University Eye Center in Durham, North Carolina. With wavefront analysis, you're also less likely to experience once-common side effects like "halos" around objects at night.

2. More of Us Qualify for Surgery

Not so long ago, you might have been ruled out for vision correction surgery if you were very nearsighted or had very large pupils or thin corneas. That's because extreme nearsightedness and large pupils raise your risk for halo vision—and if you have thin corneas, it's a bad idea to shave off some of your corneal tissue, which happens with LASIK. If that's you, surgeons can now correct nearsightedness with an implantable lens that leaves the cornea intact—the FDA approved Verisyse in 2004 and Visian ICL a year later. "The halo effect of LASIK is virtually unheard of with Visian ICL," Dr. Boxer Wachler says. There's a quicker recovery time, too—just a few hours with Visian ICL versus a full day with LASIK.

3. The Surgery Itself Is Less Stressful

The idea of someone poking at and messing with your eye while you're wide-awake (LASIK and implantable-lens patients get only numbing drops in the eye before the operation) isn't exactly relaxing. "In the past, people were afraid the procedure wouldn't work if they moved their eyes during the surgery," Dr. Boxer Wachler says. Now you can ask your surgeon to use an eye tracker, new technology that follows your eye movements during the procedure. So even if you can't stay perfectly still, the surgery will be accurate.

End Eye Irritation

YOU DON'T HAVE TO LIVE WITH DRY EYES AND BLURRY NIGHTS. PUT THESE NEW FIXES FOR EVERYDAY VISION GRIPES TO WORK TODAY.

Problem: Blurred vision in dim light, especially when driving at night
What it is: Diurnal shift, nearsightedness increasing throughout the day, affects everyone to one degree or another. Some doctors think it's caused naturally by eyelids flattening the cornea with each blink and by early vision-correcting surgeries.
What's new for it: **Alphagan (brimonidine)**, eyedrops usually prescribed for glaucoma, can also help with night-vision problems by preventing your pupils from dilating in dim light, says Andrew I. Caster, MD, an ophthalmologist in Los Angeles and author of *Eye Laser Miracle*. The drops work for about 6 hours.

Problem: Persistent dryness
What it is: Dry eye results from tear ducts not making enough tears, or producing enough but draining too many. The condition regularly affects an estimated 3.2 million American women. Its causes include hormone imbalances, contact lenses, certain medicines, and vitamin A deficiencies.
What's new for it: **Restasis**, prescription eyedrops, act as an anti-inflammatory and stop the triggering of T cells that disrupt normal tear production.

Problem: Eyestrain, blurring, dryness, and headaches after computer use
What it is: Computer vision syndrome affects more than half of America's 75 million regular computer users.
What's new for it: **Prescription lenses designed for computer use** eliminate eyestrain by reducing monitor glare and improving focus.

Problem: You see halos around lights or fuzzy-edged objects in dim light
What it is: Spherical aberration causes less-than-sharp vision, but it's not a disease. It affects an estimated 70 percent of people to some degree.
What's new for it: **Silicone hydrogel contact lenses** allow oxygen to pass through the lens. If you wear glasses, a special coating can be applied to your lenses to reduce glowing objects, such as street lights.

Problem: You use redness-reducing eyedrops habitually—and they seem to cause a rebound effect that actually makes your eyes even redder a short time after use
What it is: Your body can build up a tolerance to eyedrops that contain vasoconstrictors (marked "tetrahydrozoline" on the label)
What's new for it: **Use preservative-free artificial tears** such as Moisture Eyes, GenTeal, Systane, or Refresh Tears as your go-to eyedrops, recommends New York City optometrist Susan Resnick, OD.

Improve Your Outlook

TIPS FOR PICKING THE PERFECT SPECS.

*I*f having your corneas pulverized by a laser makes you nervous, you may want to consider a less invasive eye-opener. "The right pair of glasses can shave years off your face," says Paul Pinkham, regional manager and spokesman for Voorthuis Opticians in Washington, DC. But with the walls of optometrists' shops stacked with frames from floor to ceiling, picking out a pair of glasses (or shades) can leave you completely cross-eyed. And since they're going to sit front and center on your lovely face, they'd damn well better make you look even more gorgeous than you already do. To avoid throwing yourself at the mercy of just anyone behind the counter, here are the best styles for six of the most common face shapes.

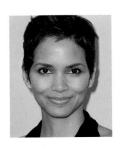

Oval

The oval face is longer than it is wide and has balanced features (think Halle Berry). Start gloating—you can wear almost any frame style without throwing your well-proportioned features out of whack. Just be sure to choose frames that are as wide as or wider than the broadest part of your face; narrower ones can make your mug look as if it goes on for miles. Try cat-eyes, wraparounds, and frames with oversize square lenses.

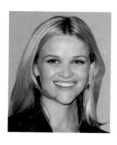

Heart

The heart-shaped face is broadest at the forehead and narrowest at the chin. (Think Reese Witherspoon.) With its delicate jaw, this face shape is the most feminine of all. Big, heavy glasses will obliterate your features, so don't even look at cat-eyes or wraparounds. Instead, opt for thin, light metal or clear plastic frames that have broader bottom halves, or choose a translucent or rimless style.

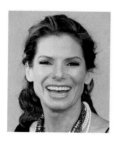

Square

The square face has a strong jawline and equally broad forehead. Like Sandra Bullock, your square jaw and brow make you look tough, trustworthy, and maybe just a little bit stubborn. Rectangular frames will exaggerate those qualities, which is fine if you happen to be a superhero or TV detective. To soften your image and balance your features, pick frames that are slightly rounded at the edges.

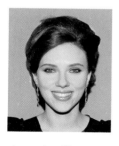

Diamond

The diamond face has high, dramatic cheekbones and a narrow brow and jawline (think Scarlett Johansson). Your to-die-for cheekbones make your face exotic, so you can choose to either complement them with equally dramatic frames or contrast them with a quiet, rimless style. To make sure the frames fit right, smile wide when you're trying them on—if the bottoms of the lenses make contact with your cheeks, you need a narrower pair.

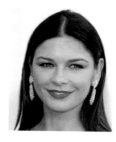

Round

Congratulations! The round face has soft curves with similar width and length (think Catherine Zeta-Jones), which we tend to associate with youth—you'll probably always look a good 5 years younger than you are. But to command respect, you might want to contrast those sweet cheeks with some sophisticated angles. Choose narrow frames with angular edges.

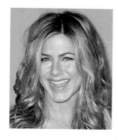

Triangle

The triangular face has a narrow forehead and prominent jaw (think Jennifer Aniston). Your goal here is simple: Enhance your subtlest features and deflect attention from your prominent ones. Since you have an impressive jaw, shift focus upward by wearing frames that have broader and/or more colorful upper halves, such as cat-eyes or aviators.

More Face Fixes

Wide-set eyes: Go with a darker, thicker bridge. This will draw the attention inward and make your eyes seem closer together than they really are.

Flat or low bridge: Adjustable nose pads are a must. (Custom-added to frames, they cost $20 and up.) They'll lift the glasses up and off your cheeks.

Close-set or narrow eyes: Glam it up with a posh design on the outer edges of the frame and temples to draw attention outward.

Small face: A modified aviator with slightly shorter lenses is best. Also, look for glasses made of lightweight metals and thinner plastics.

Long nose: Choose a straight brow bar (the metal strip running across the top of the lens). This will visually cut the bridge of your nose in half.

Get Healthy Teeth for Life

A GUIDE TO A BEAUTIFUL SMILE AND
PROBLEM–FREE DENTIST APPOINTMENTS.

O f all the health issues you could face, dental problems are among the most preventable, says Sally Cram, DDS, a periodontist in Washington, DC, and a consumer advisor for the American Dental Association. Getting your teeth cleaned twice a year and brushing and flossing twice a day is usually enough to keep your pearly whites intact. It's putting off dental cleanings and fillings—or avoiding major work like having a crown inserted—that dramatically increases your risk of losing your teeth, according to Kenneth S. Magid, DDS, clinical associate professor at the New York University College of Dentistry. It also ups the odds of cavities and decay, which is what leads to a lightning bolt of pain while eating hot or cold foods. Let

400
Number of medicines linked to dry mouths

your dentist know if you're pregnant (the extra hormones slightly raise your risk for gum disease, which affects up to 75 percent of pregnant women), or if you're taking meds. Some can cause dry mouth, making it harder for you to break down plaque. (Your dentist can take special steps, like giving you extra fluoride treatments, to help reduce damage.) And take note of headaches and jaw pain, signs that you may be clenching or grinding, which can erode your teeth; your dentist can make you a special protective mouth guard. Here, some warning signs to watch for—and fixes that will keep your smile healthy.

Twinges

With age, teeth become vulnerable to cracks. And those are prime breeding grounds for

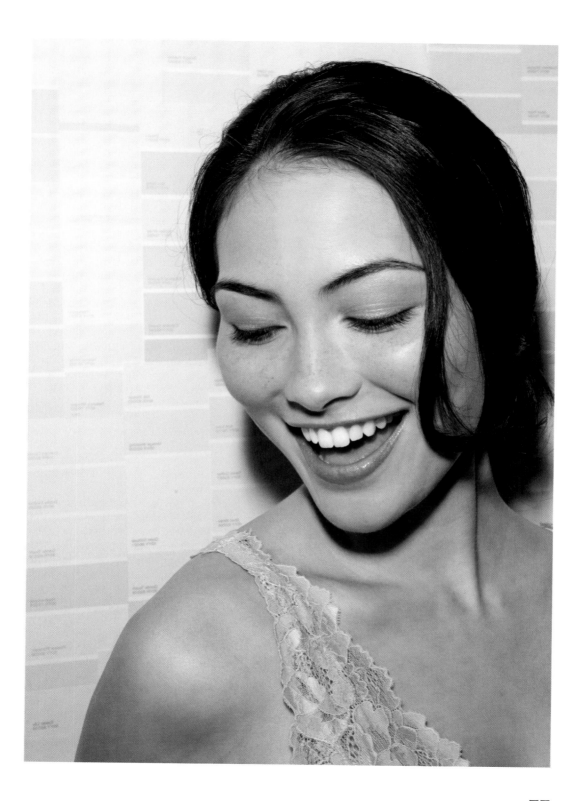

No-Tech Tricks

IF YOU'D RATHER PASS ON THE PEROXIDE, CHECK OUT THESE OTHER OPTIONS TO WHITEN YOUR SMILE.

Bring on the Baking Soda

The refrigerator deodorizer also removes discoloration on your teeth. The abrasive particles polish the surface while a chemical reaction between baking soda and water lightens stains, says Jonathan B. Levine, DMD, an associate professor at the New York University School of Dentistry and a cosmetic dentist in New York City. But don't do it more than once a week: You can damage your enamel with the scrubbing.

Feel the Crunch

"Foods that are high in cellulose—a strong, starchlike compound found in celery, carrots, and apples—act as natural abrasives, cleansing teeth and removing surface stains naturally," says Jeff Golub-Evans, DDS, a cosmetic dentist in New York City. And greens such as spinach, broccoli, and lettuce contain mineral compounds that form a film over the teeth, so pigments from other foods can't stain.

Be a Little Shady

"Stick with blue-based red and pink lipsticks," says Pia Lieb, DDS, a cosmetic dentist in New York City. Warm colors (orange, brown, warm shades of red) will only bring out the yellow in your teeth.

bacteria. Another common entry point: the gum line, where tissue recedes with age. "Decay here can become serious quickly because it's close to the tooth's nerve," says Kimberly Harms, DDS, a dentist in Farmington, Minnesota, and a consumer advisor for the American Dental Association. "If you don't prevent or catch it early, you could need a root canal."

Fix it: Call your dentist if you feel even a slight twinge. It may take an x-ray to pinpoint the crack, which can be smoothed or filled. Larger breaks often require a full crown or cap.

Prevent it: Your best defenses are brushing, flossing, and using a fluoride rinse. (In one study, twice-daily rinsers had nearly one-third the risk of root cavities as did people who used fluoride toothpaste and a placebo rinse.) But avoid rinses with alcohol, says Margaret Lappan Green, RDH, past president of the American Dental Hygienists' Association, as they can irritate gums.

Sensitive Teeth and Painful Gums

Periodontal disease erodes gums and often causes sensitive teeth. As bacteria build up at the base of your teeth, you may just notice a little bleeding when you brush. But as the microbes multiply, they loosen gum tissue, eating into underlying ligaments and bone that hold teeth in place.

Fix it: Halt early gum disease with professional deep cleaning, daily antibacterial rinses, and dental visits at least every 6 months. If you have sensitive teeth, ask your dentist about topical fluoride or other prescription desensitizing agents. Over-the-counter fluoride rinses or toothpastes such as Sensodyne can also help. And go easy on bleaching, which can temporarily increase sensitivity. (Always check with your dentist before beginning to bleach.)

Prevent it: "Get religious about flossing," says Dr. Harms. Choose a toothbrush with soft, rounded bristles, or try a rotation oscillation electric brush; research shows that they reduce plaque and gum inflammation better than manual types.

Dryness

Saliva is a magical elixir: It's antibacterial, acid neutralizing, and full of minerals that strengthen enamel. But if you don't produce enough, you can end up with bad breath, or more serious problems down the road.

Fix it: If your tongue or lips are often dry, tell your doctor. More than 400 medicines are linked to dry mouth, including antidepressants and blood pressure and bladder medicines. A Tufts University study showed that patients taking at least one dryness-causing medication developed three times as many cavities as those not on a drug. Your doctor may be able to switch your prescription as well as check for other causes of dry mouth, such as Sjögren's syndrome or sleep apnea.

Prevent it: For minor dryness or bad breath, Robert Palmer, MD, head of geriatrics at the Cleveland Clinic, suggests sucking on sugarless hard candy or chewing on gum sweetened with xylitol. Daily tongue cleaning also helps. Brush on top, underneath, and as far back as you can reach, or buy an inexpensive tongue-scraping device to make the job easier. The gunk it removes prevents your mouth from feeling fresh.

Whiten Up

TAKE YOUR CHOPPERS FROM DULL TO DAZZLING AND GIVE YOURSELF SOMETHING TO SMILE ABOUT.

*I*f you've toyed with the idea of whitening your teeth, consider this: "Since teeth naturally yellow as we age, whitening them will automatically make you look younger," says Kimberly Harms, DDS, of the American Dental Association. A 2008 Columbia University study even found that women with healthier-looking teeth earn more than those with less-sparkling grins.

How Whiteners Work

All bleaching methods use peroxide—whether in gel, strip, or liquid form—to dissolve surface stains, according to Debra Glassman, DDS, a cosmetic dentist in New York City. Teeth surfaces are made up of thousands of tiny dentinal tubules—hollow structures stacked horizontally, like thin straws. They're extremely porous and absorb pigments from food and drink. (Anything that can stain a white T-shirt can discolor your teeth, Dr. Glassman says.) Peroxide bubbles into the tubules and lightens those pigments.

Before You Bleach

A first-timer should always consult her dentist before trying any tooth whitener, even an over-the-counter product, because not all teeth react to whitening the same way. Some types of dental work (like caps, crowns, and veneers) don't take to lightening because peroxide can't penetrate them. Stains caused by antibiotics, like tetracycline, are also tricky, because they can occur in the layers inside the tooth, which brighteners can't reach. Your dentist will be able to advise you about the best method for you.

Go to a Pro

The whitening agents dentists use are up to three times more powerful than at-home versions. If you're looking for a dramatic, fast solution, consider power whitening. First, a protective rubber guard or barrier gel is placed over your gums to help avoid possible sensitivity to peroxide. Then the teeth are coated with a bleaching agent and a light is aimed at them to activate the ingredients. The procedure takes about an hour and costs about $500. For about half that price, your dentist can custom-fit you with plastic dental trays similar to retainers, which you fill with a peroxide gel and wear at home.

The Lifesaving Question to Ask Your Dentist

"DID YOU CHECK MY MOUTH FOR ORAL CANCER?"

Risk of the disease rises after age 40. Half of all oral cancers are discovered in an advanced stage, when survival odds are low. If caught early, though, it's one of the most curable cancers—so make sure your dentist is on the lookout. If you notice any lumps or bumps inside your mouth, or persistent sores or discolorations, be sure you voice your concern—especially if you've ever been a smoker.

Chapter Five

Stoke Your Sexuality

HOW TO KEEP PASSION ON THE UPSWING — FOREVER!

INVESTMENT: 4 WEEKS
AGE ERASED: 4 YEARS

Introduction

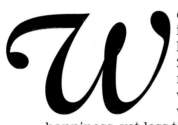e may lead the world in many ways, but when it comes to our sex lives, Americans are a little flaccid. According to the Durex 2007–2008 Global Sexual Wellbeing Survey, we rank third lowest in the world in how often we get it on. Some 81 percent of American women believe that sex is vital to health and happiness, yet less than half of us are content with our current erotic state of affairs. Less than half! That's absolutely tragic, when you think about it. But the reality is that life has a way of hijacking women's libidos—whether it's during our crazy-busy twenties with too much work and too many distractions (only made worse by all the tech interruptions), postbaby body/mind issues ("I'm too fat!" "I'm too tired!" "I'm too pissed off at him!"), the challenging nuttiness of life with kids of any age, or the hormonal shifts that start in our mid-forties and continue through menopause. So how do we go from knowing we want action to actually getting it? This chapter covers all the ways— physical and psychological—to keep the home fires cookin'.

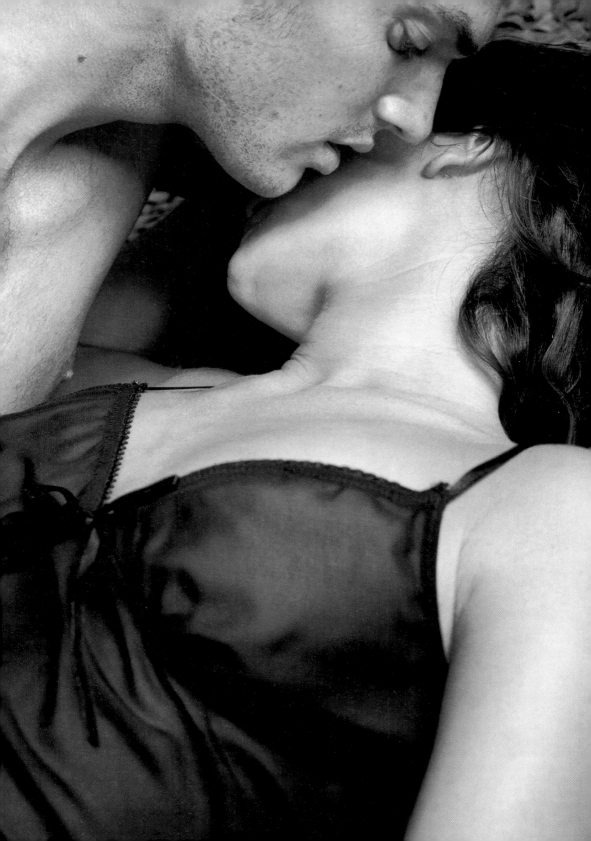

The Ultimate Guide to Your Vagina

SEX ED DIDN'T COVER THE HALF OF IT. FROM LITTLE-KNOWN ANATOMY TO TIPS ON SAFE HANDLING, HERE'S WHAT YOU NEED TO KNOW ABOUT THE SWEET SPOT BETWEEN YOUR LEGS.

*T*hat's right, we're shining a spotlight on the almighty vajayjay. And it's about time. Given the ridiculous amount of maintenance it requires—gynecologist visits, bikini waxes, yeast infection creams, and more—you'd think we'd know everything about this attention-getting organ's intricate design and how to keep it running smoother than a top-of-the-line Lexus. Yet even women who feel perfectly comfortable in their skin don't give much thought to the nooks and crannies of their nether regions. "Many women never connect with their sexual anatomy because of our society's 'keep away' attitude toward the vagina and vulva," says Elizabeth Stewart, MD, author of *The V Book*. The following guide to a healthy honeypot explains a few things you might still wonder about, like the secret to finding the nerve-packed hot spots that make intercourse feel as good as a clitoral rubdown.

The VIP Lounge

Most people call the whole kit and caboodle between a woman's legs the "vagina." But the compendium of visible outer parts is technically the vulva. Meant to keep dirt and bacteria out while providing a welcoming environment for worthy partygoers, the vulva is like a VIP lounge where the clitoris is the DJ. "The labia majora [outer lips] are a protective layer of fat covered by skin and hair," says Lillian Schapiro, MD, an Atlanta ob-gyn. Their job is to keep sex comfy even if your partner's pelvis is bonier than Iggy Pop's. Located inside the labia majora (though sometimes extending beyond them), the labia minora, or inner lips, act like a pair of swinging doors guarding the entrance to the vagina and the urethra, the tube that leads from the bladder. "The labia minora are much thinner than the labia majora and even more sensitive," Dr. Schapiro says. Plus, they contain erectile tissue made up of clusters of tiny blood vessels, which means they become slightly

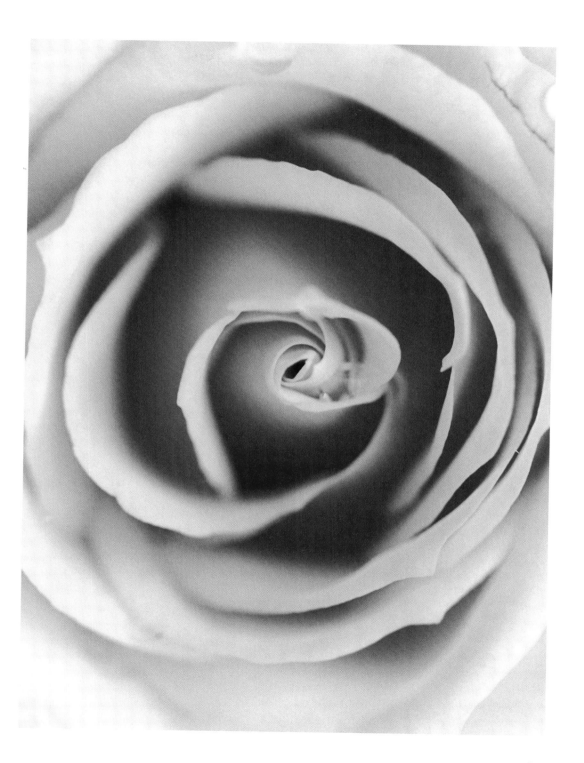

stiffer (though not as stiff as the clitoris) during arousal. The anatomist who named the parts of the vulva must have found it loungelike too, because the area between and including the inner folds of the labia minora is called the vestibule.

Your Sprinkler System

Hiding just below the skin of the labia and clitoral hood (called the prepuce) are hundreds of small glands that secrete oil and sweat to protect these delicate areas from friction and overheating. That means it's normal if the crotch of your yoga pants is soaked by the end of a workout. The inside of the vagina also stays moist to maintain healthy tissue, but as you've no doubt noticed, it gets wetter when you're turned on. That's because the lining of the vagina fills with blood during arousal, causing the saltwater in blood plasma to push through the vaginal wall. The Bartholin's glands—on either side of the vaginal opening—also pump out a few beads of slippery mucus. In the missionary position, most of this fluid collects in the back of the vagina and fails to lubricate the opening, making sex uncomfortable. And in some women, lubrication occurs for only a few moments, then stops. In both cases, a water-based personal lubricant is key to ensuring a smooth entry.

8,000
Nerve endings at the visible tip of the clitoris

Pleats and Ruffles

Like an haute-couture handbag, the vulva and vagina feature a variety of textures. Most of the vulva is smooth, but some women's labia minora have a ruffled appearance. "Labia come in all shapes and sizes," Dr. Stewart says. "The tips of the nipples and labia are similar because they both contain small, bumpy-looking glands." Examine your labia minora closely (using a hand mirror) and you may see the glands, which sometimes look like tiny pimples. Separate the labia minora and you may notice that the entrance to the vagina also has a ruffled border or just a few irregular bits of skin. Those are the remnants of the hymen, a thin membrane that once partially

covered the entrance but has been torn or pushed aside by sexual intercourse. As for the texture inside the vagina, it's full of bumpy ridges called rugae. Similar to pleats on a skirt, the rugae stretch and retract to accommodate objects ranging in size from superslender tampons to roly-poly 8-pound babies.

Finding the Wishbone

In a body full of hardworking organs, the clitoris is like a trust-fund baby who does nothing but party. It's the only part of the human body whose sole purpose is pleasure. The one thing the clitoris has that a trust-fund baby lacks? Depth. "The clitoris is larger than it seems," says Laura Berman, PhD, clinical assistant professor of ob-gyn and psychiatry at Northwestern University's medical school, author of *The Passion Prescription*, and a member of *Women's Health*'s advisory board. Beneath the visible pink button, called the glans, lies a wishbone-shaped structure comprising a shaft, which extends about an inch up toward the pubic bone, and two 3-inch arms called crura that reach down and back toward the pelvic bone in an inverted V shape. Though the shaft and crura send pleasure signals to the brain during sex, the glans is more sensitive. That's why it has a hood—without it, a pair of tight jeans would send your nervous system into overdrive.

Two bulbs of erectile tissue run alongside the crura. Many experts, including Dr. Berman and Helen O'Connell, MD, a urologist at Royal Melbourne Hospital in Australia and the first person to map the clitoris using magnetic resonance imaging, believe that this tissue is part of the clitoris too. In studies, Dr. O'Connell found that the clitoris is also connected to erectile tissue surrounding the urethra and extending up to the front wall of the vagina—where the enigmatic G-spot has been known to pop up.

Over the Hedge

Before you shave or wax it into a perfect triangle, landing strip, or lucky shamrock, the hair that

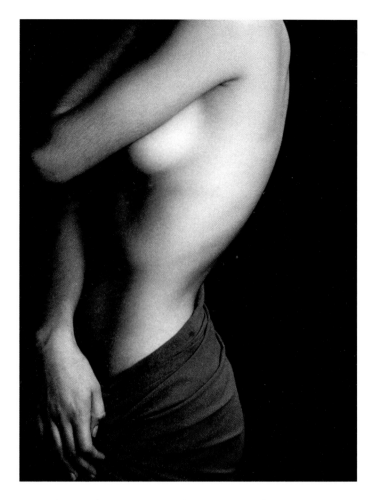

tologist and author of *Brown Skin*. "A depilatory breaks the hair at the surface, which can make ingrowns less likely, but only if the chemicals don't irritate your skin." Whenever you try a new depilatory, always spot-test the product on your inner thigh before using it on your bikini area. Another way to create an aesthetically pleasing patch is with laser hair removal, but only by a trained professional who uses a laser like the Nd:YAG, which Dr. Taylor says won't create dark spots by damaging surrounding skin.

X Marks the Spot

While the vagina is nowhere near as responsive to touch as the vulva, it does contain hundreds of nerve endings. If a woman were lying on her back with a clock placed upright inside the lower part of her vagina (don't ask how it got there), the most sensitive area would be at 12 o'clock, right behind the urethra. In a 1982 study of more than 400 women, Rutgers University sex researcher Beverly Whipple, PhD, and two colleagues found

covers the pubic mound and outer labia grows in a pattern called the escutcheon (based on the Latin term for an ornamental shield).

When allowed to grow wild, some escutcheons will wander up toward the navel and down toward the upper thighs, while others wouldn't breech the borders of a Brazilian bikini. The shape of hair shafts differs depending on ethnicity: In Asian women they're typically round, in women of African descent they're elliptical, and in Caucasians and Latinas they range between the two. "Elliptical shafts are more likely to become ingrown after shaving or waxing as the hair curls in, pierces the skin, and creates a bump," says Susan Taylor, MD, a Philadelphia derma-

that when this area was stimulated after a woman was already sexually aroused, a dime-size bump of tissue appeared and might trigger an orgasm. She named the area the G-spot after Ernst Gräfenberg, the German doctor who first documented it in 1950. Further examination of this spongy tissue found it identical to that of the male prostate gland, a well-established pleasure zone. Some doctors believe the G-spot should be renamed the female prostate. Supporting that belief is a study showing the similarity between the fluid expelled by a very small percentage of women through their urethra during a G-spot orgasm (aka "female ejaculation") and that produced by the male prostate. What if you've never

87

found your G-spot, much less ejaculated? Dr. Whipple says don't sweat it: "There are many sensitive areas inside the vagina that, when stimulated by a finger, vibrator, or penis, can contribute to sexual pleasure."

Honorable Discharge

That strip of cotton in the crotch of every panty is there for a reason—even if you don't have your period or aren't the tiniest bit sweaty, it will collect moisture. The vulva and vagina produce an average of 1 to 2 grams (about $1/4$ to $1/2$ teaspoon) of vaginal discharge every 8 hours. But even normal discharge doesn't make a pretty picture. "It may be clear, white, or yellow, and fluid, waxy, stringy, or clumpy," Dr. Stewart says. Some of it is a build-up of the oil that the glands in your vulva produce. Some is cervical mucus. Still more comes from normal vaginal secretions. Throw a sample under a microscope and you'll also find bacteria, skin cells, and yeast spores. Quantity and consistency change over the menstrual cycle. "During ovulation, secretions are thinner and more plentiful," Dr. Stewart says. "After ovulation, discharge becomes thicker. As you near menstruation, there's less." How do you keep this fluid factory fresh? Don't mess with it. "The vagina cleans itself. Over-the-counter products can make matters worse, since the protective bacterial balance will be further disrupted," Dr. Berman says. "If discharge smells bad or is accompanied by discomfort, see your doctor." Wash with water and a perfume-free, pH-balanced soap like Dove, Dr. Berman says. Always wear cotton undies and go commando at night or whenever possible. That's right: Unless you're wearing something that could chafe or otherwise irritate you down under, docs are big fans of a panty-free lifestyle.

Tilt-a-Whirl

As seen on the diagram in every Tampax box, the vagina tilts back 30 degrees from the opening, which is why you're supposed to aim toward your lower back when pushing the plunger. A side effect of this 30-degree angle is that in the missionary position, the penis has little to no contact with the supersensitive front wall of the vagina.

Sexual Healing

MORE GOOD NEWS FROM BETWEEN THE SHEETS: RESEARCH CONFIRMS THAT REGULAR SEX CAN IMPROVE OVERALL HEALTH AND MAY EVEN HELP YOU LIVE LONGER. HERE, 5 HEALTHY REASONS TO SPEND MORE TIME IN BED.

1. *Immunity:* Having sex once or twice a week increases levels of the antibody immunoglobulin A by 30 percent, which boosts your immune system.
2. *Reduced depression:* Endorphins aside, prostaglandin, a hormone found only in semen, gets into the bloodstream and may ward off depression.
3. *Pain relief:* The part of the brain activated during sex is also the body's painkilling center, which means during orgasm a woman can withstand 110 percent more pain.
4. *Weight loss:* One vigorous romp blasts about 200 calories and doubles your heart rate. Twice a week? Shed nearly 6 pounds in a year.
5. *Bladder control:* While strengthening your pelvic floor muscles will eventually lead to more powerful orgasms, it'll also help keep your bladder in good, working order.

As far as orgasm goes, this is not good. Placing a pillow under your hips, wrapping your legs around your partner's lower back, and rocking back and forth to create clitoral friction can help you get maximum bliss out of missionary, but other positions typically yield better results. "The best positions for G-spot stimulation include woman-on-top and rear entry," Dr. Berman says. Woman-on-top lets you experiment with different angles to find the most feel-good sensations. "Leaning back targets the anterior wall," Dr. Berman says. Zero in on your G-spot in rear entry by lying flat on your stomach and tucking a pillow under your hips. Or try reverse cowgirl, where you face his feet—and with that view, he'll be one very happy cowboy.

The Big Squeeze

You've heard of sex-enhancing Kegel exercises: Squeeze the muscle you'd use to stop urine in midflow (except don't actually do it while you're peeing, since that can cause bladder infections), hold it for as long as you can, release, and repeat. But perhaps you haven't seen Dr. Berman's vaginal barbells. Neither had we. For beginners, there's the Isis, which looks like a slim, clear plastic bow tie with smooth, rounded edges. And for women with power vaginas, there's the Juno, a plastic rod containing four spherical, 0.3- to 1.5-ounce weights in a row from smallest to largest (www.mypleasure.com). Start by inserting the bigger end in your vagina, tightening your pelvic floor muscles around it and holding it in place with your hand. You'll know your muscles are getting stronger when you can hold the smaller end in your vagina with no hand support. "Just like other muscles, strengthening pelvic floor muscles is more effective when you add resistance," Dr. Berman says. But even without resistance, Kegels make a real difference; according to Dr. Stewart, if you squeeze out 10 to 20 daily, you'll sense stronger orgasms in about 3 months.

Friendly Invaders

Inside your vagina reside trillions of bacteria, some friendly, some not so friendly. "*Lactobacillus* is a beneficial bacteria that keeps nastier bacteria in check," says Christopher A. Czaja, MD, an infectious diseases fellow at the University of Washington at Seattle. "Classic urinary tract infections often occur when the number of *Lactobacillus* drops and *Escherichia coli* bacteria [often present in the vagina] start to flourish and ascend the urethra." Yech. To prevent *E. coli* from migrating into the vagina from the other side of the 'hood, always wipe from front to back after going to the bathroom. Besides bullying bacterial bad boys like *E. coli*, *Lactobacillus* also crowds out yeast spores, another normal inhabitant of the vagina, which can otherwise grow to the level of an itchy infection. Keep your *Lactobacillus* count up by eating a daily cup of yogurt that contains the bacteria and avoiding unnecessary antibiotics, which kill off the good guys along with the bad.

Strings Attached

As tender as the vagina may seem, it's actually a pretty tough cookie. When it sustains small scrapes from, say, enthusiastic booty, the vaginal lining can heal surprisingly fast. Another way it gets beat up is by improper use of superabsor-bency tampons. This is different than scary toxic shock syndrome (TSS), a rare, dangerous condition (odds of getting it are about 1 in 100,000) that results from an overgrowth of *Staphylococcus aureus* bacteria. The staph bug can be exacerbated by wearing the same tampon for longer than 8 hours, but it is not actually caused by tampons themselves.

What tampons can give you are vaginal ulcers that don't cause any discomfort but do make you more vulnerable to sexually transmitted infections. "Using a high-absorbency tampon during light flow days or when spotting can draw too much fluid out of the vagina, damaging cells and causing them to erode," Dr. Stewart says. The good news is that the vaginal lining is quick to produce new cells, allowing ulcers to heal completely in as little as 48 hours.

Vagus, Baby

Many lucky-as-hell women report experiencing three different kinds of orgasms (four if you include the faux-gasm): one that radiates from the clitoris and feels a little bit superficial, a more satisfying one that happens deeper inside the vagina, and an even bigger bang that's a divine blend of the two. Makes sense, considering that our brains receive pleasure signals through as many as four sensory fields. According to *The Science of Orgasm,* a book coauthored by Dr. Whipple, Barry Komisaruk, PhD, and Carlos Beyer-Flores, PhD, clitoral stimulation sends tingles up the pudendal nerve; sensations inside the vagina travel up the pelvic nerve; and pleasurable contact with the cervix activates the pelvic, hypogastric, and vagus nerves.

That last link—between the cervix and the vagus nerve, which controls activities as seemingly unrelated as swallowing and sweating—is a new one that Dr. Whipple's team discovered during a clinical study of women with spinal cord injuries. "We don't yet know if it's a supplemental tract that the genitals normally use to send messages to the spinal cord or if it's activated only if the spinal cord is cut off by injury," Dr. Stewart says. But one thing the involvement of the vagus nerve makes clear is that female orgasm is just as mysterious on the inside as it can seem from out here.

Anatomy of an Orgasm

WANT IT, NEED IT, GOT TO HAVE IT—BUT WHAT PRECISELY
IS HAPPENING IN YOUR BODY DURING THAT CLENCH–THE–SHEETS
MOMENT? A BLOW–BY–BLOW LOOK AT HOW AND WHY WE COME.

*I*t's the only thing that feels better than diving into a cool lake on a sweltering day, biting into a juicy cheeseburger when you're starving, or even getting your wallet back after losing it on vacation abroad. An orgasm is that good. Which is why it bites that it doesn't happen more often. According to several major surveys, only 25 percent of women always climax during sex with a partner. The rest of us either hit—or miss—depending on the night, or never orgasm during intercourse at all. Compared to the male version (more than 90 percent of men get their cookies 100 percent of the time), the female "O" is a fleeting phenomenon. The question is: Why? What the hell was Mother Nature thinking?

That's what evolutionary biologists have been trying to figure out—with little success. *The Case of the Female Orgasm: Bias in the Science of Evolution* by Elisabeth Lloyd, PhD, a biology professor at Indiana University in Bloomington, shoots holes in virtually every theory that has ever attempted to pinpoint an evolutionary purpose to the female climax. "The clitoris has the indispensable function of promoting sexual excitement, which induces the female to have intercourse and become pregnant," Dr. Lloyd says. "But the actual incidence of the reflex of orgasm has never been tied to successful reproduc-

tion." Translation: Because women can and do get pregnant without climaxing, scientists can't figure out why we orgasm at all.

The good news is that most scientists do agree on the how. Here's what they know, so far—and how that knowledge can help the average girl hit her peak more often. Because even if orgasms do turn out to be pointless in terms of sustaining the species, they still feel pretty damn good.

While You Were Blissing Out . . .

When in the throes of an orgasm, you wouldn't notice if your dog, your cat, and your cockatiel started rearranging the furniture. Which makes it unlikely that you could track all the subtle changes that are happening in your body. Luckily, famous sex researchers William H. Masters and Virginia E. Johnson have done it for you in their seminal work, *Human Sexuality*. Here's what they found:

• That warm rush you feel during foreplay is the result of blood heading straight to your vagina and clitoris. Around this time, the walls of the vagina start to secrete beads of lubrication that eventually get bigger and flow together.

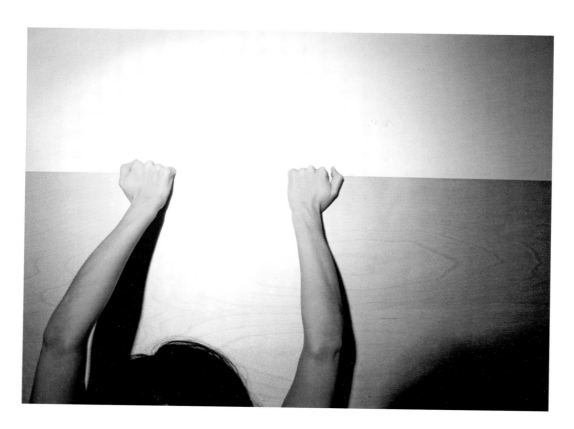

As you become more turned on, blood continues to flood the pelvic area, breathing speeds up, heart rate increases, nipples become erect, and the lower part of the vagina narrows in order to grip the penis while the upper part expands to give it someplace to go. If all goes well, an incredible amount of nerve and muscle tension builds up in the genitals, pelvis, buttocks, and thighs—until your body involuntarily releases it all at once in a series of intensely pleasurable waves, aka your orgasm.

The big bang is the moment when the uterus, vagina, and anus contract simultaneously at 0.8-second intervals. A small orgasm may consist of three to five contractions; a biggie, 10 to 15. As we mentioned earlier, many women report feeling different kinds of orgasms—clitoral, vaginal, and many combinations of the two. According to Dr. Whipple, coauthor of *The G-Spot: And Other Discoveries about Human Sexuality*, the reason may simply be that different parts of the vagina were stimulated more than others, and so have more tension to release. Also, muscles in other parts of the body may contract involuntarily—hence the clenched toes and goofy faces. As for the brain, a recent small-scale study at the Netherlands' University of Groningen found that areas involving fear and emotion are actually deactivated during orgasm (not so if you fake it).

After the peak of pleasure, the body usually slides into a state of satisfied relaxation—but not always. "Like their male counterparts, women can experience pelvic heaviness and aching if they do not reach orgasm," says Ian Kerner, PhD, a certified sex therapist and author of *She Comes First*. In fact, Dr. Kerner says, "many women complain that a single orgasm isn't enough to relieve the buildup of sexual tension," which can leave us with our own "blue balls." (Your call if that's a good or bad thing.)

Big "O" Blockers

So what goes wrong when the fuse gets lit but the bomb never explodes? "Nine times out of 10 it's because [the woman isn't] getting enough continuous clitoral stimulation," Dr. Kerner says. Often, "A woman will get close to orgasm, her partner picks up on it, and [then he either] orgasms or changes what he was doing."

That's why Dr. Kerner frequently recommends the woman-on-top position. Because you control the angle and speed of the thrusts (try a back-and-forth motion so that your clitoris rubs against your partner's abdomen), it allows for the most constant clitoral stimulation. Another solution is to find a position that mimics how you masturbate. If you have solo sex by lying on your belly and rubbing your clitoris with your hands tucked beneath you, then your man can enter you from behind in that position. By watching you he'll also get a better sense of the stimulation you need.

"Spectatoring" is another problem that can trip women up. "It's when a woman is too concerned with her appearance and/or performance to actually enjoy herself," Dr. Kerner says. There's no way you're going to have an orgasm if you're fretting or stressing. Instead, let the erotic sensations register in your mind. Focus. Breathe. Let go. "It may seem counterintuitive," he says, "but you need to relax to build sexual tension."

The best preparation for a big orgasm is probably a long, steamy shower, full-body massages, or 10 minutes of oral sex. It's not so much your body that needs the R&R as your mind. "Many women need a transition period between dealing with the stress of everyday life and feeling sexual," Dr. Kerner says. "A few minutes of foreplay usually isn't enough." Doing something ritualistic and soothing that will clear your head of to-do lists, work issues, family problems, and whatever else might be distracting you from connecting with your body is essential to feeling ecstatic.

A Hormone Worth Getting Excited About

The most fascinating orgasmic side effect of all happens in the brain. During the big moment,

Thanks, Mom

WHEN YOUR JEANS COME OFF, YOUR GENES COME INTO PLAY.

Your ability to reach orgasm isn't just a product of your mother's liberal or conservative views about sex—her genes play a hefty role, too. Two recent studies showed that identical twins experienced a significantly similar rate of orgasmic success or failure. Based on surveys of hundreds of twin sets, scientists at St. Thomas' Hospital in London concluded that the genetic influence on orgasm was a whopping 34 percent. Meanwhile, psychologists at the University of Chicago determined that genes were responsible for 31 percent of how frequently women orgasm during sexual intercourse. Still, simple math reveals an encouraging detail: The majority of climax control remains all yours.

the hypothalamus releases extra oxytocin into your system. Called the "cuddle hormone," oxytocin has been correlated with the urge to bond, be affectionate, and protect. Since an increase in oxytocin has been shown to strengthen the uterine contractions that transport sperm to the egg, those findings are giving evolutionary biologists new hope. According to Dr. Lloyd, it's conceivable that the additional oxytocin gives enough of a boost to contractions that orgasm could play a part in conception after all. "Of all the avenues of orgasm research, I think the oxytocin avenue is the most promising," she says.

The latest news is that this cuddle hormone might also be linked to our ability to trust. In a recent study at the University of Zurich, scientists asked 178 male college students to play an investment game with a partner they'd never met. Half of the students used an oxytocin nasal spray (not yet available in the United States) beforehand; half used a placebo. Those with the spray containing oxytocin were more than twice as likely to feel comfortable giving all of their money to their anonymous (but legitimate) partner. If oxytocin can help women feel more at ease about letting go and intensify orgasmic contractions, we might all want a bottle of the stuff stashed in our bedside drawers someday soon.

The Better Sex Workout

ENLIGHTENMENT IS GREAT AND ALL, BUT DOING YOGA WILL ALSO PAY OFF IN A VERY IMMEDIATE, EXTREMELY EARTHY WAY: IN THE SACK.

*I*n ancient times, yogis practiced celibacy so that all of their energy could be directed toward spiritual advancement. Makes you wonder: How could these supposedly wise guys have gotten it so wrong? Today yoga lovers are finding that more time on the mat means more—and steamier—time spent reveling in their newly toned bodies. Here's why.

It Helps You Flow

Yoga increases your overall bloodflow, and some positions, such as the eagle pose (see page 95), direct it straight toward your pelvis. When all that blood rushes to your privates, it literally makes you hot. That heat, combined with a Viagra-like stimulation (as the blood swells your button), heightens your sensitivity and increases desire.

It Makes You Stronger Down Below

Yoga tones and strengthens your entire core—which includes your pelvic floor. "The more you work these muscles, the greater range of motion you have," says Becky Jeffers, fitness director at the Berman Center for female sexual health and menopause management in Chicago. "This gives you stronger contractions and releases, which can help you experience a more intense orgasm."

It Breeds Confidence

Quieting your mind and focusing on your breath during a pose help you become more aware of yourself and your own needs. "When you're present, you know what you need to feel fulfilled by your partner," Jeffers says. "You can then translate and communicate this deeper understanding to your partner during sex." Knowing and expressing your desires will make you feel good—psychologically as well as sexually.

It Eases Pain

For some women, especially runners, hip and thigh tightness can make sex tough, but yoga eases pain by releasing that tension and relaxing your hips. "Tension in your hips can affect how your pelvic floor works," Jeffers says. One tight muscle can lead to another, making your chances of orgasm remote and your love session about as sexy as a sweaty round on the rowing machine. Relax, and everything gets easier, and better.

93

It Gives You Mojo

Yoga moves like triangle and seated open-angle pose stimulate your chakras. According to Eastern philosophy, your sex life is governed by these chakras—your body's energy centers surrounding your spine, in yoga-speak. "When your chakras are in healthy working order, you'll find your sexual relations to be vibrant and healthy, too," Ellen Barrett, author of *Sexy Yoga*, says. Your three "sexiest" chakras are the root chakra (located at your perineum—the area between your pubic bone and anus), the sacral chakra (in the center of your lower abdomen), and the heart chakra (in the center of your chest). Yoga enriches these critical areas with blood and "prana," the life force, according to Barrett. That promotes openness and decreases sexual inhibition, which make you a more game sex partner and, in turn, a much happier person.

To take a walk on yoga's carnal side, read through the following pointers, and then try the poses in "Make Your Move" on the facing page.

1. Flex Time Is Sex Time

Having more flexible muscles and joints definitely helps in assuming those compromising positions. Opening your hips in particular gives you a wider range of motion in your nether regions, allowing for more direct stimulation in just the right spots. After all, one micromovement in missionary is sometimes all it takes to ring the bell.

Try Bound Angle: In a seated position, bring the soles of your feet together, put your hands on your ankles, allow your knees to relax toward the floor, and hinge forward at the hips as far as is comfortable. Hold for 10 to 15 complete breaths (inhales and exhales).

2. Power Up the Pelvis

Strengthening one key muscle helps you engage and lift the pelvic floor, bringing you more sensation and control during those hot times.

Try Root Lock: You may also hear this referred to by its Sanskrit name, "Mula Bandha." Seated or standing, contract and then release the pubococcygeus muscle located between the pubic bone and the tailbone, as if you wanted to stop the flow of urine. You can even do this at your desk, say, 10 times at three intervals during the workday.

3. Sex Goddesses Go the Distance

Shake-the-headboard sex is hard work. "The better shape you're in, the more pleasure you have and the longer you can do it," says Kimberly Fowler, owner of Yoga and Spinning Studio in Venice, California.

Try Yoga Pushups: Start in the pushup position, arms extended. Engage your abs as you lower your body slowly toward the floor. Stop when your torso is about 2 to 3 inches away. Keeping your elbows in, hold there for five breaths, then lower to the floor. Repeat 3 times at first and build up to 5.

200
Calories burned during a vigorous romp

4. Charge Up the Bed Batteries

A killer day at work can leave you too beat to boogie. But a few minutes of nonstrenuous yoga when you get home can mean one less night with Netflix and one more erotic evening entwined with your sweetie.

Try Legs Up the Wall: Change into some yoga-friendly clothes. Lie on your back with one hip touching a wall. Swing your legs up and turn your body so you face the wall, legs resting against it from heels to butt, arms at your sides. Bring your awareness to your breath and focus on it for 5 minutes. This position allows more oxygen-rich blood to flow from your lower body back up to the heart and the brain, so you'll get up reenergized, refocused, and ready to rumble.

Make Your Move

GET LOOSE—AND LET LOOSE—WITH THESE 7 SEXY YOGA POSES.

Yoga expert Ellen Barrett recommends the following exercises in this order, twice a week, after a 10-minute cardio warmup.

Eagle Pose
Pushes fresh blood to your root chakra and your privates. Stand with your feet together. Extend both arms as you inhale, then exhale as you move the right arm under the left, twisting them so that your palms meet. If you can't wrap your arms, hold your palms together as if in prayer. Then bend your knees and cross your right leg over your left, tucking your right foot behind your left calf. Pull your elbows down and balance on your left leg. Hold for five full breaths, then repeat on the other side. Modification: If you feel off-balance, keep your arms out to the side like airplane wings.

Forward Hero's Pose
Relieves bloating and improves pelvic circulation. Sit on your heels, then slide your heels out to the side so your butt is touching the floor. Sit upright, inhale, and raise both arms, bringing your elbows up by your ears. Keeping your butt on the floor, reach forward with your torso and drape your body over your knees. Hold for 10 full breaths. Modification: If you feel pinching in your knees, sit on a yoga block or folded towel.

Plow Pose
Improves spine flexibility and releases tension in hips and pelvis. Lie on your back, arms at your sides and legs straight up, so your body forms a 90-degree angle. Squeeze your abs, keep your knees straight, and bring your legs back overhead. Try to touch the floor with your toes. Keep your chin away from your chest and breathe freely. Hold for 1 minute. Modification: If tight hamstrings prevent you from fully straightening your legs, simply remain at the 90-degree angle pose.

Frog Pose
Relaxes and stretches hips and groin. Bend forward with your legs spread and walk your hands away from your body until your belly touches the floor. Prop up on your forearms and, keeping your legs wide apart, press the insides of your feet and knees to the floor. Gently press your hips as close to the floor as possible. Hold for 10 full breaths, push up to your hands, and work back to the start. Modification: If your knees hurt, place a blanket or towel underneath them for padding.

Triangle
Opens all three of the sexual chakras (root, sacral, heart) simultaneously. Stand with your feet about 1 yard apart and extend your arms to the sides. Turn your left foot out about 90 degrees, and pivot your right foot slightly to the left. Keeping your knees and arms straight, bend at the waist and tilt your body to the left until your left hand rests on your shin. Look up to your right thumb and hold for five full breaths. Return to start, switch legs, and repeat. Modification: If you have tight hamstrings or a sore lower back, slightly bend your front knee.

Seated Open-Angle Pose
Increases hip, thigh, and groin flexibility and stimulates root and sacral chakras. Sit on the floor with your legs straddled wide and your feet flexed. Contract your thigh muscles to lift your kneecaps up toward your hips. Next, place your hands on the floor behind you, fingers facing forward; your arms should support your straight spine like a kickstand on a bicycle. Hold for 10 full breaths. Modification: If your hips are painfully tight, bring your legs a bit closer together and bend your knees slightly.

Lying-Down Leg Raises
Releases hips. Lie on your back and raise your right leg. Hold your right big toe with the first two fingers of your right hand, and lower your leg smoothly toward your right shoulder. Go as far as you can, and then hold this pose for five full breaths. Gently release and repeat with your left leg and hand. Modification: If reaching your toes is difficult, use a yoga strap.

5. Breath of Desire

While most poses help prepare you for a libidinous rendezvous, this breathing exercise can actually heighten your pleasure in flagrante.
Try Breath of Fire: While you're in the act, take rapid, forceful, and rhythmic breaths through the nose with the mouth closed. Don't worry if your partner thinks you're hyperventilating; he'll forget all about it when you reach a spine-tingling climax (and no doubt take credit for your fulfillment).

6. Double Your Pleasure

Practicing with your man is "like foreplay," says Jacquie Noelle Greaux, creator of the *Better Sex Through Yoga* video series. "You start to breathe together, sweat together, and move together. It gets your energy synced up." Some mat work might make him more sexually imaginative as well. "Yoga sparks creativity," Fowler says. "Women don't want bang-boom from a man, they want an explorer—and yoga invites you to explore."

The 8 Sexiest Foods on Earth

FORGET LINGERIE — EAT THESE
FOODS TO FEEL FRISKY FROM THE INSIDE OUT.

By Morgan Lord

Sex-starved humans have been hunting get-in-the-mood grub for thousands of years. Romans slurped shellfish while splashing around in public baths, and the Marquis de Sade downed untold quantities of Spanish fly as he boinked his way through 18th-century France. Of course, finding libido boosters with scientifically proven positive effects on sexual health is a different story (oysters, yes; Spanish fly, no). We tracked down eight foods that will increase hormone levels and get your blood pumping.

1. Bananas

If you want sex to go the extra mile, fuel up for foreplay just as you would for a marathon. A big banana is the perfect food for bedroom endurance: Bananas contain B vitamins, which are key for converting carbohydrates into energy and are believed to help manufacture sex hormones such as testosterone. Munch on one a few hours before getting busy to make the most of your monkey business, says Hilda Hutcherson, MD, author of *Pleasure*.

2. Celery

Serve your guy celery sticks and he may suddenly seem more irresistible than Leonardo DiCaprio. "Raw celery contains the male hormone androsterone, which can act as a pheromone to trigger female attraction," says Ava Cadell, PhD, author of *Passion Power*. After a few bites, his sweat glands start releasing the pheromone. If you're feeling too cranky to fool around, nibble a stalk yourself—androsterone has mood-elevating effects in women, according to the *Journal of Fertility and Sterility*. Your man not a celery fan? Add a few truffle shavings to his meal. (Who can dislike those?) Truffles boast even more androsterone—enough for female pigs to detect the precious mushrooms growing as deep as 3 feet underground.

3. Dark Chocolate

An Italian study found that women who report eating chocolate on a daily basis claim to have more satisfying sex lives. Coincidence? We think not. Willy Wonka's favorite raw material contains a cocktail of chemicals linked to relaxation, intoxication, and pleasure, Dr. Hutcherson says. Like other sweets, chocolate triggers the release of feel-good endorphins. It also provides small amounts of anxiety-quelling tryptophan, arousing caffeine, and a few substances—anandamide and theobromine—that, in large quantities, work like a psychedelic drug and an opiate, respectively. You'd have to down several pounds of chocolate to feel the funky effects, but simply nibbling a few squares after dinner can help transform your mood from stressed to saucy.

4. Flaxseeds

Just 1 tablespoon of flaxseeds a day helps increase testosterone—the chemical with the most direct libido-boosting effect, according to Helen Fisher, PhD, author of *Why We Love* and a *Women's Health* advisor. Besides enhancing sex drive, these nutty-flavored seeds contain essential fatty acids, including omega-3 and omega-6, which are the major building blocks of all sex hormones. "If you don't have enough fatty acids, your hormone levels may decrease, and so will your desire," Dr. Hutcherson says. To rev your engine, sprinkle a tablespoon of flaxseeds on your cereal and salads every day. If seeds aren't your thing, opt for walnuts, which contain about 90 percent of your omega recommended daily intake.

5. Ginger

Wondering what to cook for your anniversary dinner? Make it an Asian stir-fry with loads of fresh ginger. The powerful root stimulates the circulatory system, increasing bloodflow to the genitals. Fresh ginger has a more "pungent smell" than the stuff in a jar, Dr. Cadell says. So? Smelling ginger has a stronger effect on penile and vaginal bloodflow than actually eating it. When a food or aroma raises blood pressure, vessels in the genitals admit a rush of blood that inflates erectile tissue. The vessels then close off, preventing blood from exiting the erogenous zones, keeping sensitivity levels high. Only powdered ginger on hand? It will also boost bloodflow a bit, but the effect won't be as intense.

6. Honey

No wonder newlyweds' sweaty getaways are called honeymoons. The sticky sweetener contains simple carbohydrates that provide instant energy and fuel for working muscles. "Honey is rich in B vitamins, which are needed for testosterone production, and it contains boron, which helps the body metabolize and use estrogen—an important part of bloodflow and arousal," Dr. Hutcherson says. Use a few teaspoons as a natural sweetener in tea or spread it on toast with peanut butter.

7. Nutmeg and Clove

Researchers have found that nutmeg and clove, both from evergreen trees, bolster the sexual activity of rats. Each stimulates the parasympathetic nervous system—helping the little critters, and you, relax—but the effects were greater with nutmeg. Just don't eat too much of the magical spice, as it also has hallucinogenic properties, Dr. Cadell says. A sprinkle on your cappuccino or hot cocoa should do the trick; as with chocolate, you'd have to eat a lot (about 2 tablespoons' worth on an empty stomach) before the walls would start melting.

8. Oysters

Ancient Romans pegged this shellfish as a sex-spurring food, and they were definitely on to something. Oysters contain high levels of zinc, a mineral required for the production of testosterone. A team of American and Italian researchers recently found that mussels, clams, and oysters deliver two types of amino acids that spark a rush of sex hormones. Be sure to chew your shellfish thoroughly before swallowing—you'll extract more of the mojo-cranking mineral.

Part Two:
The Art of Hormone Management

Has Anyone Seen My Sex Drive?

YOUR LIBIDO CAN BE A SLIPPERY LITTLE SUCKER—AND FOR
SOME, ALWAYS ELUSIVE. WE WENT UNDERCOVER
TO FIND OUT WHERE YOUR DESIRE MIGHT BE HIDING.

By Jennifer Benjamin

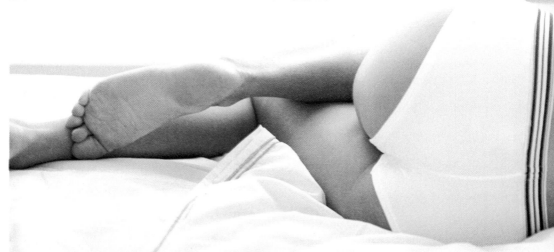

We all want to be that woman— at least for a night. The naughty little sex glutton who grabs her guy mid–cocktail party for a quickie in the coatroom, who plans entire vacations around the ideal skinny-dipping spot, who actually has tried all 69 of the moves "guaranteed to drive him wild"

and loved every one of them. But even if you were a Lusty Lana once upon a time, these days your libido may be more lifeless than a dorm-room houseplant. Or maybe it's always been a bit limp.

Either way, you're not alone. In a recent survey published in the *Archives of Internal Medicine,* more than one in three women admitted

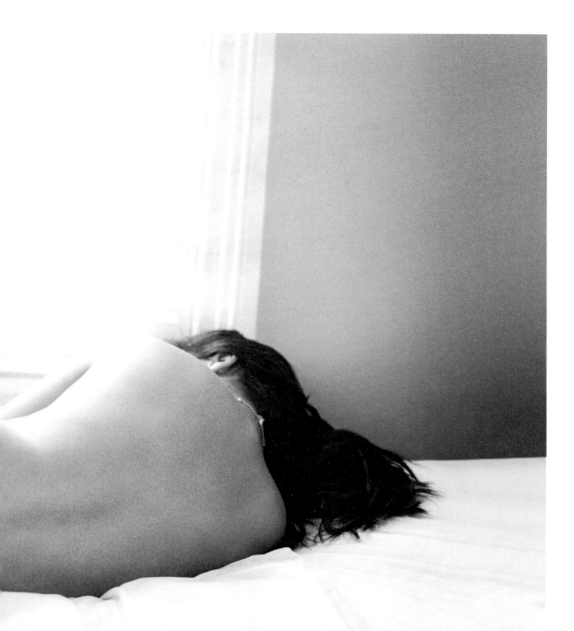

to experiencing low sexual desire in the past month. Hello—that's more than 40 million of us! While men can pop Viagra (those lucky bastards), women can't quick-fix their sexual desire with a magic pill. For us, there's more to it than bloodflow.

But there's good news: According to experts, once you ID the possible causes of your luke-warm libido, you can start homing in on a solution. "Take the time to assess yourself—not just physically but emotionally and mentally—and you'll be able to see what might be holding you back," says Patti Britton, PhD, a Los Angeles sexologist and author of *The Art of Sex Coaching*.

To help you reconnect with your saucy side, we asked three women to share their struggles with low desire and then turned to top sex therapists for their analyses. This may not turn you into the woman who speeds home for a lunch-hour power romp, but the following insights and advice will help make you hungrier for lovin' than you may have been in a long time.

Trust Is the Best Aphrodisiac

Guys seem to have it pretty easy when it comes to sexual arousal: Man gets turned on. Penis takes over. Brain shuts down. Enjoyment ensues. For most women, it's more complex. To feel even the slightest bit of desire, our heads have to be in the game. A 2003 study at Chicago's Northwestern University found that even when women show the physical signs of sexual excitement below the belt, if they're not mentally turned on they won't feel a damn thing.

Now, imagine you're busy trying to muster desire, but your brain—the main factor in the equation—won't stop analyzing, fretting, or planning. For Kira Barnes* that kind of overall anxiety has left her with "zero sex drive." After working 12-hour days, she comes home exhausted and way too preoccupied even to consider sex. "I'm always stressing about my job—I even have nightmares about it," she says. Work concerns aside, Kira describes herself in general as a very anxious person, a perfectionist who's always making to-do lists on paper and in her head.

Though the flip advice might be to tell Kira that she just needs a hearty hump session (or a strong cocktail) to feel right as rain, we know it doesn't work that way. For Kira, sex is just one more thing to worry about. "I'll have sex because

Names changed to protect identity.

I know it's important to the relationship, but I never feel a desire for it," she says. Kira describes her boyfriend as a sweet, supportive guy, understanding about the fact that she isn't exactly likely to swing from the chandelier. Besides, he leaves for work at 6:00 a.m. and often doesn't return home until midnight, after she's already asleep (they have sex two or three times a month). "The pressure to have sex, or the guilt over not wanting it, isn't there because, logistically, we can't really have it that often."

When Kira's alone and it's time for a little self-lovin', on the other hand, it's a whole other ball game. "I find that I'm more in the mood," she says. "I'm able to just clear my mind and get into it."

According to experts, if a woman masturbates regularly, she doesn't actually have a low libido. So what's going on? Probably trust issues, says sex therapist Gina Ogden, PhD, author of *The Return of Desire*. "You're at your most vulnerable—body, mind, and heart—when you're naked with a man," she explains. "If you're afraid of that kind of intimacy, you're going to subconsciously avoid sex, and you certainly won't have a desire for it."

For many, that fear of intimacy can stem from early sexual experiences. If they were filled with angst or with emotional or even physical pain, they can leave women with an underlying sense of "I don't want to go through that again," Dr. Ogden says.

Kira's issues could be traced back to a high school boyfriend who couldn't keep it in his pants. "In the four years we were together, I always thought he was cheating. I remember feeling self-conscious about hooking up, like he was getting it better somewhere else," she says.

Then in college, she dated a guy who was all about pleasing her. The only problem was that he wanted it morning and night and would get upset if Kira refused him. Around the same time, she

Even when women show the physical signs of sexual excitement, if they're not mentally turned on they won't feel a damn thing.

Shy No More

WANT TO BE BOLDER BETWEEN THE SHEETS? TAKE THIS EXPERT ADVICE ON GETTING OVER COMMON BEDROOM INHIBITIONS.

Stop Worrying about Hygiene
Men are hardwired to be turned on by your natural smell and taste, says Joy Davidson, PhD, a sex therapist in New York City and the author of *Fearless Sex*. If you still feel funky, make showering with your guy part of the foreplay.

Start Asking for What You Want
To take the pressure off, "try to talk about it when you're not in bed," says Pepper Schwartz, PhD, author of *Prime: Adventures and Advice on Sex, Love, and the Sensual Years* and the relationship expert for www.Perfectmatch.com. Once you're between the sheets, "turn requests into erotic expressions, not instructions," Dr. Davidson says. "Saying 'Oh, baby, do that slower' isn't an order, it's sexy."

Do It with the Lights On
There's nothing sexier than a woman who lets her guard down in bed. "He loves when he can see and feel your body, and the biggest turnoff for him is your acting embarrassed," Dr. Schwartz says. "So create an environment where you can enjoy yourself—candles, lingerie, whatever you need to relax and feel beautiful." Trust us, he's not worrying about anything other than the parts that give him pleasure. Neither should you!

went on antianxiety medication to help her sleep and noticed an upswing in her sex drive as a result. She didn't stay on the pills for long because her health insurance wouldn't cover the cost; her sexual urge has been pretty much MIA ever since. The few relationships Kira's had in the past several years have been short-lived. "Either the guy would get annoyed with my lack of sex drive, or, since we weren't having that sexual connection, I would end up just viewing him as a friend," she says.

Kira's experience, though more extreme than that of most women, is not uncommon. For many women, anxiety and low libido go hand-in-hand, explains sex and relationship therapist Laura Berman, PhD, director of the Berman Center and author of *Real Sex for Real Women*. "If you're not able to quiet your mind, you can't be present in the moment, you can't connect with your partner, feel desire, or achieve orgasm—it's practically impossible."

The first step for women like Kira is to unplug the mental ticker tape. "It's important to redirect the brain away from outside stresses and issues and connect the mind back to the body," Dr. Britton says. She suggests taking a warm bath every night before bed to help you feel good in your skin. She also recommends audio therapy three times a week. "It sounds corny, but just lying in bed listening to a CD of nature sounds—waterfalls, birds chirping, wind in the trees—is really good for shutting out the noise in your own head."

After Kira has tuned out her worries, she needs to tune in to her partner. "He probably doesn't know what's going on, much less how to help her fix it, because she doesn't really know herself," Dr. Ogden says. "They may want to consider a session or two with a therapist, where she can explain to him what's going on in her head and what's keeping her from feeling desire." Meanwhile, Dr. Britton recommends that Kira and her boyfriend undress and try this: "Get into a position where they're really body-to-body, heart-to-heart, with their legs and arms wrapped around each other, like a seated position with her facing him on his lap. Then they can work on breathing in sync, not only to help relax, but to feel more connected." When Kira's mind starts to wander, Dr. Britton says, she should redirect her thoughts to her physical self—what she's feeling, how her body is responding—to try to truly enjoy every skin-on-skin sensation.

The Confidence Cure

Not all psychosexual blocks are anxiety-related. For many women, low self-esteem can be the biggest booty buzzkill. Caroline Burns,* has always struggled with a lack of confidence. "Growing up, my brothers and my dad were pretty brutal with the way they would tease me about my weight. Plus, I always had a sense that my dad was not being faithful to my mom during their marriage. I think he had a few affairs with different women, who were usually thin and blonde; that didn't make me feel any better about what men were looking for," she says. "Even though my family and I have better

Ultimatums—especially those bred from frustration—only add more pressure to an already tense situation.

relationships now, these self-esteem issues have been a running theme for me." In her early twenties, Caroline turned to sex as a way to feel validated, attractive, and loved. But hookups were never fueled by good old-fashioned desire. "I enjoy the cuddling and the closeness, but the act itself just doesn't do it for me," she says. "And I've never been able to orgasm during sex."

Many women like Caroline approach sex from the wrong direction. "We've been fed these messages that sex is supposed to be for him and about his needs," Dr. Ogden says, "and has nothing to do with our own pleasure, bodies, or desires." And for Caroline, who was raised in a strict, religious household and spent 12 years in Catholic school, there was plenty of guilt surrounding sex. "For a long time there was a part of me that felt that sex was wrong," she says. "That feeling has almost disappeared now, though."

Adding to her cycle of shame, Caroline feels insecure about being so "nonsexual." For reasons she can't figure out, she says, "I just don't have the urge to have sex or even masturbate." It probably doesn't help that her boyfriend of 2 years has a crazy-high sex drive. "He wants sex in the morning and at night, and is really into trying new things," she says. Although she usually has sex with him when he wants it, Caroline says, her inability to orgasm creates even more tension between them. For the most part, he's been patient and supportive of her, she says, but one time his frustration boiled over and he threatened to break up with her if she didn't take more aggressive steps to fix her sexual issues.

Ultimatums—especially those bred from frustration—only add more pressure to the situation, says sex therapist Ian Kerner, PhD, author of *Sex Recharge*. Caroline needs to have honest conversations with her guy, Kerner says, and remind him that, although she realizes this is difficult for him, she is doing "everything she can to improve her sexual response." His patience and understanding will help her achieve that goal faster.

And her boyfriend will really need to put that patience into practice because, in Caroline's case, the best solution is to stop having sex for a while. "She's overwhelmed with her sexual insecurities and needs a serious break," Dr. Kerner says. "Instead of having intercourse, she and her partner need to focus on sensual touch, without the pressure to have an orgasm." Caressing each other, trading massages, kissing—they're all ways for women like Caroline to operate outside of the sexual sphere but still feel tenderness, love, and validation. To sell the "no-sex" idea to her man, Dr. Kerner suggests explaining that in addition to clearing out the muck in her own head, she wants to focus on finding fun new ways to get him off that don't involve intercourse.

Finally, Caroline also has to address her body-image concerns. She needs to adjust her perception of what's sexy, Dr. Britton says, so she can start feeling sensual and sexual. For starters, she could ask her boyfriend to tell her why he finds her so attractive physically. Then she should "find an image of a woman in a magazine that reminds her of herself and that she believes is sexy," Dr. Britton says. "She should keep that image in her head when she thinks about her body." Over time, the idea that she's just as sexy as the woman in the photograph will start to sink in.

Bonding Leads to Booty

Sometimes it's not anxiety or hormones but life's rough patches that contribute to a sex-drive nosedive. Last August, Sarah Arnold,* went through a debilitating period of grief after the death of her mother. "Imagine your best friend, just gone," she says. "I went completely numb. I lost my interest in and motivation for everything." She also felt consumed with feelings she didn't know how to deal with. "I was pissed off at the world for taking away my mother," Sarah says. "And the person I took it out on was the person closest to me: my boyfriend. I put walls up just to keep an emotional distance from him."

Before her mother's death, Sarah had had a healthy libido and wanted sex every day—sometimes twice a day. But in her grief, the sex dwindled to once every week or two. "For me, sex had always been so much about connection, but I was so closed off, I didn't want to be intimate with my boyfriend." Although she'd lost her desire, Morgan still tried to have sex when she could, thinking that the act itself would make her feel better and perhaps make her relationship stronger. "Everyone is different, but for some, it can be very therapeutic to do things that remind you that you're alive, that reconnect you with the joys of life," Dr. Ogden says.

After several months, Sarah began to bounce back. "I started really dealing with my grief, talking about what I was going through, talking about my mother with my boyfriend and my friends. That really helped," she says. "My boyfriend and I also started to understand each other better, to communicate and see where the other was coming from, and really be sensitive and sympathetic." As Dr. Kerner points out, "Sex for many women is such an emotional experience that in order to really boost your desire for it, you have to nurture that connection with your partner."

*Names changed to protect identity.

Another big help: They started working out together. "We signed up for a triathlon," Sarah says. "I thought that if we were spending time together training, running, and raising our serotonin, it would enhance our sex life." She was right. Studies have shown that exercise is both a mood enhancer and a libido booster. It increases endorphin levels, Dr. Kerner says, and gets you in touch with your body. In Sarah's case, working with her boyfriend toward a shared goal also reinforced their bond.

Sarah also realized that in order to start having more sex, she would have to make it a priority again. "No one wants to schedule sex," she says, "but I've found that if I carve out time for that purpose, I end up looking forward to it." According to Dr. Berman, for many women, sex often begets more sex. It's not necessarily going to be the hot-and-heavy, spontaneous variety, she says, but a roll in the hay—even when you don't think you're in the mood—can actually make you want sex more.

If you can scrape up some extra cash, consider getting away to get it on. A 2006 national study conducted by the Berman Center found that couples who vacation together once or twice a year actually have more emotional intimacy than those who do a weekly date night. "That time away from your life can be rejuvenating," Dr. Berman says. "And there's a dopamine effect you get from being in a new environment, with new experiences, and that can also increase your sex drive." (Lounging under a giant palm tree on a white-sand beach while the sun's rays warm your skin and a frosty piña colada slides down your throat will send your mind straight to the gutter.)

While Sarah's sex life hasn't returned to what it was in its heyday, things have definitely improved. Resuscitating a lackluster libido, or just trying to dig it out from under piles of emotional baggage, takes time and energy. Much the way forcing yourself to do 100 crunches a day will get you closer to an enviable six-pack, doing what it takes to stoke your sex drive has a life-enhancing payoff that's worth every bit of effort—and sweat.

24

Percentage of couples who report having a sexual drought in the last 3 months

The Sneaky Libido Stealer

IF YOU'RE STILL AT A POINT IN YOUR LIFE THAT BIRTH CONTROL SEEMS LIKE A GOOD IDEA, KNOW THIS: IT MIGHT BE MESSING WITH YOUR MOJO. HERE'S HOW TO GET IT BACK.

By Lauren Russell Griffin

For nearly 50 years, the Pill has given women the freedom to knock boots without getting knocked up. And while popping hormones does have its cons (like a slightly higher risk of blood clots), you can't deny the perks: the convenience, the protection against uterine and ovarian cancers, the 99.7 percent effectiveness rate. But it turns out your trusty little OC can come with a caveat that might make you think twice about swallowing those little pills every day.

In the past decade, researchers have found that hormonal contraceptives—including the Pill, the Patch, and the vaginal ring—can dampen how often women want, think about, and even respond to sexual stimulation. And an online *Women's Health* poll backs that up: We found that 36 percent of you firmly believe the Pill muffles your mojo.

Unfortunately, no official stats are available on how prevalent this problem really is. When asked to estimate how many of their patients on the Pill have suffered a blow to their sex lives, doctors' answers range from 10 percent to 40 percent—though some sexual-health specialists argue that 40 percent is a lot closer to reality. The phenomenon may be underestimated because many docs simply aren't clued in to the, well, ins and outs of their patients' sex lives. "Sex drive is not a subject most doctors are comfortable discussing, because it's not something they learn about in detail in medical school," says Irwin Goldstein, MD, director of sexual medicine at Alvarado Hospital in San Diego. And while some European countries, including Germany, list decreased desire as a side effect on birth control pill packages, there are no printed warnings about it in the United States.

There Are Reasons We Bonk . . .

So, what drives your love machine? A key component is testosterone. As a woman, you don't have enough juice to grow a goatee or develop a burning desire for an Xbox 360, but the amount you do have plays a role in your randiness, espe-

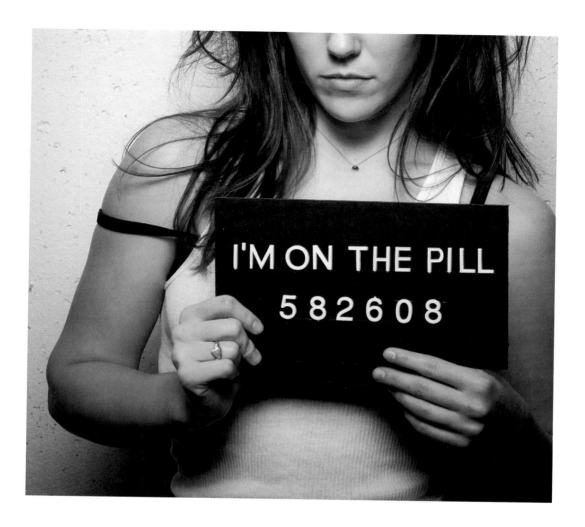

cially just before ovulation (when you're most likely to get pregnant). Every month at midcycle, women's brains signal their ovaries, which create 50 percent of the body's testosterone, to produce a surge of the lust-stimulating stuff. That makes perfect sense, given that our main biological goal is to propagate the species.

Testosterone also initiates bloodflow that causes your girly parts to become plump and sensitive. This leads to lubrication and, with any luck, one hell of an orgasm. According to an article in *Hormones and Behavior,* Canadian researchers report that women with higher levels of testosterone climax more often than those with lower hormone levels.

The problem is that daily contraceptives alter the body's testosterone production—and not in a good way. This occurs for two reasons. First, the hormones in the Pill put the ovaries to sleep, halting ovulation. Conked-out ovaries can't produce testosterone.

And what about the other 50 percent of your body's testosterone, which is produced by the adrenal glands? The Pill renders it useless, thanks to the superpotent synthetic estrogen it contains. After you take each pill, your liver—convinced that you've consumed a potentially toxic amount of estrogen—starts pumping out a protein called sex hormone–binding globulin (SHBG). It works by glomming onto sex hormones (including estrogen, but also testosterone) like a mosquito onto flypaper. As more of your testosterone glues itself to

SHBG, less of it is available for your body to use. This "free" testosterone—whatever's produced that SHBG doesn't swallow up—partially determines your sex drive. In fact, a 2004 Boston University study found that subjects who reported the greatest sexual desire had higher levels of free testosterone.

...And Reasons We Don't

Now, even if you've been popping Ortho-Cyclen since puberty, the artificial flux might never affect your sex drive. That's because the Pill lowers testosterone in all women, but it lowers libido only in some. To demo the discrepancy, experts cite a 1995 study in which British scientists gave 150 women either an oral contraceptive or a placebo for 4 months. (All subjects were unable to conceive, either because they'd had their tubes tied or they had partners with vasectomies.) For nearly half the women taking the Pill, sexual interest and intercourse frequency took a nosedive. However, sex drive did not stall for the others who took the drug.

"Unfortunately, we really don't know what the discriminating factor is," says Claudia Panzer, MD, a female sexual dysfunction specialist and endocrinologist at the Canterbury Wellness Center in Denver. But theories exist. The most popular is that nonhormonal factors help keep your sex drive in high gear. For instance, not having to worry about getting pregnant may increase your arousal and, in effect, cancel out the Pill's libido-squashing potential, says Cynthia Graham, PhD, a researcher at the Kinsey Institute for Research in Sex, Gender, and Reproduction in Bloomington, Indiana. The adrenaline rush of a budding relationship can also override the effects of low testosterone.

But Nobody Likes a Lazy Libido

If your life's missing more booty than the TV cut of *Basic Instinct*, we say it's time to play the field (of options). Ask your doctor to prescribe a different hormonal contraceptive: a new brand, a lower-estrogen pill, or the Patch. "Despite the fact that all forms of hormonal birth control increase SHBG levels, 30 percent of women who switch somehow get their sex drive back," says Alan Altman, MD, a sexual dysfunction specialist and assistant clinical professor of obstetrics, gynecology, and reproductive biology at Harvard Medical School. "We don't know why this happens; it may be just a placebo effect."

Or you can simply chuck your pills and see what happens. While it may not sound like the most cutting-edge remedy, it is what many doctors prescribe. "If you've determined that there's nothing else that might be impacting your sex drive, certainly the first thing I would recommend is a hiatus from the Pill," Dr. Altman says. Of course, ditching your birth control pills is no trivial decision. Some women need the hormones to help treat medical conditions such as endometriosis or ovarian cysts. IUDs can be a long-term commitment, and messy barrier methods like condoms and diaphragms put an end to spontaneity faster than an 80-hour workweek.

But if you decide that having a hotter sex life is worth a little trial and error, consider shelving your pills for 3 to 6 months, which should allow time for you to notice changes in your libido. With no artificial hormones swimming through your bloodstream, your ovaries will wake up from their snooze and start producing testosterone again.

If you go OC-free and your libido's still in low gear, then the Pill probably isn't your problem. "Your sex drive is like a big pizza, and just one slice is hormones," Dr. Panzer says. Other common mood killers include depression, stress, and other prescription medications, such as some antidepressants and drugs to treat hypertension. Even antihistamines can dry out the vagina, making for painful intercourse. "And why would you be interested in sex if it hurts?" Dr. Goldstein asks.

Find yourself a sexual medicine specialist to help you discern the exact catalyst. Just knowing what's wrong can be enough to help ease your frustration and get you excited about the prospect of putting the *whoop!* back in your whoopee. Once you're in the habit of generating some heat between the sheets, you'll feel more relaxed and confident—not only sexually, but mentally as well. Just think of it as the sweet feeling of sex-cess.

The Back-on-Track Sex Plan

SIMPLE STRATEGIES FOR BUSTING OUT OF A LUST RUT NO MATTER WHERE YOU ARE IN YOUR RELATIONSHIP.

By Margo Trott

Despite the endless hype about how crucial hot sex is to a happy relationship, few couples on the planet actually do the deed every night. In fact, most couples go through periods when one or both partners would rather watch Animal Planet than make the beast with two backs. One study published in the *Journal of Marriage and Family Therapy* found that 24 percent of couples reported having had a sexual drought in the past 3 months. Whether you're stressed, he's tired, or you both have something else on your minds, it's perfectly normal to have the occasional sex-free period. But if you've been low on lust for a little too long, there are plenty of ways to reignite the flames. We identified four phases in relationships when sex drives typically fizzle and asked top experts for the best strategies to get you both back into a steamy groove.

Lackluster Phase #1
The Novelty Has Officially Worn Off

When you first met, your mattress springs squeaked on a regular basis and you always had that dewy glow. That's because infatuation triggers the release of extra dopamine, a brain chemical that fuels your libido, says our go-to expert, Laura Berman, PhD, director of the Berman Center for sexual health and menopause management in Chicago and author of *The Passion Prescription*. When the initial attraction begins to wane, so does the dopamine boost, Dr. Berman says.

Scare your pants off. Dopamine also kicks in when you're taken by surprise. "Do things that are new and different together, even a little scary," Dr. Berman says. Even a relatively tame act can be a thrill if it's unexpected, says Sherry Amatenstein, relationship expert for iVillage.com and author of *Love Lessons from Bad Breakups*. Pick up a box of drugstore hair color (the kind that eventually washes out) and go to town on each other. You'll get that sexy hands-on-the-scalp feeling along with the risky excitement of not knowing quite how it's going to turn out.

Reset boundaries. Sometimes people get so comfortable together they forget that sexual attraction requires a little mystery and excitement, says Mary Ann Donohue, PhD, assistant vice president of patient care services at Clara Maass Medical Center in Belleville, New Jersey. Maybe it's time to start closing the bathroom door, burping under your breath, and getting dressed up for bed

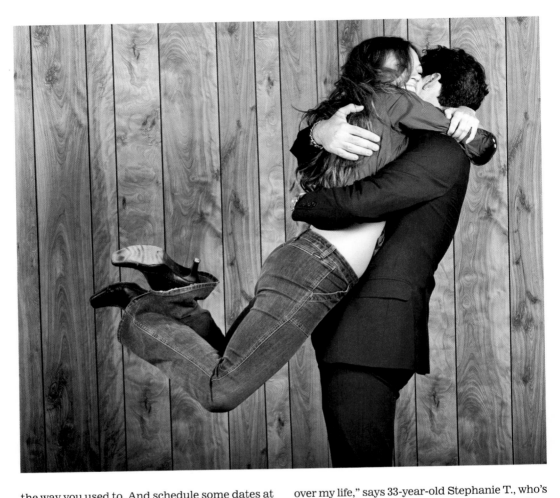

the way you used to. And schedule some dates at swank venues—cocktails at a posh hotel bar or a night at the opera—where you have to dress up and act formal. Seeing each other looking your best and surrounded by lights, music, and other couples can bring back the thrill of dating, which will segue into livelier sex when you get home.

Lackluster Phase #2
You're about to Forsake All Others

And one, or both, of you is freaking out. Before her wedding, "I was so stressed about losing control over my life," says 33-year-old Stephanie T., who's been married to Joel for 10 years. For some of us, the idea of having one sexual partner for a lifetime makes walking barefoot over thumbtacks sound more appealing than sauntering down the aisle.

Just do it. Sex is how guys say "you're the center of my universe" without having to utter the actual words. "Women may want to shoot me for this, but in an otherwise good relationship, if you sometimes go ahead with sex even when you're not in the mood, the benefits can be significant," Dr. Berman says. Stop addressing those envelopes and undress each other instead. That 5-minute nooky break tells him he's more important than the florist or the caterer, Dr. Berman says. And it releases oxytocin, a hormone that makes you feel bonded and attached—so you'll remember the reason for those 200 invites in the first place.

Look beyond the big day. Odds are on your side: Married women are more than twice as likely as single ones to have sex two or three times a week, according to a survey by the National Opinion Research Center. And that marriage bond will actually bring you closer. "These last few years we've been very sexually connected," Joel says. What's different? He and Stephanie know each other better. "Now we communicate about intimacy; we make time to do that. We've grown to understand the other person's sexuality and needs better, too."

Lackluster Phase #3

One of You Gets Pink-Slipped

"We'd been dating for a year when Matt got fired," says Cynthia B., 41. "He responded by withdrawing; he didn't want to sleep with me." Stress—financial or otherwise—can cause levels of libido-stoking testosterone to drop, says Beverly Whipple, PhD, a neurophysiologist and coauthor of *The G-Spot: And Other Discoveries about Human Sexuality*. And when a guy loses his provider status, it's a blow to his ego and manhood—not exactly the feeling he wants to bring into the bed. If you've been canned? Research reported in *JAMA*, the *Journal of the American Medical Association* shows that when a woman's income is reduced by just 20 percent, her self-worth and sex drive can plummet.

Tackle it together. When he's the one taking the hit, form a united front, says Yvonne Thomas, PhD, a psychologist in Los Angeles. Refer to the issue as "ours" instead of "his," which lets him know you don't blame him. Also make it clear that he hasn't lost any status in your eyes. Remind him how talented and capable he is. Then break out the massage oil and offer to rub his worries away. No, you're not his geisha girl, but playing that role for a night or two will pump up his self-esteem.

Think dirty thoughts. When it's you in the stress-

induced slump, talking about sex in a positive way can be powerful, Dr. Berman says. She suggests saying something like "I miss being intimate with you." It can help you recall your last intimate encounter—and all the delicious details—reminding you of how good getting naked can make you feel.

Lackluster Phase #4

You're Baby Bombed

Sometimes just trying to get the sperm to sidle up to the egg can be enough to make your inner horndog hibernate. Janine L., 34, and Roger L., 35, tried for about a year to have a baby and wound up seeing an infertility specialist. "When you're dealing with a fertility schedule, sex stops being fun," Roger says. "He felt so much pressure that a couple of times he couldn't 'finish,'" Janine adds. "He'd feel guilty and embarrassed."

Do it when it doesn't count. When sex's end result is pure pleasure instead of pregnancy, you have fewer expectations and less likelihood of disappointment. So sneak in nonbaby-making sex when you're not ovulating, Dr. Berman says. And if your bedroom has become "fertility central," take the fun-only sex on tour. Your best bet? The closet—where, according to a University of California–Berkeley study, clothes emit a potent chemical from men's sweat, hair, and skin that arouses women. Who knew?

Schedule a grown-ups–only playdate. Once kids arrive, "getting regular alone time gives you a chance to talk like adults about intimate things," Dr. Whipple says. This may seem obvious, but as Rebecca admits, "We're so busy, it wouldn't happen if we didn't plan it." Sneak away for a day or two every few months. If you've got weather (and geography) on your side, head to the ocean. You'll have uninterrupted time for conversation in the car and—dopamine booster!—you can jump in for a late-night skinny-dip. Even the local Starbucks makes for an easy getaway. Talk like adults over cappuccino and use the caffeine perk for that crucial extra hour after the kids go to bed.

Can an Orgasm a Day Keep the Marriage Counselor Away?

SWINGING FOR THE FENCES IS A GOOD WAY TO FIND OUT.

By T. Edward Nickens

*W*hen Charla Muller's husband, Brad, turned 40, she could have given him a custom split-cane fly rod. But instead, she decided on a more interesting gift: sex every day for the next 12 months.

Pressure much? But what they learned during a year of loving copiously, Muller writes in *365 Nights: A Memoir of Intimacy*, "transformed" their marriage. And not just that aspect that involved bedsheets.

Muller is no fishnet-clad sex addict. She's a sensible mother of two and a former corner-office public relations executive who downsized her career to part-time status once the kids were born. She's a fortysomething woman who attends a weekly women's Bible-study group. "Our marriage was in a really good place," she says. "But I was up to my eyeballs in kids and carpools and keeping up the house, none of which had any-thing to do with the one thing my husband and I could do for each other."

In the end, after factoring in sick days, out-of-town business trips, and other chinks in the schedule, the Mullers figured they got things done an average of 27 times a month. Off goal, perhaps, but still damn impressive. Here, her top five tips for improving every aspect of your marriage, culled from what she learned from every-day lovin'.

Nourish kindness

"I can't roll in the hay with someone I'm mad at or irritated with," says Muller. "We had to nurture each other throughout the day so that we could come together in the evening and be able to find worthwhile intimacy." Phone calls, compliments, helping around the house . . . an overall increase in niceness paid dividends in nookie.

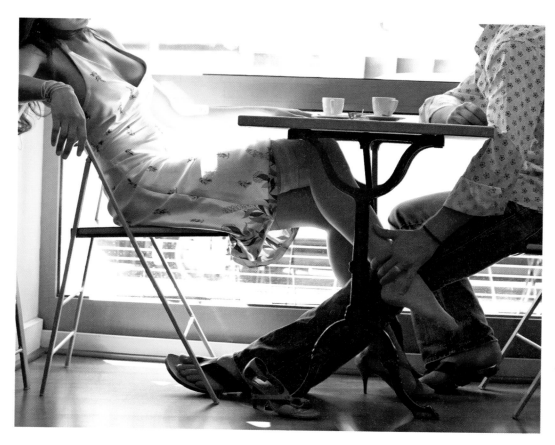

Kill your television

Nothing siphons off the opportunities for bare-naked gestures of appreciation more than the tube. Banishing the remote until after lovemaking was a key decision. "After all," says Muller, "that's why the digital video recorder was invented."

Make a game plan

Time-strapped couples must be intentional. "We had to plan by the day and by the week," says Muller. "Initially, Brad felt that talking about sex so straightforwardly distracted from its allure. But it's a lot easier to negotiate intimacy when you're talking about it."

Establish house rules

As we've established, finding the time and space for sex is a serious issue when you have kids.

Muller laid down the law with her then 5- and 7-year-old children: A closed door is a closed door. Just like the kids have their nap time, Mommy and Daddy have quiet time. (Turn to page 117 for more useful tips on this topic.)

Don't take all day

Quickies count. "Real life begets real sex," says Muller. "It's not like every night is a three-course gourmet meal, but we have to eat."

Keep it exciting

Couples who are sexually adventurous—role-playing, sex toys, acrobatics (if that's your thing)—are 26 percent more likely to have sex several times a week than are their more conservative peers, who, according to the Kinsey Institute, may have sex just twice a month.

The New Rules of Sexuality

UPGRADE YOUR RELATIONSHIP BEHAVIOR.

By Jill Waldbieser

*T*hink about it: You wouldn't be caught dead using a dinosaur of a cell phone or wearing the hairstyle you sported in 10th grade. So why would you continue to follow love rules that have expired? "The realities of dating change all the time," says Pepper Schwartz, PhD, chief relationship expert at www.Perfectmatch. com. "So there's a lot of folk wisdom about relationships that doesn't hold true anymore." To make sure that you're armed with modern information, we tweaked four traditional pieces of advice.

1. Don't Have Sex If You're Not in the Mood.

New rule: Getting Busy Gets You in the Mood.

"The whole idea that you have to be 'in the mood' for sex is a fallacy," says Sandra Leiblum, PhD, author of *Getting the Sex You Want: A Woman's Guide to Becoming Proud, Passionate, and Pleased in Bed*. Women often think that to have sex, the stars need to align—it has to be just the right moment in just the right place, and they need to be crazy turned on. But according to Dr. Leiblum, fooling around often is the very thing that triggers desire. The act of hooking up pumps out oxytocin—the bonding and attachment chemical—and testosterone, which boosts arousal. And studies have shown that testosterone lev-

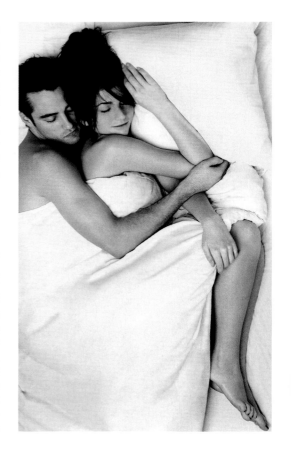

els can stay elevated in women after intercourse. So the next time he rubs up against you just as you were about to get in the shower, opt to get dirty instead.

2. You Need to Say "I Love You" to Each Other Every Day.
New rule: Verbalizing Feelings Should Be More Than Just a Habit.

When those three little words are mumbled through mouthfuls of cornflakes every morning or tossed out absently at the end of every phone call, their importance becomes diluted. The trick to keeping them meaningful: Say "I love you" only when you're really feeling it. Better yet, say it in new and interesting ways. For example, try a

Staying Power

WANT TO MAKE YOUR MARRIAGE LAST? TURN CONVENTIONAL WISDOM ON ITS HEAD.

Talk less. "Love is not all about talking," says Patricia Love, coauthor of *How to Improve Your Marriage without Talking about It.* "It's about connection." Her research reveals that while women release the bonding hormone oxytocin through talk, "men need physical stimulus to feel connected," she says. Touch him a lot a few hours before tackling big relationship issues. And don't hold back. "Men need two or three times more touch than women do to feel bonded," she says. Even if it's not sexual. "Stroke him on the arm or brush him as you walk by," she says.

Go to bed angry. Seeing red at midnight? Sleep on it. "The worst time to resolve conflict is when you're angry," says Terri Orbuch, PhD, a marriage and family therapist. Marriage researcher John Gottman, PhD, discovered that conflict causes hormones to "flood" the body, which encourages us to fight harder against a perceived threat. The results—pounding heart, shallow breathing, that overheated feeling—make it tougher to concentrate on the conversation at hand. "The body needs at least 30 minutes to return to normal levels," Dr. Orbuch adds. So suck it up, tuck in, and calmly continue the discussion tomorrow.

Sweat the small stuff. Fostering a constant curiosity about each other keeps relationships growing. "And by slowing down and noticing interactions, our partners become richer and more complex," says James Cordova, PhD. "Cultivating curiosity about your partner is the same cognitive trick as slowing down to appreciate a delicious food." Just as savoring a juicy bite of steak lets you taste its complex flavors, relishing a detail about a joke your husband made or asking about his day helps you appreciate him.

compliment ("You're seriously the greatest husband on earth"), a term of endearment ("honey" or "babe"), or a statement of appreciation ("It was so thoughtful of you to fill up the tank of my car."). They all send the same message of affection without becoming rote, says Yvonne K. Fulbright, PhD, author of *Touch Me There!* and a *Women's Health* relationship advisor.

3. If You Cheat, You Should Confess.
New rule: Honesty Is Not Always Best.

Cheating on your guy is almost always a selfish act—and so is telling him about it. "Revealing an affair can be damaging to everyone involved," says Robi Ludwig, PsyD, a New York City-based psychotherapist. Sure, it might relieve your guilt short-term, but you have to weigh that against the consequences: Confessing an indiscretion can shatter your man's trust in you and make him feel inadequate and insecure. More often than not, it also results in an ugly breakup. So unless you get caught with your pants down, stay mum. "If you're at a point where you can stop cheating and are ready to deal with the dissatisfaction in your relationship that likely caused you to stray, you may not need to burden your partner with your impulsive, regrettable choices," Dr. Ludwig says.

4. You Should Never Fake an Orgasm.
New rule: It's Okay to Pull Off an Oscar–Winning Performance Every Once in a While.

Those in sexually gratifying relationships are perfectly entitled to fake it from time to time. "Women usually fake an orgasm because they're tired and want to go to bed, and that's fine, on occasion," Dr. Fulbright says. It's also a convenient way to please your partner without getting into a potentially complicated and ego-bruising conversation about how, though you're thoroughly enjoying the ride, there's no way you're going to make it to O-Town tonight. "But if you don't have orgasms on a regular basis, never fake it," Dr. Fulbright says. You'll only encourage him to keep doing whatever he's doing that isn't working. Instead, show him how to get you off—guide his hand to your hot spots during sex or initiate a position you know is a sure thing for you.

10 Tantalizing Tricks He'll Remember

TAKE THE NOOKIE POSITIONS YOU LOVE AND KICK 'EM UP A NOTCH.

By Celeste Perron

It's so easy to get lazy in bed. When the mood strikes, why contort like a Cirque du Soleil acrobat when 1) the fact that you're already having satisfying sex is more than most people accomplish and 2) a simple you're-on-top-tonight position can get the job done fine? But like anything easy—an energy bar for lunch, the treadmill at the gym, shopping on www.Bluefly.com—before long, you feel like you're missing out on the really fun stuff. So every once in a while, liven it up a little (seriously, even just once a month will do the trick). For the best way to do that naked "thing that you do," we asked experts and real women to share their proven strategies for getting new thrills out of those same old positions you know and love.

Missionary

Gripe #1: "I can't move the way I need to for an orgasm."
Upgrade: To get more wiggle room—for hip grinding or to reach your clitoris with your fingers—start by having him sit back on his heels on the bed. Then lie back against a couple of pillows, place your legs on either side of his thighs, and have him grasp your hips and pull your pelvis toward his, er, crotch. You can rest the bottoms of your feet on the bed for balance and leverage or

wrap them around his waist. Stack those pillows up high behind you to prevent all the blood from rushing to your head. Then again, that might just add to the excitement.

Gripe #2: "I can't breathe when he's on top."
Upgrade: It's impossible to get swept away by passion when you're oxygen deprived. For more breathing space, ask him to support his weight on his forearms, suggests David Taylor, MD, who teaches a sexuality class for couples at Arizona's Miraval Life in Balance Resort. Put your hands on his chest to keep him there—guys get even lazier than we do. Because his body is now at a different angle than yours, his penis moves down more toward your tailbone, so the shaft can rub against your clitoris when he thrusts.

Woman on top

Gripe #1: "I don't get the G-spot stimulation that I crave."
Upgrade: Being on top is the best way for you to control the rhythm and level of penetration, and it's ideal for clitoral contact. But if you're looking for the almighty G-spot power-gasm, it's not going to do much for you. That's because your G-spot is located a few inches up the front wall of the vagina, Dr. Taylor says—meaning just out of

thrusting range if you're leaning forward or sitting upright, which most of us tend to do. Instead lean back, placing your hands behind you on his quads if you need the support. "From that angle his penis hits me in just the right place," says Amy K., a lab technician from Maplewood, New Jersey.

Gripe #2: "When I start to move, everything jiggles and I don't feel sexy enough to enjoy myself."
Upgrade: Forget everything you've heard about how empowering and intimate it is to have sex with the lights on and just shut the damn things off—even the night-light. "If the reality is that you feel too self-conscious about your body to really let go in bed, then having sex in the dark will allow you to forget all about what you look like and just have some fun," says Ian Kerner, PhD, author of *She Comes First*. "There's no point in doing the empowering thing if it's not making you happy." When you're ready, fire up a candle and see how that makes you feel. Then light two, then three . . . until you feel comfortable doing it in broad daylight. On the beach!

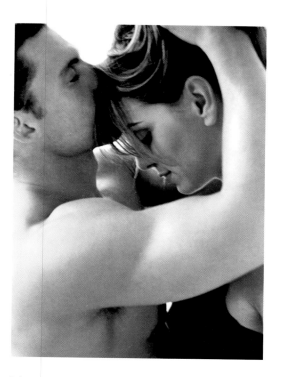

Hands and knees

Gripe #1: "It's a turn-on, but it doesn't give me the clitoral contact I need and want."
Upgrade: No amount of wrangling the classic from-behind positions is going to move your clitoris to a different anatomical location. But you can free it up—along with your hands—if he kneels and rests his butt on his heels and then you lower yourself onto his lap, like you're sitting on a chair. Place your feet flat on the floor for balance and support—and so you can move up and down. If it sounds kind of like a workout, well, it is. But it feels so good you won't even notice that you're toning your calves and thighs.

Gripe #2: "It feels really impersonal because I can't see his face or touch his body."
Upgrade: The thing about having sex with your partner behind you is that it exposes the back of your body to a host of erotic sensations usually only played out in front. Plus, you tap into a naughty feeling that can be insanely hot. To get all of that without sacrificing any intimacy, try lying on your stomach and have him lie flat on top of you (with some of his weight on his arms so he doesn't squash you). "It's more intimate because it provides lots of skin-on-skin contact," Dr. Taylor says. Even if you can't see him, you can hear his breath in your ear and feel the warmth of his body.

Side by side

Gripe #1: "We have sideways sex when we're both too tired to move. It's not very erotic."
Upgrade: Sleepy sex is so underrated, especially first thing in the a.m. Make the relaxed side-by-side position more exciting but just as effortless with what Julie D., a personal trainer from Lakeville, New York, calls the "sideways split." You lie on your back and he lies on his side perpendicular to you so that your bodies form a T shape, where your torso is the stem of the T. Drape one leg over his shoulder and the other over his calf. "I can control how much stimulation I'm getting by spreading my legs farther [for more] or closing them a bit [for less]," Julie says.

Gripe #2: "It's hard to figure out what to do with all our limbs."

Upgrade: Damn those pesky arms and legs. To get them out of the way, try spooning, suggests Patti Britton, PhD, clinical sexologist and author of *The Art of Sex Coaching*. You both lie on your sides, but your back is to him and he enters you from behind. Since you're facing away from him your limbs don't get so tangled up. "This variation makes it easier for him to touch your breasts and clitoris, and it's still very intimate," Dr. Britton says.

Standing up

Gripe #1: "We're about the same height, so standing-up sex works if I stand on my tiptoes, but then my calves get tired!"

Upgrade: Orgasms are elusive enough without having to maneuver around on your tippy-toes. To double the surface area you stand on and still get the extra few inches you need for the perfect pelvic matchup, break out the highest heels you own—platform boots, wedges, pumps, doesn't matter. Don't have any heels that high? Buy a cheap (but stable) pair for this purpose alone. You never have to wear them out of the house, and he'll get an extra thrill from seeing you in a pair of stilettos—which, for some still-a-mystery-to-us reason, guys seem to find hot.

Gripe #2: "I'm shorter than he is, so he needs to lift me. But then his arms get tired and I feel like he's going to drop me."

Upgrade: Lisa G., a copywriter from Houston, solves that problem by perching her butt on the edge of the desk in her home office (a sturdy table, window sill, or kitchen counter will also work). "It has the spontaneous quality of standing-up sex, without him having to lift me," she says. To make the most of the countertop approach, stick to the very edge of it so your clitoris stays front and center for maximum contact with his penis.

Knocked Up? Knock the Boots!

Those giant boobs aren't the only sexual perks that come with pregnancy. Being in full-on pod mode is like living in a constant state of semiarousal. Really. To nourish the fetus, bloodflow increases by 50 percent, and your blood vessels dilate more quickly and with less stimulation. When the highly sensitive cells around the vaginal opening become engorged with blood, they also become extra-responsive to pressure and vibration, says Trina Read, PhD, a sexologist in Calgary, Alberta. And, she says, when you're pregnant, the uterus tightens more powerfully during orgasm, making those waves of joy even more intense. Here are four of the best ways to have prenatal nookie.

Side by Side
Best for when you need high-intimacy sex.
Tip: Lie facing your partner on your left side to avoid pressure on the vessels taking blood back to the heart, which doesn't hurt the baby but does make you short of breath. Toss your right leg over his hip to give him access. As your midsection gets bigger, he can scoot his body down a fraction so his penis can get under your belly.

Woman on Top
Best for taking pressure off your abdomen. Being upright means you won't feel pinched or squashed, and "it gives you the ability to shift positions and control depth of penetration," says Jennifer Berman, MD, cofounder of the Female Sexual Medicine Center at UCLA.
Tip: Have him support your belly with one hand as you grind away and use his other hand on your clitoris.

Spooning
Best for when you'd rather be sleeping. Because he does most—okay, all—of the work.
Tip: Lie facing away from him on your left side—it will be easier to breathe. Place a pillow or two under your belly for extra support. Try adjusting your angle by leaning forward or back until his penis hits your G-spot.

Edge of the Bed
Best for when the sheer size of your belly makes you feel like you're having the wrong kind of threesome. Because it's like having sex in a Barcalounger.
Tip: You lean back on a pile of regular pillows or a wedge pillow like the Liberator Ramp ($140, www.liberator.com) and bend your knees so your feet rest on the edge of the bed. He kneels or stands in front of you. Try to block out the image of your feet in stirrups.

Postnatal Nookie

YOUR 5-STEP PLAN TO GETTING OUT OF THE NURSERY AND BACK INTO THE BEDROOM.

By T. Edward Nickens

The arrival of a child is a whirling vortex of change. Gone are leisurely Saturday mornings filled with coffee and lingerie piled on the living room floor. A baby demands all: time, energy, attention, space. Despite knowing that, most couples enter a complete state of denial about the impact a baby will have on their physical relationship, according to John Gottman, PhD, and Julie Schwartz Gottman, PhD, authors of *And Baby Makes Three* and founders of the Seattle-based Relationship Research Institute, where they run workshops to help new parents preserve intimacy. "Sexual intimacy is directly related to relationship satisfaction," says Dr. John Gottman, "and research shows that two-thirds of women become unhappy with their relationship within 4 months of the birth of a child." But there are ways to keep the home fires burning. After all, most couples have a baby to bring more love into the family, not less. One solution whose simplicity belies its efficacy: Designate one room in the house as the sex room. Rig it up with a baby monitor and head down the hallway two or three nap times a week. Here are five prescriptions for reinvigorating intimacy once your love bears fruit.

Create a timetable

"Men and women start back on the road to physical connection from very different places," says Carolyn Pirak, director of the Gottmans' intimacy workshops. "For that first 6 months, most women experience a sharp decrease in desire. That's just the way it is."

Ask for foot massages

"Sexual intimacy arises from emotional intimacy," says Dr. John Gottman, "and after a baby's birth, physical intimacy needs to be reheated slowly." Find little ways to reintroduce physical touch, like asking him for a foot massage.

Win the mind game

Relationships are built through a bidding process of small gestures that seek attention. Say your partner is reading the newspaper and murmurs, "Hmm." "Responding positively to a bid for attention is a foundational behavior for successful couples," says Dr. John Gottman.

Mop it up

Once a baby arrives, tell your husband that housework is a sort of Foreplay 2.0. "Our research shows that men who help around the house more often have more and better sex," says Pirak. "The key to the bedroom could be the vacuum cleaner." (Or the iron, or the dishwasher, or, or, or. . . .)

Schedule sex

Just as you had to overhaul your home for the baby, you need to reconfigure your physical relationship with a greater degree of intentionality. One idea: Alternate responsibility for initiating intimacy. "It's like movie night," says Pirak. "Take turns choosing the time and place for sex once a week. It sounds crazy, but it works."

A Better Kind of PlayStation

BRING THIS SEX PILLOW INTO THE BEDROOM AND YOU MIGHT NEVER LEAVE.

By T. Edward Nickens

How does one scratch a little 15-year marital itch without leaving the house? By ordering the Wedge. It's a sex toy, yes, but it's about as nonthreatening a device as you can imagine. There are no batteries required, no need to stress test the wall studs behind your headboard. It's a pillow. But it's a pillow with a purpose, and sleep ain't it.

At first glance, the Wedge looks like something you'd prop your head on to watch TV in bed. It is 14 inches long and 7 inches tall, comes in five colors, and is cut to a precise 27-degree angle. Made of firm, high-density polyurethane foam, the pillow is stain resistant and clad in a velvety, washable microfiber cover.

But the geometry is what makes it a hip rest, not a headrest. That 27-degree angle, say its designers, raises a woman's pelvis just enough to bring man and G-spot consistently together. "Testers started at 45 degrees and worked their way down," explains Frank DeMarco, vice president of product design for Liberator, the manufacturer of the Wedge. "There was a lot of trial and error. But after a lot of sex, they figured it out." They also figured out that this seemingly innocuous hunk of upholstery performed well as the foundation for numerous sexual positions.

You can buy the Wedge as a stand-alone for $85 at large pharmacies and at www.liberator.com, or packaged with the Ramp, a larger pillow that comes in three sizes to "strategically lift" your hips to the appropriate rear-entry altitude, according to the instructions. The pillows have been lauded by physical therapists for people with disabilities; they relieve lower-back pain, according to many users; and they have been profiled positively in that subversive kinky-sex journal *Arthritis Today*.

Is the sex that much better when going Wedgey? In short, yes. There are more possibilities afforded by a firm 27-degree angle than you would have ever imagined—and you'll probably find yourself thinking about geometry more than anytime since 9th-grade math. The trick, then, is just finding a secret hiding spot for it.

The Best Feel-Young Sex Games

ADD A LITTLE FUN TO YOUR USUAL ROUTINE.

Most sex games for couples are hokier than a Love Boat episode, and every box we found that had the words "great for parties" scrawled across it involved ridiculous dares ("Show a stranger your thong!") that made us cringe. But these six, we're happy to say, are fun, creative, and guaranteed to lead to an inspired night of naked coed wrestling.

1. *Strut Your Stuff*
Okay, so this isn't actually a game, but it'll definitely make you want to play. The Striptease Kit in a Box packs pasties, body glitter, a sheer scarf, and illustrated instructions on how to give your partner a variety of old-school stripteases. We doubt he'll put on the pasties, but there's absolutely no reason why he can't strip for you too. $25, www.goodvibes.com

2. *Get into Bonding (Emotional, That Is)*
If you're looking for something softer, slower, and more romantic and don't mind a little "cosmic energy" talk, the Tantric Lovers game by sex educator Ava Cadell is perfect for getting your om on. Bonus prize: Practicing tantra can lead to greater intimacy and prolonged orgasms. $30, www.drugstore.com

3. *Try Some Sexperimentation*
Way wilder than strip poker, Nookii takes card playing to a whole new level. You simply take turns picking a card and following the extremely racy, step-by-step instructions. It's a brilliant way to orchestrate foreplay. $40, www.mypleasure.com

4. *Roll—er, Shake of the Dice*
Victoria's Secret Play with Me massage oil contains snake eyes printed with dicey instructions. Give the bottle a shake, and follow the rules to foreplay. $15 for 5 ounces, www.victoriassecret.com

5. *Ante Up, Boys*
Agent Provocateur Strip Poker recalls a more genteel time of party-rotica, when guests enjoyed "cerebral games of logic, memory . . . and patience." AP's kit includes chips, playing cards, and a book about groping strangers who get busy at a London party. $30, www.mypleasure.com

6. *Harness the Tension*
The game Seduction has three levels: desire, arousal, and release. You choose the activities—blindfolding, nibbling, etc.—that move you through the different levels, while building sexual tension and intensity. $20, www.funlovinggames.com

Chapter Six

Trim, Tone, and Gravity-Proof Your Curves

EVERYTHING YOU NEED TO KNOW ABOUT SCULPTING
YOUR BACKSIDE, MINIMIZING CELLULITE,
SLIMMING YOUR LEGS, AND CARING FOR YOUR PAIR

INVESTMENT: 3 WEEKS
AGE ERASED: 3 YEARS

Introduction

Introduction

T housands of years ago, when our female ancestors roamed forests and savannas, it made sense to have an extra helping of heft around the hips and a bit of bounce in the butt. During droughts, famines, and long winters, women burned additional fat to fuel both pregnancy and lactation. (Childbearing also provided a boon to our breasts' size, though they weren't getting much support back then—the brassiere as we know it only began to emerge in the last few hundred years.) As a result, women with more lower-body fat tended to survive harsh conditions and consequently passed on their genes to their children, whereas women with more slender proportions did not. So congratulations, kid: You're a survivor.

Your great-great-great-great-great-grandmother's ability to carry around a week's supply of calories under her loincloth, however, isn't doing you any favors today; in America, food is hardly scarce and body fat is plentiful. And upstairs, bras have ultimately helped transform our thinking about breasts, elevating expectations to unnatural levels even though they're an aspect of our anatomies that's largely outside our control (without surgery, that is). But there's no need to despair. The secret to thinner thighs, for one, is to stop obsessing about them and start using them. Same thinking applies to your butt. According to scientists at the American Council on Exercise—who apparently get a kick out of sticking electrodes on people's bums—squatting, lunging, and lifting your legs behind you are the most effective ways to perfect your rear view. In other words, you can buy all the expensive jeans you like, but a simple, easy-to-use plan that concentrates on your lower-body muscles is the most effective way to kick your ancestor's gift to the curb.

The lessons in this chapter will reveal the best ways to sculpt every inch of your lower body—even those particularly troublesome spots like your inner thighs—and regain confidence in your cleavage. It's time to get started!

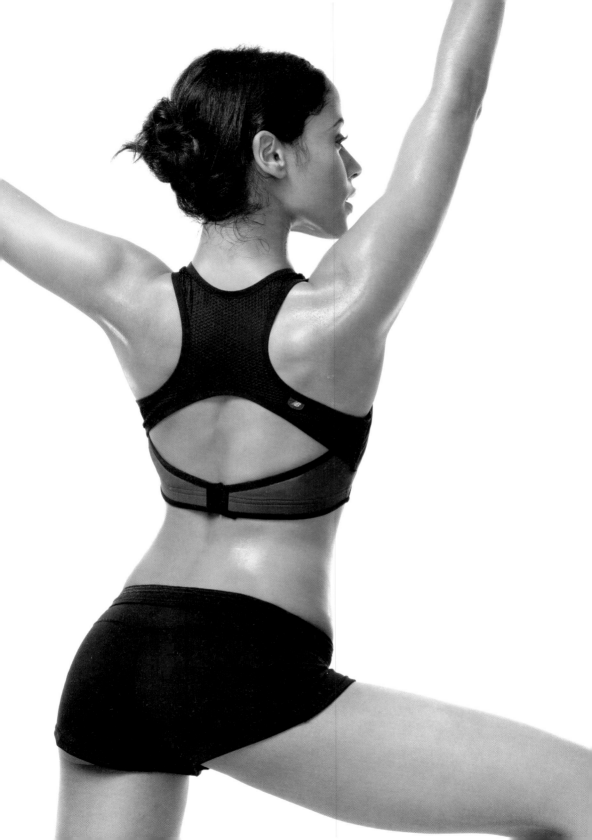

A Guide to Your B-Side

ALL YOU NEED TO KNOW ABOUT THE MUSCLES THAT SURROUND YOUR BUM.

By Yelena Moroz

You want your butt to have more perk than a sorority pledge on a latte bender, but no matter how many glute moves you do, your junk still jiggles. Working the following muscles—what physiologists call the posterior chain—is the only way to a ripple-free rear end.

Erector Spinae

What they are: The cablelike muscles that line your spine and extend to the base of your skull
What they do: Support your spine when you bend and twist
What it means for your b-side: Weak erector spinae can lead to poor posture—and when you slouch, your lower back and upper bum become indistinguishable. Not hot.

Glutes

What they are: The gluteus maximus is the body's largest muscle. Beneath it are the medius and minimus—a pair of deeper-set, fan-shaped muscles that attaches to the side of each hip.
What they do: The maximus generates the power to sit, stand, or run, while the smaller two keep you from tipping to the left or right.
What it means for your b-side: Working all three parts of your glutes adds roundness and ensures that your cheeks are wider near the top and narrower at the, er, bottom.

Hamstrings

What they are: Three muscles that run diagonally across the back of your leg, from the inside of your sit bone to the outside of your knee
What they do: Stabilize the hip and knee joints so you can bend over and kick without getting injured or landing on your face
What it means for your b-side: You need strong hamstrings for deadlifting—the absolute best exercise for your bum because it works not only the butt itself, but also the prone-to-droop area beneath your cheeks. (More on that in a few.)

Calves

What they are: The muscles that run down your lower leg. They're thicker near the knee and get thinner as they approach the Achilles tendon.
What they do: These are the muscles involved in lifting your heels and flexing your knees, which means they're crucial for explosive power.
What it means for your b-side: When you lean forward, you put pressure on your delicate knees. Strong calves keep you upright and stable.

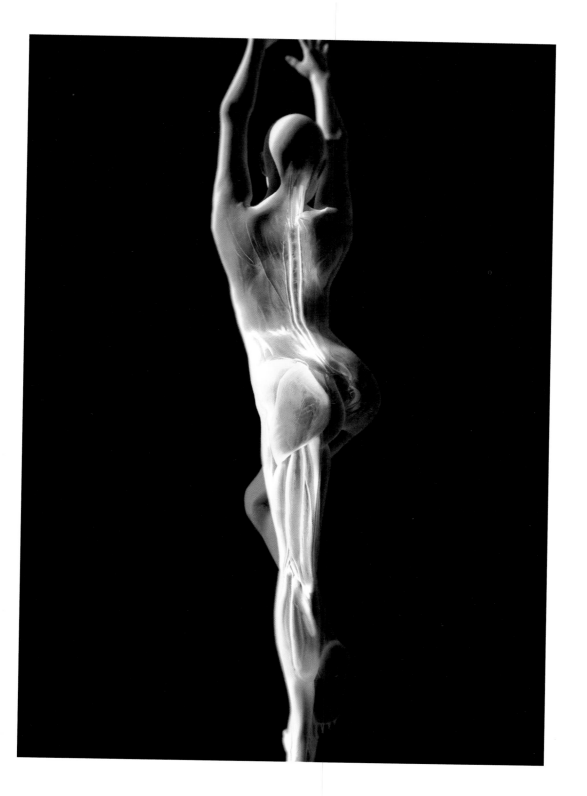

The A**-Kicking Workout

GET A REAR THAT WILL TURN HEADS.

By Mike Mejia, CSCS

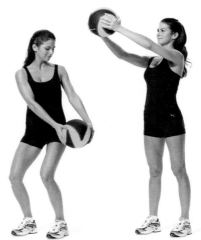

*A*s we've just established, the key to a beauteous gluteus is a workout that targets your back, calves, and hamstrings. When you strengthen this supporting cast— and you can always make it stronger—your butt looks better and can work even harder. Stick with our program and you'll start seeing results after just 10 workouts—at which point, you may want to consider investing in one of those dressing room–style mirrors that lets you check out that fine-looking specimen you've created. After all, admiring your own ass 24-7 can be a pain in the neck.

PHASE ONE:
Support Your Assets

Spend 2 to 4 weeks building the supporting muscles in your back, calves, glutes, and hams to stay injury free in Phase 2—and get more bang for your butt.

Perform three sets of 12 to 15 reps, resting for up to 60 seconds between sets, 2 or 3 nonconsecutive days a week.

Reverse Woodchop
Works Calves, Glutes (Gluteus Maximus, Medius, Minimus), Hamstrings

Grab a 4- to 8-pound medicine ball and stand with your feet shoulder-width apart. Hold the ball with both hands outside your left hip, then perform a half squat (so your legs lower by 45 degrees). Keeping your chest up and arms straight, stand up as you "chop" the ball up and across your body until it's above your right shoulder. Pause, then lower the ball back to your left knee. Complete all reps before repeating on the other side. That's 1 set.

Butt-kicker: Rather than using your arms, brace your core and push up with your legs as you drive the ball upward.

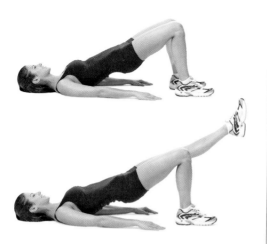

Walking Supine Bridge

Works Glutes, Hamstrings

Lie on your back with your knees bent and your feet flat on the floor. Lift your hips until your body forms a straight line from your knees to your shoulders. Slowly extend your left leg until it's in line with the rest of your body. Pause, then lower it and repeat with your right. That's 1 rep. Don't drop your hips until you've completed all reps.

Butt-kicker: Pressing through your heels will isolate and maximize the involvement of your glutes and hamstrings.

Reverse Hyperextension

Works Erector Spinae, Gluteus Maximus, Hamstrings

Lie facedown on an exercise bench so your head, chest, torso, and hips are on the bench but your legs are mostly hanging off. Wrap your arms around the bench and brace your abs. Lower your legs as far as possible, then, keeping your legs straight and together, lift them until they're just past parallel to the floor. Pause, then lower and repeat.

Butt-kicker: Place the entire bench on a step or other stable platform to increase your range of motion in the targeted muscles.

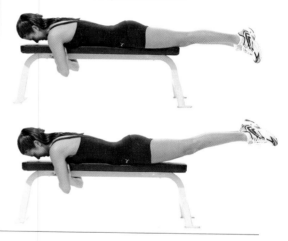

Hydrant Extension

Works Glutes

Get on all fours with your knees directly beneath your hips and your hands under your shoulders. Keeping your knee bent, lift your left leg up and out to the side as high as possible. Next, extend your leg straight back so it's in line with your torso. Pause, then bring it back to the starting position. Repeat with your right leg. That's 1 rep.

Butt-kicker: Keep your lower back as still as possible throughout the exercise.

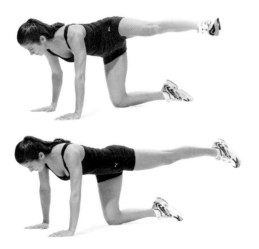

PHASE TWO:
Sculpt a Superior Posterior | Workout 1

Phase 1 has prepped you to shape your butt as quickly as possible. For the next 4 weeks, 3 nonconsecutive days a week, alternate between Workout 1 and Workout 2 (you'll do one of the workouts twice each week). Do three sets of 10 to 12 reps of each exercise, resting for up to 60 seconds between sets.

1 ¼ Barbell Squat

Works Erector Spinae, Gluteus Maximus, Hamstrings, Quads

Place a barbell across your upper back and stand with your feet hip-width apart. Lower your hips until your thighs are parallel to the floor. Push back up a quarter of the way, then pause before going back down to parallel.

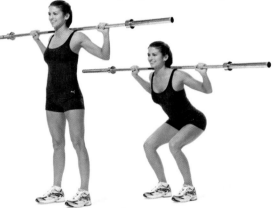

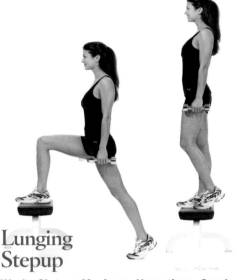

Pause again, then return to start. That's 1 rep.
Butt-kicker: Do this move first. It's a killer: If you wait until the end of your workout, you'll be too burnt to maintain good form.

Lunging Stepup

Works Gluteus Maximus, Hamstings, Quads

Grab a pair of 5- to 10-pound dumbbells and stand 2 to 3 feet from an exercise bench. Place your right foot on the bench. Drive your right heel down and pull your left leg up. Allow only your left toes to touch the bench. Lower your left leg first and then your right. Repeat, lunging up with your left leg. That's 1 rep.

Modified Glute-Ham Raise

Works Calves, Erector Spinae, Gluteus Maximus, Hamstrings

Wrap a towel around the middle of a loaded barbell and place a mat under it. Kneel with your back to the bar and your ankles anchored beneath it. Keeping your hands at your sides as you start, slowly lower your torso. Use your arms to catch yourself when your legs give out. Return to start by pushing up with your arms and raising your torso until you're kneeling again.

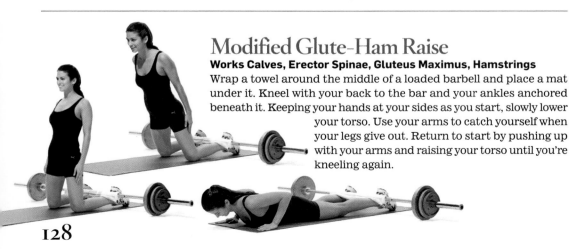

Workout 2
Romanian Deadlift
Works Erector Spinae, Gluteus Maximus, Hamstrings

Grab a barbell with an overhand grip (add weight plates once you can do all sets of all reps with perfect form), hands shoulder-width apart, and stand with your feet hip-width apart and knees slightly bent. Hold the barbell with straight arms in front of your thighs. Without rounding your back or changing the bend in your knees, lean forward from your waist while lowering the bar until your torso is parallel to the floor. Pause, then rise to start.

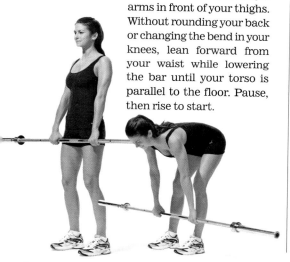

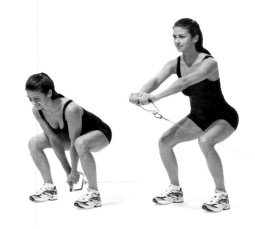

Cable Pull-Through
Works Glutes, Hamstrings, Quads

Stand about 2 feet from a pulley station set at a very light weight (increase it only once you've nailed the form), with the cable on the setting closest to the floor. With your back to the station, position your feet shoulder-width apart, then bend from your hips as you squat until your thighs are nearly parallel to the floor. Reach back through your legs and grab the handle. Keeping your head up, drive your heels into the floor and straighten your legs to standing. Pause, then lower the weight and repeat.

Offset Squat
Works Glutes, Hamstrings

Grab a 5- to 8-pound dumbbell in your right hand, hold it at your right side, and lift your right foot so you're balancing on your left. Raise your right arm straight out in front of you until it's at shoulder level and squat down until your thigh is as close to parallel to the floor as possible. Pause for a second and then push back up to start.
Butt-kicker: Keep the dumbbell as far from your body as you can throughout the squat to work your glutes harder.

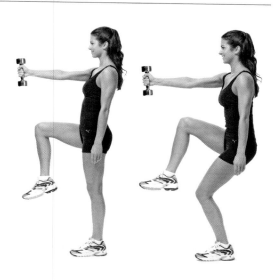

Burn More Fat!

TIGHTEN YOUR BUTT BY ADDING THESE SMALL BUT POWERFUL CHANGES TO YOUR CARDIO WORKOUT.

By Dimitry McDowell

Familiarity might be comfortable, but it's not always effective—certainly not when it comes to your workout. Doing the same thing over and over lulls your muscles into an I-can-do-this tedium and lessens your calorie burn. The good news: You don't need to ditch your current workout to see more results. You just need to learn how to rev it up. Follow these tips from some of the top trainers around the country for an ultraefficient workout that zaps more calories and burns more fat.

The Treadmill
YOUR COMFORT ZONE

Flipping channels on the tube, you lope along, either running or walking, at the same ho-hum speed you were at yesterday. And the day before. And the day before that. Yet beneath your feet is a machine with endless potential.

BLAST MORE FAT
Don't Bounce.

You're not in an allergy-drug ad, running through fields of blossoming flowers. So stop bounding around like you don't know what you're doing. Keep your movement forward, not up and down, says Beverly Hills, California-based personal trainer Gunnar Peterson. "Anything vertical is wasted energy: It doesn't help you." By focusing on what's ahead, you'll go faster and burn more calories in a shorter period of time.

Squeeze Your Glutes.

"Do it as you push off your toes," says Jan Griscom, a personal trainer at New York City's Chelsea Piers. By focusing on your backside, you'll contract—and tone—the muscle (and make it, not the fat surrounding it, the star attraction). And the more muscle you have, the more calories you'll need to maintain it—and the more fat you'll burn.

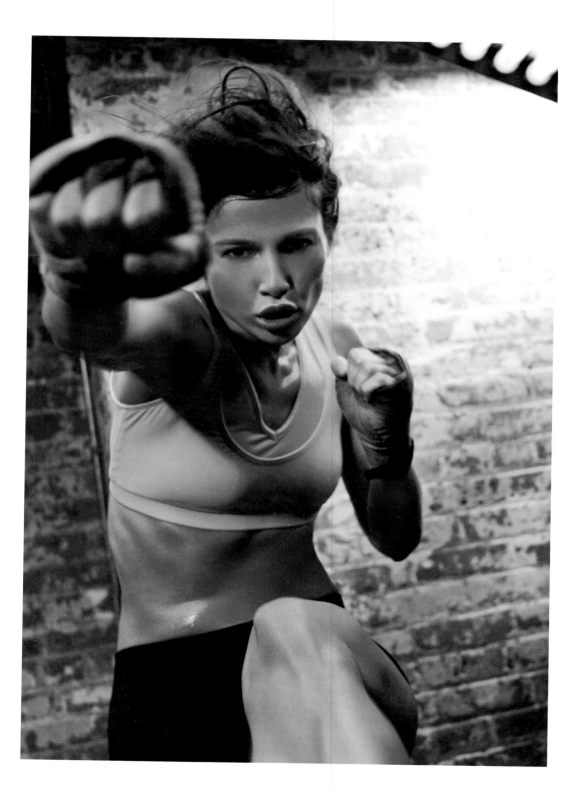

Challenge Your Muscles.

At the end of a workout, slow your speed to $2\frac{1}{2}$ to $3\frac{1}{2}$ miles per hour. Skip for 30 seconds, walk for 30; walk backward for 30, forward for 30; stand sideways and shuffle with your right foot leading for 30 seconds, walk for 30, and repeat with left foot leading. "You'll call into action other muscles that don't work while going forward," Peterson says. "Which means they'll be surprised"—as will the person on the treadmill next to you—"and add to the calorie burn."

Elliptical Trainer

YOUR COMFORT ZONE

Gliding along at a medium pace, your legs are on autopilot. And, if the machine has arms, your upper body is too. Yet few cardio machines can help you achieve such a full-body workout.

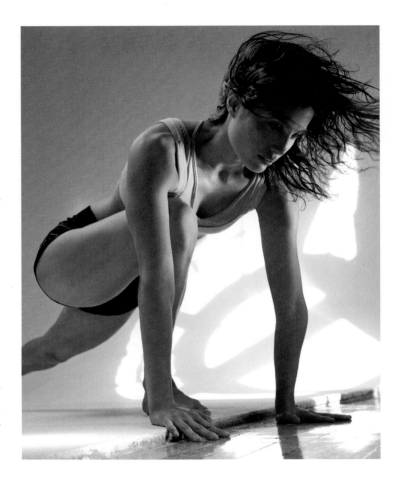

BLAST MORE FAT
Never Stop Working.

To maximize fat burning, don't let the machine's gliding momentum dictate your pace. Your leg muscles should push the pedals around. If there are rails, lightly rest your hands on them—but no white-knuckling, since you may end up supporting your body weight that way.

Use Intervals.

During every third song on your MP3 player or every commercial break, ramp up the intensity and go as hard as you can. "A steady pace at a sustainable speed burns calories consistently, but intervals blast up the count," Peterson says. Back off after 2 or 3 minutes.

Use Your Whole Body.

Every other minute, concentrate on strengthening your arms or core—you'll recruit more muscles and incinerate more fat. For example, if you're on a full-body machine, consciously engage your arms; push and pull with the same intensity as you're using for your legs. If it's a lower-body machine, put your arms in an athletic position—elbows bent, upper arms close to your ribs—to strengthen your core.

Stairclimber

YOUR COMFORT ZONE

You're bent forward at the hips, elbows locked, hands on the rails to ease your load on your beloved hills program, where you've been slogging away at level 7 since Christmas.

BLAST MORE FAT
Stand Up Straight.

Pretend you're squeezing a balloon between your shoulder blades, says Brooke Siler, author of *The Ultimate Pilates Body Challenge*. Use the rails for balance only, not support. Picture-perfect posture forces your core and back muscles to contract—great for toning. And engaging more muscles means burning more fat.

Mix up the depth of your climbing.

In doing so, you'll surprise your muscles, which leads to an increased calorie burn. If you're a short climber, add 1 minute of long, slow steps every 5 minutes. "Challenge your leg muscles in a way that they're not used to being challenged," Peterson says. If you usually go long and slow, pick up the pace and shorten the step to about 6 inches to make your muscles react and therefore adapt—that's where the change comes in.

Tuck your glutes under your hips.

And make sure your feet are flat on the pedals. If you originate all movement in your core, not your legs, it will (a) hurt like a bitch and (b) work new muscles hard (see [a]), giving you—you guessed it—a more intense burn.

Spinning Class
YOUR COMFORT ZONE

Forget sweating—you haven't even started glistening yet. And you're about to start the cooldown. What was that about indoor cycling being such a good workout?

BLAST MORE FAT
Crank it up.

God created the resistance knob for a heavenly reason. Use it, especially on hills, to whittle your thighs to swimsuit-worthy slimness. Dixie Douville, RN, a master spinning instructor in Flanders, New Jersey, advises a pace of 60 to 80 revolutions per minute (rpm) on hills. Find yours by counting how many times one foot goes around in 15 seconds and multiplying by four.

A 10-Minute, Butt-Blasting Routine

THE ABSOLUTE BEST TONING EXERCISES, BASED ON NEW RESEARCH

Research from the University of North Carolina reveals that the exercises below activate muscles up to 30 percent more than traditional moves. Complete 8 to 12 repetitions of each exercise on each side, and do the entire routine twice through, three times a week on nonconsecutive days (add in regular cardio for or five times a week). For quicker results, do 3 sets of 10 to 15 reps every other day. Researchers say you'll start noticing a firmer, shapelier rear in as little as 2 to 4 weeks.

Side Leg Lifts
Lie on your right side with your legs stacked, right arm bent and right hand supporting your head, left hand resting on the floor in front of your chest for balance. Raise your left leg about 2 feet, keeping your foot flexed and squeezing your butt. Pause, then slowly lower. Complete all reps, then switch sides. To make it more difficult, once your top leg is lifted, raise your bottom leg to meet it, pause, and then lower one leg at a time.

Banded Shuffle
Stand with your feet a few inches apart with an elastic band (www.spriproducts.com) tied in a taut loop around your shins, hands extended to the front at shoulder level. Step about 3 feet to your right, then bend your knees and sit back until your thighs are almost parallel to the floor, keeping your knees behind your toes. Staying low, step with your left foot to follow. Take two more shuffle steps to your right, then switch directions and repeat. To make it more difficult, bend your knees only 45 degrees and step out just slightly more than hip-width.

Balancing Squat
Balance on your right foot with your left knee bent and your foot lifted a few inches off the floor in front of you. Keeping your back straight, slowly sit back into your right leg, bending your right knee about 45 degrees. Pause, then press into your right heel to stand up. Complete all reps, then switch sides. To make it more difficult, complete the move while holding a dumbbell in each hand.

Single Leg Deadlift
Balance on your right foot, keeping your knee soft and your hands on your hips, and lift your left leg behind you. With your abs tight and your back straight, hinge forward from the hips, lowering your left hand toward your right foot. Pull through your right leg to return to standing. Complete reps on your right leg; switch sides. To increase difficulty, reach both hands to the floor, holding a dumbbell in each hand.

And keep it there.
On flat terrain, aim for 80 to 110 rpm. That way, you'll use your muscles, not the momentum of the weighted front wheel, to power the bike. Go faster and you risk momentum taking over. "If you're going above 110, you need to increase resistance" until you're back in the 80 to 110 range, Douville says. "That makes the workout much harder and the calorie burn more significant than just pedaling faster."

Sit when you climb.
This increases your muscular endurance and incinerates more fat. When you stand, you can use your whole leg for leverage and your body weight for momentum; sitting means you have to push more weight around with less help. "Unless you increase the resistance significantly, standing is basically bailing out of a climb," Douville says.

Running
YOUR COMFORT ZONE
You pass the yellow house 7 minutes into your run, the coffee shop 10 minutes later. Thirteen minutes after that, you're home—where you take off your shoes so you can find them tomorrow to do the exact same route.

BLAST MORE FAT
Run tall.
"Doing that immediately stops you from slouching and forces your arms to go front to back, not side to side," says Greg McMillan, a personal trainer and running coach in Austin, Texas. "Your hips stay tucked under, your butt doesn't stick out, and as a result, your stride is much more effective: You go farther with less energy expended." The result? You can suddenly run longer— and burn more calories.

Mix it up.
Run your regular route in the opposite direction so your body doesn't know when to expect the hills. Better yet: Change your speed. "People shuffle when they run at the same pace all the time," McMillan says. "The body gets very efficient and doesn't have to work." If you typically run for 30 minutes, try this 3-day routine: Day 1,

Rump Shakers
AMP UP YOUR CARDIO WORKOUT WITH THESE BUTT-TARGETING STRATEGIES.

Researchers at the Madonna Rehabilitation Hospital in Lincoln, Nebraska, recently set out to learn which machines kick your ass the hardest. Here's how their findings shake out, as well as a few glute-blasting pointers from Lindsay Dunlap, a personal trainer at the Sports Club/LA in New York City.

THE MACHINE	PERCENTAGE OF GLUTEUS MAXIMUS ACTIVATED
Treadmill (jogging)	48.9
Elliptical	32.6
Treadmill (walking)	24.3
Stairclimber	24.0
Recumbent Bike	6.0

Jogging
Bum Spanker: Make sure your heels, not the balls of your feet, hit the ground first.

Elliptical
Bum Spanker: Ease your hips back so your butt sticks out a bit, and push down with your heels as much as possible.

Walking
Bum Spanker: On a treadmill, increase the incline. On the road, try walking sideways: This will work your bum from a different angle as you pull your leg away from your body.

Stairclimbing
Bum Spanker: Lean forward slightly at the waist and take larger steps, as though you're climbing two at a time. Let go of the rails, forcing your glutes to take the brunt of the stabilization duties.

Biking
Bum Spanker: Ditch the recumbent ride for an upright one. Then sit a little farther back on the seat and focus on pushing the pedals down forcefully.

go slower than your usual pace, but run for 40 minutes. Day 2, speed it up a notch, but run for only 20 minutes. Day 3, throw in some intervals: Run fast for 1 minute, easy for 2, and repeat 6 to 10 times. "Not only does that make the workout go by fast," McMillan says, "but it also burns more calories."

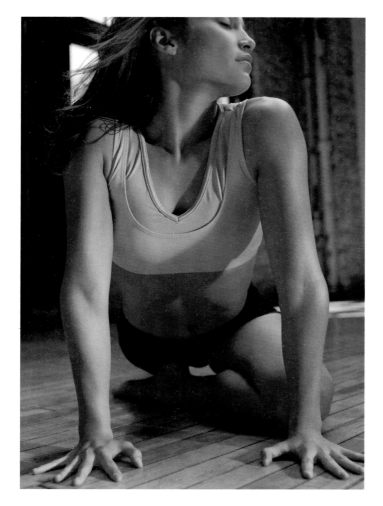

Weight Training

YOUR COMFORT ZONE

Intimidated by heavy metal, you stick to the light stuff—nothing more than 10 pounds, please—then saunter over to the watercooler for a drink. Your rest period there lasts more than a few minutes.

BLAST MORE FAT

Pop some veins.

Forget vanity. The weight you're hoisting should leave you red-faced and weak. "By the last rep, you should feel as though you have to put the weight down," says Brad Jordan, a personal trainer in Dayton, Ohio. "Three sets are plenty." Each day you lift, change it up. On one day, choose a weight you can lift for 8 to 12 reps; the next session, go with a lighter weight and lift 12 to 15 reps; on the last session, increase the load and lift only 6 to 8 reps. It will build more muscle, which (all together now) burns more fat, and it won't make you huge.

Drill it in.

At the end of a workout, slim down your legs, bump up your heart rate, and build speed by doing drills. For 15 seconds, do knee pulls: Lift one knee high until your quads are parallel to the ground, then alternate with the other knee in rapid succession. Jog for 1 minute. Do 15 seconds of butt kicks: Try to hit your glutes with your heel. Jog for 1 minute. Finally, do grapevine (moving sideways, step your left foot over your right foot, then your left foot behind your right foot). Do 15 seconds leading with one foot, then 15 seconds with the other. Jog for 1 minute, then cool down. As your strength increases, add sets.

Minimize downtime.

Give yourself 1 minute of rest between sets for maximum burn. You'll keep your heart rate elevated and your metabolism juiced, both calorie-burning boosts.

Recruit all your muscles.

To use as many muscles as possible, stand instead of sitting. Or, even better, stand on a Bosu or balance board. Don't let machines be an excuse to rest, Griscom says. For example, on the chest press machine, don't let your back touch the seat (or drop the seat all the way down). Get into a squatting position and do the reps from there.

Jump Your Way into Sleeker Stems

TONE TROUBLE SPOTS WITH A LOWER–BODY ROUTINE THAT MAKES YOU LEAVE THE GROUND.

By Dimity McDowell

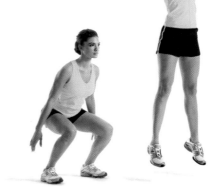

*T*he key to hotter legs, it seems, is to spend more time in the air. A 2007 study found that dancers who did plyometric exercises (moves that require leaping, jumping, or skipping) twice a week for 6 weeks increased their strength by 37 percent and their jump height by 8.3 percent. "Plyometrics are a good alternative to strength training on machines," says Patricia Fehling, PhD, the study's coauthor and chairperson of exercise science at Skidmore College in Saratoga Springs, New York. "The change in movement from static [say, the bottom of a squat] to dynamic [exploding into the air] shocks your muscles, so you see results quickly." This workout burns calories and builds lean muscle fast. For 2 weeks, do it once a week, then increase to twice a week. Start with one set of 10 reps of each exercise, then add one set of each exercise weekly until you reach the max: three sets of 10 reps twice a week. Finish each session with the two kink-busting stretches.

Squat Jumps
Works Glutes, Hamstrings, Quads, Calves
Stand with your feet shoulder-width apart, your arms hanging at your sides. Squat down until your knees are bent at about 90 degrees. Immediately swing your arms overhead and jump upward as high as you can. As you land, gently bend your knees and sink back down into the squat position. That's 1 rep. Do 10.
Trainer tip: Swinging your arms will give you momentum so you can catch more air.

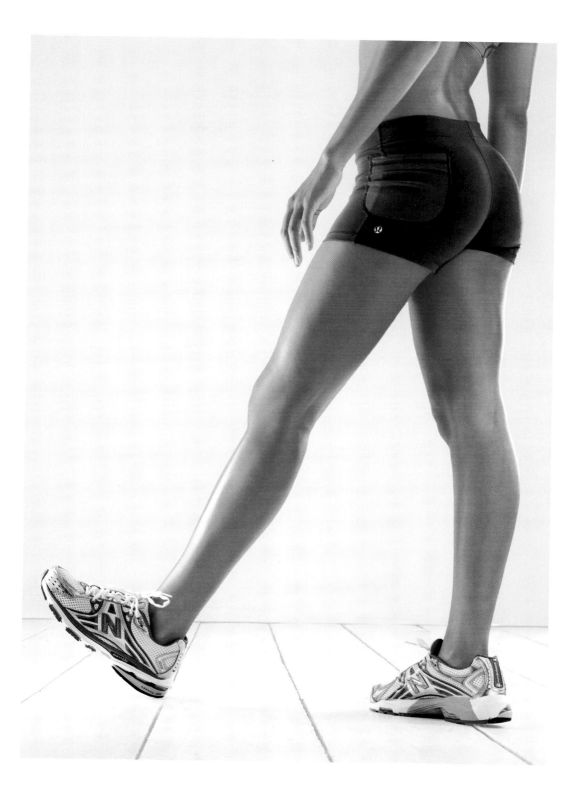

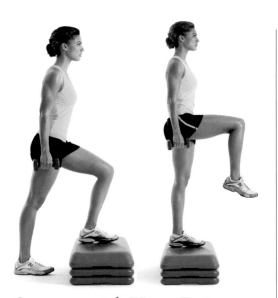

Stepups with Knee Raise

Works Abs, Hip Flexors, Glutes, Hamstrings, Quads

Place a 12- to 24-inch-high step in front of you. Step up with your left foot, bringing your right leg forward and up and bending your knee until your thigh is parallel to the floor. Lower your right leg back to the starting position, then the left. Repeat with the other leg. That's 1 rep; do 10.

Trainer tip: For a tougher challenge, hold 5- to 10-pound dumbbells.

Wood Chopper

Works Shoulders, Abs, Glutes, Hamstrings, Quads

Grab an 8- to 10-pound dumbbell with both hands and stand with your feet shoulder-width apart. Let the dumbbell hang naturally in front of your thighs. Squat down until your knees are bent at about 90 degrees. Keeping your elbows slightly bent, brace your abs and press up to standing, swinging the dumbbell up until it's directly overhead. Lower the dumbbell back toward the floor. That's 1 rep; do 10.

Trainer tip: Keep your movement controlled to work the most muscle.

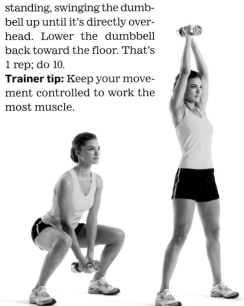

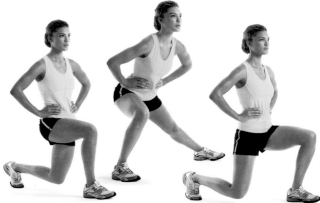

Clock Lunge

Works Glutes, Hamstrings, Quads, Inner and Outer Thighs

With your hands on your hips, lunge forward with your right foot, sinking down until your right knee is bent to 90 degrees. Return to standing. Take a big step to the right and lunge again. Step back to center. Lunge back with your right leg. That's 1 rep. Do 10, then repeat with your left leg.

Trainer tip: Keep your neck in line with your spine throughout the move.

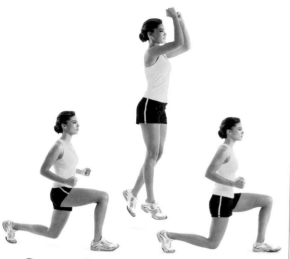

Lunge Jumps
Works Hip Flexors, Glutes, Legs

Stand with your feet together and your elbows bent to 90 degrees. Lunge forward with your right foot. Jump straight up as you thrust your arms forward, your elbows still bent. Switch legs in midair, like a scissor, and land in a lunge with your left leg forward. Repeat, switching legs again. That's 1 rep; do 10.

Trainer tip: Try to land as softly as possible.

Inchworm Stretch
For Lower Back, Hamstrings

Standing with your feet hip-distance apart, slowly bend at the waist, keeping your legs as straight as possible, until your hands touch the floor about 8 to 12 inches from your feet. Walk your hands out to the pushup position, then walk your feet in toward your hands. Work up to two sets of 8 reps.

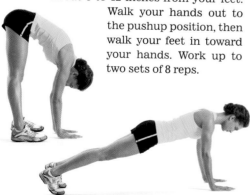

Figure 4 Stretch
For Hip Flexors, Glutes

Starting out on all fours, cross your left leg under your body so you are almost resting on your left hip. Extend your right leg directly behind you. Lower your upper body over your left leg, placing your forearms on the ground in front of you. Hold for 30 seconds, then switch sides.

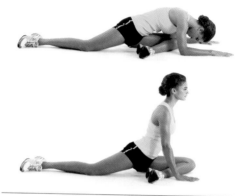

Power Skips
Works Hip Flexors, Glutes, Quads, Calves

Skip as high as you possibly can by raising your right knee to hip height and simultaneously extending your left arm straight overhead. Land, and then repeat with your opposite arm and leg. That's 1 rep; do 10.

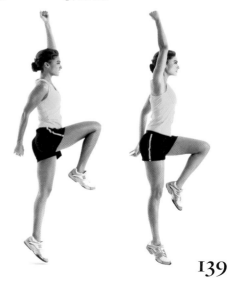

139

The Cellulite Solution

HOW TO DISGUISE IT—AND FIGHT IT.

By Selene Yeager

Your nemesis, cellulite, doesn't discriminate. It can show up on girls in their teens—or younger. That's because, despite what you've heard about cellulite being some mysterious condition linked to "trapped toxins" or poor circulation, cellulite is simply old-fashioned fat. It just looks different because of how it's arranged.

Everyone has strands of connective tissue that separate fat cells into compartments and connect fat to skin. In women, these fibers form a honeycomb, so any increase in fat tends to bulge out like stuffing in a mattress. You see less cellulite in men because their fibers run horizontally, forming a crisscross pattern that prevents bulging or dimpling.

Though cellulite can pop up any time, it is true that cellulite does seem to appear out of nowhere and get worse with age. That's because our tissues change. Those strands of connective tissue thicken with age, and our skin gets thinner, making cellulite more noticeable. More importantly, we gain fat with age. The average woman loses 5 pounds of muscle and replaces it with about 15 pounds of fat in every decade of her adult life, says Wayne Westcott, PhD, fitness research director at the South Shore YMCA in Quincy, Massachusetts.

"Because fat is exceptionally soft, it doesn't keep our skin taut like muscle does. It also takes up more space, so it bulges out," he explains.

Before you're duped by an infomercial, though, there are no proven permanent cures for cellulite, only temporary treatments. Even liposuction can't remove it. But adding more muscle tone to your legs and butt will make the skin look firmer. Try a routine that focuses on low weight and high repetition, says Robert Weiss, MD, associate professor of dermatology at Johns Hopkins University medical school in Baltimore. "The more you build muscle, and stretch and loosen the fibrous bands that squeeze the fat, the less puckery your cellulite will look," he says.

Dr. Westcott agrees. With the right exercise plan, you can reduce your cellulite and make your lower body look smoother and firmer, he says. The trick is to work all your lower-body muscles from every angle, reducing the underlying fat stores and replacing lost muscle tissue to give the area a taut, toned appearance throughout.

Perform one set of 10 to 15 repetitions of the following exercises 3 days a week. Lift slowly, counting 2 seconds to lift and 4 seconds to lower. Before starting, warm up thoroughly with walking, stationary cycling, or light calisthenics.

Side to Side
Works Quadriceps, Abductors, Adductors, Hamstrings, Glutes
Equipment: Dumbbells
You can make this basic exercise easier by doing

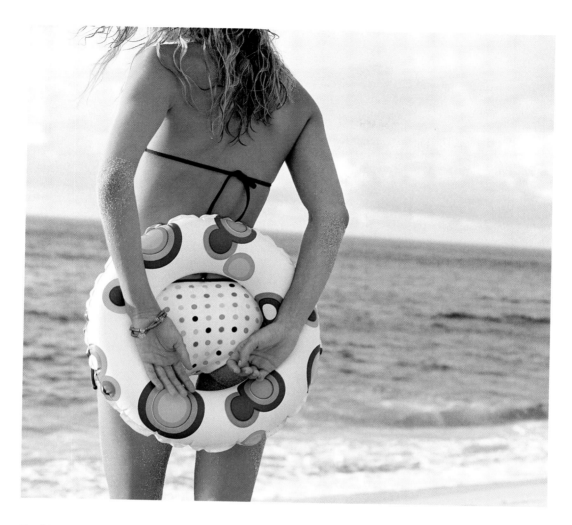

it without any weights. Just keep your hands on your hips. To make it more difficult, hold the dumbbells up at your shoulders while performing the exercise.

Step 1. Stand with your legs about shoulder-width apart, your toes pointed outward at an angle of 45 degrees, and your back flat and straight. Hold a dumbbell in each hand and rest them at your hips.

Step 2. Take a giant step to the left and bend your left knee until your thigh is parallel to the floor, keeping your right leg extended. Do not allow your left knee to jut over your toes or your butt to dip below your knee. Pause, then return to the starting position and repeat the motion to the right side without resting.

All-Fours Kickback

Works Glutes

Equipment: Ankle weights

When doing this exercise, remember not to arch or hunch your back. This will prevent you from putting stress on your back. You can make the exercise easier by doing it without ankle weights. If you don't have ankle weights, do the exercise with a light dumbbell held behind the knee in the crook of your working leg.

Step 1. Wearing ankle weights, get down on your forearms and knees (similar to the all-fours position, but bend your arms and support your weight on your forearms instead of your hands). Keep your back straight and your head in line with your back so that your eyes are looking down.

Step 2. Keeping your back straight and your leg bent, slowly swing your right leg back and lift your right foot toward the ceiling until your thigh is parallel to the ground. Your foot should remain flexed throughout the exercise. Hold for 1 second, then return to the starting position. Do one set with your right leg, then switch to your left.

Lying Inner-Leg Lift
Works Inner Thighs
Equipment: Ankle weights

By working these muscles, you can create a strong, lean line down the insides of your leg. While you're doing this exercise, keep your upper body stationary; resist the urge to sway back and forth as you lift and lower. (You might also want to do the move without weights in the beginning to learn the motion.)

Step 1. Wearing ankle weights, lie on your left side, resting your head on your upper arm, and place your right hand on the floor in front of your chest for support. Bend the knee of your top leg, placing the foot of that leg in front of your other knee. Your bottom leg should be fully extended.

Step 2. Slowly raise your bottom leg as high as is comfortably possible. Hold for 1 second, then slowly lower. Do one set with your left leg, then switch and repeat with your right.

Squat and Side Lift
Works Glutes, Hamstrings, Quads, Hip Flexors, Abductors
Equipment: Ankle weights

Wearing ankle weights, stand with your feet shoulder-width apart, your hands on your hips, your elbows out to the sides, and your toes slightly pointed outward. Remember to keep your head straight and your eyes facing forward. If you want to push yourself a bit, hold a light dumbbell in each hand as you do the moves.

Step 1. Slowly bend at the knees and squat back as though moving your butt down toward an imaginary chair. Keep your back flat, and don't allow your knees to jut over your toes. Stop when your thighs are just about parallel to the floor; don't go any lower.

Step 2. Pause, then straighten your legs, lifting your left leg off the floor and out to the side as you stand. Pause again, then return to the starting position. Repeat, lifting your right leg to the side this time. Alternate legs throughout the exercise.

V-Leg Pull
Works Outer Thighs
Equipment: An exercise band

The outer thighs are a problem area for many women. Toning these muscles will not only help with cellulite, but will also make you stronger and more stable.

When going through these moves, keep your back flat on the floor; do not arch your lower back or twist your torso. If balance is a problem, lie next to a chair and hold on to one of its legs for support.

Step 1. Loosely tie an exercise band around your ankles and lie on your back with your arms down at your sides. Extend both legs straight up directly above your hips, with your feet spread wide enough that the exercise band is slightly taut. Flex your feet.

Step 2. Slowly open your legs as far as you can. When the tension becomes too great to pull any farther, pause, then slowly close your legs to return to the starting position.

One-Legged Lunge
Works Glutes, Quads, Hamstrings
Equipment: A sturdy chair or bench

Since this is a somewhat advanced exercise, practice doing regular lunges to get comfortable with the movement before you start. To make this move even more challenging, hold dumbbells down at your sides.

Step 1. Stand about 2 feet in front of a sturdy chair or bench with your back to it. Bend your left knee and extend your left leg behind you, putting the top of your left foot on the seat of the chair. Keep your back straight, your head aligned with your spine, and your eyes facing forward.

Step 2. Slowly bend your right knee until the right thigh is parallel to the floor. Do not allow your right knee to jut over your toes. Pause, then rise back to the starting position. Do one set with your right leg, then switch and repeat with your left.

Vein Event

ARE YOUR LEGS STARTING TO RESEMBLE A STREET MAP?
HERE'S WHAT YOU NEED TO KNOW.

By Camille Noe Pagán

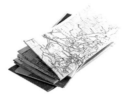

U p to half of American women have varicose veins. While that may dash your dreams of rocking a miniskirt at your 20th high school reunion, at least you won't be the only one covering up. These bumpy blue seams occur when the valves that keep blood flowing toward your heart malfunction, allowing blood to flow backward, which fills and stretches veins. Family history helps determine just who will be blessed with varicose veins, but pregnancy, extra pounds, or long hours spent standing or sitting with crossed legs raises your risk, says cosmetic surgeon Min-Wei Christine Lee, MD, director of the East Bay Laser and Skin Care Center in Walnut Creek, California.

Prevention is key. "For every 30 minutes that you're sitting or standing still, walk around for 5 minutes to increase circulation," advises Hema Sundaram, MD, a Washington, DC–based cosmetic surgeon and the author of *Face Value*. Exercising regularly and maintaining a healthy weight can also help by decreasing pressure on the veins. Already seeing blue on the backs of your calves? Technology's got you covered. Dr. Sundaram recommends the Palomar Lux1064 laser. "It generates heat that can close off superficial varicose veins, which makes them less no-

ticeable or even invisible." Treatment ranges from $350 to $1,000 per session, and most people need at least one to three sessions. Other options include sclerotherapy—injections that close small veins, making them disappear from sight—and surgery to remove large, bulging veins.

It's...Too...Tight

WHY YOU SHOULDN'T STUFF YOURSELF

Body shapers, compression garments, and girdles make cottage cheese lumps look smooth as butter in the short term. But, like aging, obesity, and pregnancy, they can create varicose veins. The problem is that your leg veins aren't strong enough to overcome their stranglehold. The force that hides bulges also restricts circulation. That causes the blood to pool, stretching your veins. "The pressure makes veins inflate like balloons," says Lenise Banse, MD, a dermatologist in Clinton Township, Michigan. Do enough time in sausage casing–like slimmers and nasty blue cords pop up in your thighs. Minimize the damage by getting your blood flowing again. Once you can wiggle free, walk briskly for 5 minutes so the muscles squeeze that venous blood back up toward the heart, Dr. Banse says. Then elevate your legs at a 45-degree angle for as long as you can.

Your Best Breasts

A LOOK AT THE LATEST NEWS ON BREAST HEALTH AND THE
UPS AND DOWNS OF SURGICAL ENHANCEMENT.

By Beth Howard

Breasts begin turning heads as soon as they make their debut. They provide pleasure, bolster body image, and inspire pride and satisfaction. They also nurture babies with milk uniquely suited to an infant's needs. But as you get older, all that front-and-center attention has a downside. Where they once heralded your youth, your breasts may now seem to announce your decline. They can be a source of discomfort—and as you enter the years of higher cancer risk, they probably cause you some worry now and then.

Despite this dramatic shift, you don't hear much about how best to cope with these changes. And except for frequent reminders about getting mammograms, there isn't even much info about how to keep your breasts healthy for the long haul. Got breasts? We've got answers.

How the Breast Ages

Your breast has more of the milk-producing glands called lobules in its upper outer quadrant. **Result:** That area is particularly prone to pre-period tenderness—and to the development of tumors. The milk ducts transport milk to the nipple. About 95 percent of breast cancers begin within the ducts. Fat fills the spaces between the lobules and ducts—more of it as you get older. That increases sag, but has a bonus: It makes mammograms easier to read.

Breast Pain

In the run-up to menopause, your breasts can feel like a battleground—the scene of all manner of lumps, pains, and general aggravations. Thank goodness, most of these breast bothers have nothing to do with cancer. (Studies show that pain is the sole symptom of breast cancer in 2 percent of cases or less.) But don't just feel reassured—feel better. Here's how.

1. Lumpiness or Thickened and Tender Areas

It may be: Fibrocystic breast changes, a condition that affects so many women (more than 60 percent, estimates say) that it's considered a version of normal. Researchers don't entirely understand the cause, although they lay blame at least partly on hormones. The thickened, rubbery feeling comes from fibrous tissue—the same sort of tissue that's in scars. The lumps are due to fluid-filled cysts. Breasts may also feel full and achy and have a clear yellow or greenish discharge.

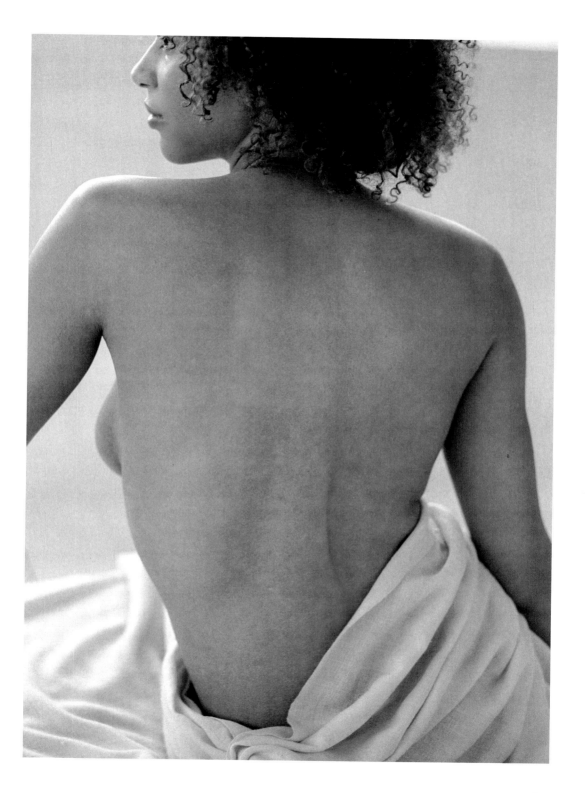

Rest easy: Fibrocystic breast changes don't increase breast cancer risk. And though the problem typically worsens in the years before menopause, most women find relief as their hormones quiet down.

Try this: Reduce your caffeine consumption—it exacerbates soreness in up to 50 percent of women. NSAIDs (nonsteroidal anti-inflammatory drugs) such as aspirin and ibuprofen help some women, as do vitamin E (800 IU daily) and evening primrose oil (1,500 to 3,000 mg daily). Research on primrose oil is mixed, but it can't hurt you. If pain is severe, your doctor may prescribe a drug to block the effect of your reproductive hormones.

2. A Single, Distinct Lump

It may be: A cyst. In 80 percent of cases, a lump is not due to cancer. Cysts are usually firm and round; they can be smaller than a BB or as big as a grape, sometimes larger. They often disappear after your period but can recur with the next cycle.

Try this: Because there's always the possibility of cancer, tell your doctor about any new or dominant lump. NSAIDs may help ease pain.

3. Thick Green or Black Discharge

It may be: Mammary duct ectasia, which just means that one of your milk ducts has become inflamed and clogged. As many as one in four women develops the condition during or after menopause. Other signs of the problem: soreness; a lump or thickening; an inverted nipple; or the pain, swelling, and redness of mastitis (breast infection).

Try this: Warm compresses, NSAIDs, and a supportive bra often help (see page 150 for a few of our favorites). But you should have your doctor take a look. Antibiotics may be necessary—and you may need to have the duct surgically removed if the problem doesn't get better.

Cancer

After years of bickering, most experts now agree that mammograms save lives for women over age 40. Yet, surprisingly, only 64 percent—barely half!—of fortysomethings show up for regular screenings, according to the American Cancer Society (ACS).

In Your Forties

Your risk of developing breast cancer in this decade: 1 in 70

YOU SHOULD KNOW: If cancer is found, be prepared for intensive treatment. Cancer in these years tends to be more aggressive and less likely to respond to estrogen-blocking therapies such as tamoxifen. But younger women typically can tolerate more treatment side effects, so you can get larger, more effective doses of chemo drugs, says Gabriel Hortobagyi, MD, chairman of the breast medical oncology department at the University of Texas M. D. Anderson Cancer Center in Houston. "On average, chemo in women younger than 50 reduces recurrence rates by as much as 55 percent, compared with 20 to 30 percent in older women," Dr. Hortobagyi says.

ESSENTIAL STEPS: Ask for a digital mammogram, which does a better job for younger women, who tend to have denser breasts. In a large, multicenter study, digital scans found 15 percent more cancers than standard mammograms in women under age 50. (Don't be dismayed if you're called back for another exam. It's harder to get a good view in women in their forties, so they're more often recalled for additional tests.)

In Your Fifties

Your risk of developing breast cancer in this decade: 1 in 40

YOU SHOULD KNOW: Breast cancer rates have declined significantly among women 50 and older since 2001, in large part because of the drop in the use of hormone therapy, says Debbie Saslow, PhD, director of breast and gynecologic cancers for the ACS.

ESSENTIAL STEPS: Don't forget your mammogram. Even with the recent drop in incidence, your risk of developing cancer remains higher than it is in younger women—yet mammography rates in this age group have fallen 7 percent since 2000. Early detection pays off: Breast cancer that develops in a woman's fifties is more likely to be estrogen-receptor positive, so there are more drugs available to treat it.

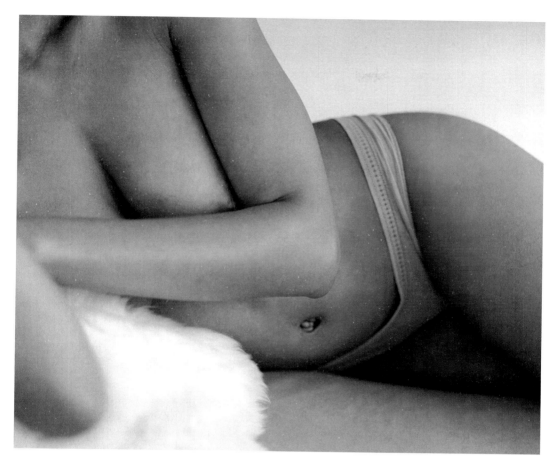

Nip/Tuck

A life well lived leaves traces on your body: laugh lines, crow's-feet, and, yes, sagging breasts. One perfectly good reaction: Shrugging at the changes. But for some women, that gesture doesn't have the desired oomph. More than 163,000 women over age 40 got gravity-defying help in 2007, spurred on by improved surgical techniques and the return of the silicone implant. Here, the benefits and downsides of nips, tucks, and more.

Lift

The rate of lift surgery has nearly doubled since 2000, according to the American Society of Plastic Surgeons (ASPS), with well over 53,000 procedures performed in 2007.

How it works: By removing excess skin and tightening the surrounding tissue, surgeons can raise and reshape the breasts. A new technique leaves a smaller scar that can be neatly camouflaged by the nipple's areola—although many factors determine whether this less conspicuous approach or the older anchor lift is right for you.

Downside: The procedure can't replace lost volume, so if breast deflation is a big issue for you in addition to sag, a lift may not be adequate.

Breast Implants

The number of women over 40 getting breast implants increased by 17 percent between 2005 and 2006; in 2007, more than 107,000 women in that age range got the procedure.

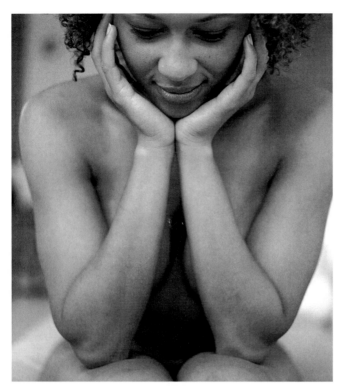

3 years after surgery and then again every 2 years (in addition to their annual mammograms). Implants can also harden—it happens with up to 80 percent of the silicone variety and 40 percent of saline ones. All told, most women need to replace or remove an implant within 15 to 20 years, says Walter L. Erhardt, MD, a cosmetic surgeon in Albany, Georgia, and past president of the ASPS. Implants can also make mammograms harder to read, though technologists who perform the exam make adjustments. A University of Washington study found that mammograms missed 55 percent of breast cancers in women with implants, versus only 33 percent among women without them. Fortunately, this doesn't seem to affect mortality. "Women with augmentation may be more breast aware and seek medical care more quickly," suggests study author Diana L. Miglioretti, PhD.

Reduction

More than half of reduction surgeries were in 40-plus women in 2007, according to the ASPS; more than 56,000 women over 40 got the procedure. Small wonder: By that age, the health effects of large breasts—chafed skin, back and neck pain, and grooves in the shoulders from ill-fitting bras—are mounting. In a recent study, discomfort was vanquished or greatly reduced 1 year after surgery for 88 percent of patients. "Women invariably say they wish they'd had it sooner," Dr. Erhardt says. Benefits go beyond comfort. Breast exams and mammograms are often easier to perform and more effective after surgery. And some research suggests it can even reduce the risk of breast cancer, especially in those over age 50.

Bonus: Because of the health problems that can result from uncomfortably large breasts, insurance often picks up the tab.

Downside: The surgery can cause a loss of nipple sensation and, in some cases, can result in asymmetry of the breasts.

How it works: Adding implants during a breast lift helps with sag and loss of volume. A 1994 study from Washington University School of Medicine in Saint Louis, Missouri, found that 95 percent of women felt better about themselves after the surgery. But it presents a tough choice: saline or silicone. Silicone implants look and feel more natural than saline, but in 1992, they were pulled off the market for use in cosmetic procedures because of concerns they might raise the risk of scleroderma or other disorders. Now, after several large National Cancer Institute studies, silicone is back. "Breast implants have been studied more extensively than any other medical device," says Donna-Bea Tillman, PhD, director of the Office of Device Evaluation at the Food and Drug Administration. "And our experts concluded that they're safe and effective."

Downside: About 10 percent of implants—saline or silicone—rupture within 5 years, and the rate goes up as time passes. To make sure ruptured implants are detected and removed, women should get MRIs

6 Habits That Can Save Your Life

SOME RISK FACTORS FOR BREAST CANCER CAN'T BE CHANGED. OTHERS FALL WITHIN YOUR CONTROL.

1. Keep Moving
"Exercise lowers levels of estrogen, which is linked to breast cancer," says the ACS's Debbie Saslow, PhD. It's best to get 45 to 60 minutes of heart-thumping activity most days of the week, but moderate levels (30 minutes, 5 days a week) can make a difference. You're never too old: A recent study in the *British Medical Journal* showed that postmenopausal women (along with those with a normal body mass index, or BMI) get more of a benefit from regular sweat sessions than other women.

2. Get—and Stay—Slim
After menopause, obese women have double the risk of breast cancer compared with women of a healthy weight. But weight gain among previously trim women also bodes ill. "Gaining even 20 pounds of weight as an adult increases risk," says Heather Spencer Feigelson, PhD, MPH, strategic director of genetic epidemiology at the ACS.

3. Take Vitamin D
More and more studies demonstrate the cancer-fighting power of this vitamin. The latest piece of evidence, reported at a recent meeting of the American Society of Clinical Oncology: Breast cancer patients who were deficient in vitamin D were 94 percent more likely to have their cancer spread than women with adequate D levels. "I advise women to take 800 to 1,000 IU a day," says Andrew Kaunitz, MD, a professor at the University of Florida College of Medicine–Jacksonville.

4. Drink Lightly, If at All
New data from the National Cancer Institute shows that women who have one or two drinks daily increase their risk of developing the most common kind of breast cancer by 32 percent—and those who drink more hike their risk by 51 percent.

5. Keep Hormones Temporary
Long-term use of hormone replacement therapy can increase breast cancer risk, the *Women's Health* Initiative demonstrated—and new research shows the heightened risk persists several years after you stop. Take hormones only if menopausal symptoms are unmanageable, and limit time on the therapy to no more than 5 years. Consider alternatives, such as certain antidepressants for hot flashes and vaginal creams with estrogen for dry genital tissues.

6. Forget Self-Exams, but Be Self-Aware
After hearing for years that you should do a monthly breast self-exam, you might be surprised to learn that it's now considered optional. Studies have found that it doesn't save lives and can increase the odds of an unnecessary biopsy. But many doctors are reluctant to completely abandon it. "About 15 percent of breast cancer is detected by women themselves," says Eva Singletary, MD, a professor of surgical oncology at M. D. Anderson. So doctors still want you to get to know your breasts—and alert your provider to anything outside the norm for you.

Invest In Your Chest

SWEAT YOUR TA-TAS OFF IN ONE OF THESE ALL-STAR ATHLETIC SUPPORTERS.

Your body, believe it or not, has its own built-in bra. Breasts, which are made of fat, milk ducts and lobules, connective tissue, lymph nodes, and blood vessels, are attached to your chest by thin, delicate bands called Cooper's ligaments. Woven throughout the breasts, the Cooper's ligaments keep the breasts standing at attention. But, like rubber bands, they wear out—and intense bouncing and movement stretch them out even more. In fact, in a 2008 study from the University of Portsmouth, United Kingdom, biomechanics experts found that breasts fly as much as 8 inches up and down regardless of size, and that they also go in and out and left to right in a sort of figure-eight pattern. (If you're intrigued, go to www.shockabsorber.co.uk/bounceometer to watch an animated version of your bouncing boobs.) Because you can't rebuild ligaments the way you can increase muscle mass, exercise will not reverse the damage once the sag has set in. All the more reason to shell out some coin on a well-constructed, properly fitting, supportive sports bra. A sports bra should perform like the man of your dreams: hug you close, get physical when you want, and provide plenty of unconditional support. Thanks to cutting-edge engineering, space-age fabrics, and ingenious design details, you're bound to find the perfect match on the following page.

Note: Low-impact activities include cross-country skiing, inline skating, meditation, tai chi, walking, weight training, yoga. Medium-impact activities include cycling, skiing, elliptical training, golf, hiking, most martial arts, rowing, snowboarding, spinning, stair-climbing, tennis. High-impact activities include basketball, boxing, horseback riding, mountain biking, racquetball, running, soccer, volleyball

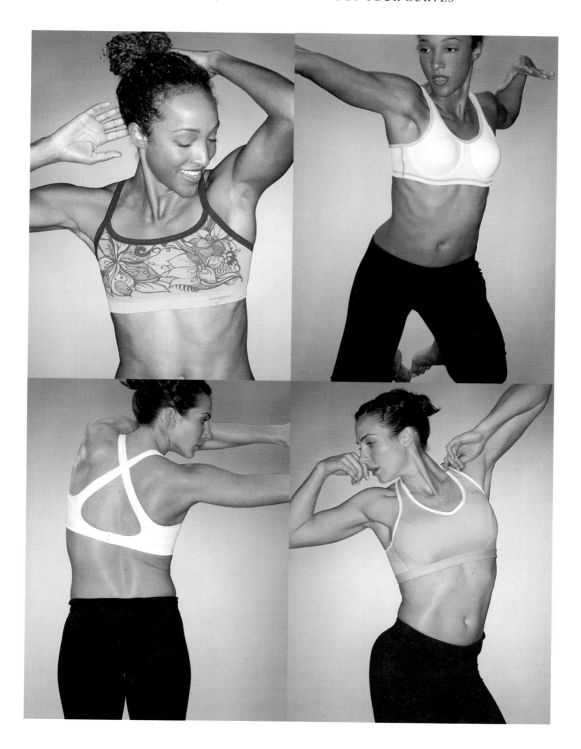

A Boob-by-Boob Guide to Sports Bras

	A—B CUP	B—C CUP	C—D CUP
LOW IMPACT	*Eco Chic* Our tester, a yogini, designated the Patagonia Active Mesh bra her "go-to choice for low-impact activities." Pretty floral graphics in front and supportive straps that contour to a slimming V in back guarantee unobstructed movement. www.patagonia.com	*Living Color* The Asics Renah seamless bra, available in four high-volume colors, looks good anywhere. Our tester said: "I'd totally wear this without a shirt." Quick-dry fabric controls sweat. Spandex hugs the body (our tester even wore it to bed!). www.asicsamerica.com	*Full Package* The built-in shelf bra in the Free Motion Fitness Sport Tank 5.6 keeps you locked and loaded while the seamless stretch fabric construction hugs your curves. Our tester said you'll feel "pulled together but not strapped in." www.nordictrack.com
	All the Right Notes The Lululemon Athletica Flow Y bra is the ultimate overachiever: A mesh insert wicks sweat from your upper back, flat seams eliminate chafing, and the garment's X-shape construction between your shoulder blades permit a full range of motion. www.lululemon.com	*A Full Tank* The clever Champion Powerlite Empire Tech tank has a double-layer bra for extra holding power and an empire waist that sveltefies anyone. Tip: Avoid activities that turn you upside down unless you like flashing your tummy. www.championusa.com	*Technical Support* Uniboob, begone! The Isis C/D sport bra, with its encapsulated double-layer cups, "felt like it was supporting me rather than smashing me down," our tester said. Bonus: none of her usual postworkout breast pain. www.isisforwomen.com
	Cheery-O! Available in an array of vivid colors and a sleek racerback design, the Champion Shape Vented Cami sports bra just begs you to pull a Brandi Chastain. Our tester raved about the "fabulous fit," and the moisture-control band kept her dry. www.championusa.com	*No Shake with That, Please* Our tester swears the Saucony Motion Sensor bra is "the only bra I'm comfortable wearing in front of guys at the gym." Built-in cups, made of a stain-resistant stretch polyester-spandex blend, hold you firm. www.saucony.com	*Air Ride–Equipped* Made of lush cotton, the Natori Sport underwire sports bra makes you feel as if "your boobs are on air," our tester said. Wide straps don't dig into shoulders, and the hard-ware and elastic are hidden away—so no pinching or pulling. www.freshpair.com
	Fab Figure No more "meet the pancakes." Our tester, who compares her chest with a 12-year-old boy's, declared the Moving Comfort Alexis bra "the Wonderbra of sports bras!" The cups are lightly padded to prevent "high beams." www.movingcomfort.com	*No Sweat* Bring on the humidity! Stay dry this summer in the lightweight CW-X Ventilator Support Bra. Mesh vents below the bustline and between the breasts keep you cool, and star-shaped webbing in the cups reduces jarring and bouncing. www.cw-x.com	*Shock-Proof* The New Balance Versatility Cami top, best for medium-impact activities, has a nifty internal stabilizer to absorb shock and adjustable Velcro straps with extra padding to prevent annoying indentations. www.newbalance.com
	Dry, with a Twist Our fussiest tester loved the Lily of France In Action sport underwire bra. The breath-able fabric sucked up moisture like a sponge, and the underwire "disappeared into the supportive structure with no discomfort." www.shoplilyoffrance.com	*Drop and Do 20* Your buff upper bod will look fab in the Under Armour Strength 2 bra with HeatGear fabrication and mesh side inserts that enhance breathability. Our tester loved the full cups, which gave her more coverage than most sports bras do. www.underarmour.com	*Know When to Hold 'Em* The Anita molded sports bra's outer cups separate while retaining your breasts' natural shape; its inner cups are lined with nonchafing microfiber. Triple clasps give an extra-secure fit. www.herroom.com
HIGH IMPACT	*Place Keeper* Not even a 2-hour run will budge Bestform High Impact's bras. One model—the two-ply micro crop for powerful support—features a stay-put ribbed band, no-slip straps, and chafe-safe fabric. www.bestformintimates.com	*Black Beauty* Even an intense cardio workout couldn't shake our tester's love for the Shock Absorber Support Level 3 sports bra, with a protective layer in each cup for support. www.figleaves.com	*Ironclad* Our full-busted tester said "breasts have no chance of moving" in the Bendon Sport Max Out bra's molded cups. With its satiny feel, you may want to wear it when you're not in workout mode. www.bendonsport.com

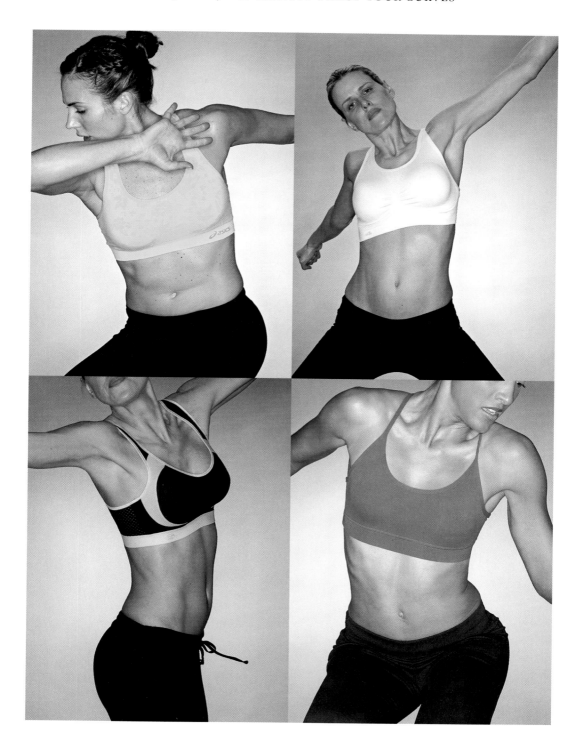

Chapter Seven

Boost Your Brainpower

HOW TO SHARPEN YOUR MIND AND PROTECT YOUR MEMORY

> INVESTMENT: 2 WEEKS
> AGE ERASED: 5 YEARS

Introduction

D o you remember when your high school biology teacher grimly pronounced that once you destroy a brain cell, it's gone for good? Half the class traded "I know what you smoked last night!" looks. But these days, the idea that you're born with finite neurons is as outdated as the yearbooks you stashed in your parents' attic. In recent years, revolutionary noggin-scanning technologies such as functional magnetic resonance imaging (fMRI) have allowed researchers to observe living brains at work, and they've found that your 3-pound blob is a dynamic organ that changes more often than the cast of *Saturday Night Live*. In the past decade, plasticity—the theory that the brain changes and grows throughout our lives, creates new cells, and even repairs itself after trauma and illness—has become the hot topic around neurobiology labs.

Every time you move or think, neural connections are made, reinforced, or lost. The average brain cell makes about 10,000 connections with other cells. But to keep them firing, you have to abide by a crucial neuro motto: "Use it or lose it." Brain researchers know that just about everything you do—or don't do, for that matter—contributes to your brain's long-term well-being (or its descent into decrepitude). And they've discovered a number of ways you can help fire up mission control.

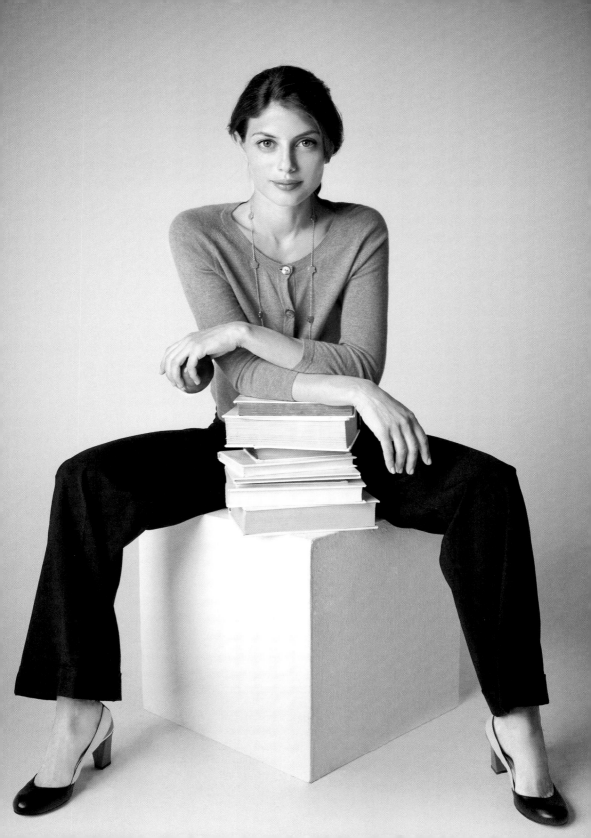

Part One:
Secrets of a Keener Mind

Stay Sharper Longer

WIN ANY BRAIN GAME WITH THESE SIMPLE STRATEGIES.

By Matthew Sloan

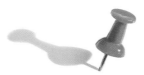

At one point in your life, your mind was a steel trap. But the stress of modern life can make anyone's brain more closely resemble a colander. Life keeps pouring in, but you retain less and less of it. Fear not: We've created a cheat sheet that will give you the mental edge you need to survive in this cut-throat job market, plus the brain strength necessary to keep your wits years from now when you're a grandmother. The key to all this is simple: Stop taking your gray matter for granted, says P. Murali Doraiswamy, MD, chief of biological psychiatry at Duke University's medical school in Baltimore. "You can add 10 or more years to your brain's useful life just by paying some attention to it." If that doesn't sound like a fantastic return on an investment, then, well, you may already have lost your mind.

Break a Mental Sweat

Just as exercise builds endurance, bolstering your neurological connections creates a reservoir of stamina that you can tap later in life. To bulk up your neurons, study another language. *Parlez-vous français? Non?* Then you may find yourself less able to stave off dementia when you're older. In a 2007 study at York University in Toronto, bilingual seniors kept the worst effects of the condition at bay 4 years longer than those who'd never ventured beyond their native tongue. Learning a second language appears to increase the density of gray matter in the areas of your brain that govern attention and memory, says researcher Ellen Bialystok, PhD.

During your commute, play some language-instruction CDs, such as one from Macmillan's *Behind the Wheel* series (www.macmillanaudio.com, or download the MP3 version from www.audible.com).

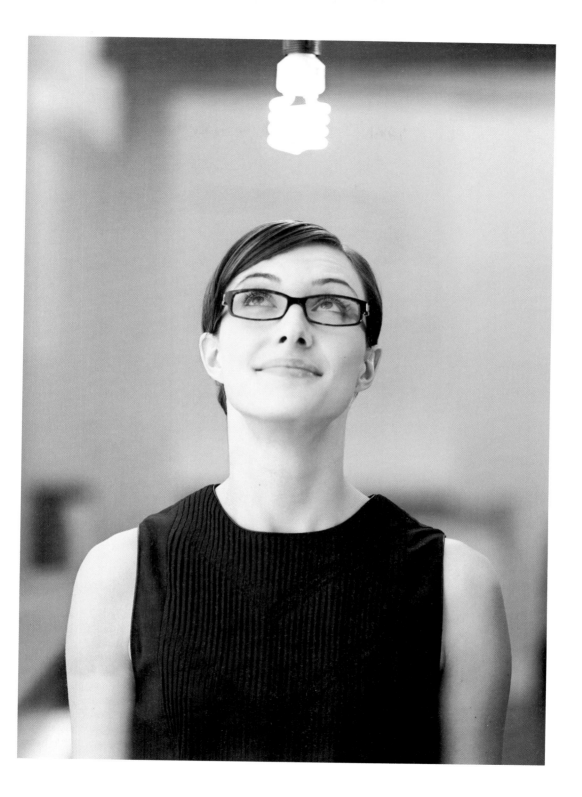

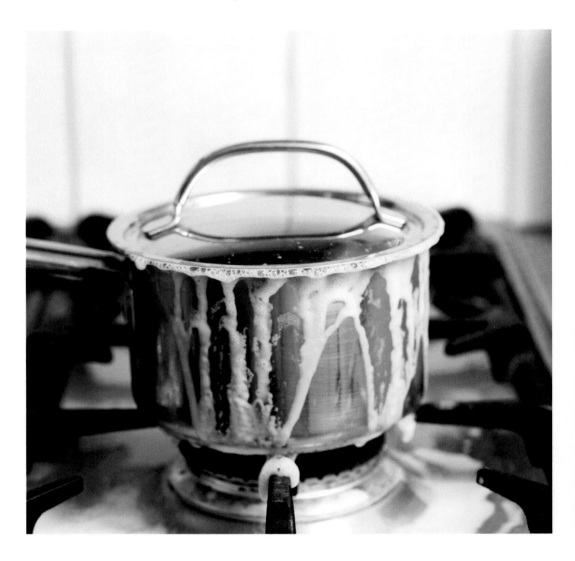

Eat and Drink Smarter

"Food affects your brain like a drug," says Fernando Gómez-Pinilla, PhD, a professor of neurosurgery at UCLA. The right nutrients will fire up neurotransmitters, strengthen communication between brain cells, and stimulate the production of neuron-protecting proteins. But a diet heavy in calories from sugar and saturated fat not only slows overall brain functioning, but also makes your brain more vulnerable to free radicals—molecules that can damage tissue and ultimately lead to disease. Change your habits now to bring an end to this slide.

• **Fish for omega-3s.** Thirty-five percent of your brain consists of fatty acids such as docosahexaenoic acid (DHA), an omega-3 that helps nerve cells communicate with one an-

30
Age at which you begin to lose brain tissue

other. Another omega-3 called eicosapentaenoic acid (EPA) increases your brain's sensitivity to serotonin, a hormone that produces feelings of happiness. Both of these fats can decline as the years stack up. A 2008 University of Cincinnati study, for instance, found that the brain tissue of 65- to 80-year-olds contained 22 percent less DHA than the brain tissue of 29- to 35-year-olds. "If you want to keep your wits about you as you age, start consuming omega-3s now," says William Harris, PhD, a nutrition researcher at the University of South Dakota in Vermillion. Dr. Harris recommends taking an omega-3 supplement. Nordic Naturals Omega-3 (www.nordicnaturals.com) is good for 330 milligrams of EPA and 220 milligrams of DHA in a two-capsule serving, and it contains lemon oil to mask the fishy taste. Ocean Nutrition (www.ocean-nutrition.com) is another good brand to look for.

• **Raid the spice rack.** Sprinkle some rosemary on your entrées and side dishes. The carnosic acid found in this spice has been shown to reduce stroke risk in mice by 40 percent, according to a new study published in the *Journal of Neurochemistry*. Carnosic acid appears to set off a process that shields brain cells from free-radical damage, which can worsen the effects of a stroke. It can also protect against degenerative diseases like Alzheimer's and the general effects of aging. But rosemary is not the only "mind spice" on the shelf: Cinnamon, turmeric, basil, oregano, thyme, and sage can all protect your brain from inflammation, says neurologist Eric Braverman, MD, a clinical assistant professor at Weill Cornell Medical College. Shoot for 3 to 7 teaspoons of any combination of these spices each day. "Add a teaspoon of cinnamon to your morning yogurt or coffee," says Dr. Braverman. "Sprinkle basil and oregano on a sandwich, or stir a teaspoon of rosemary into tea. It'll add up."

• **Raise a glass of the good stuff.** In a 2006 University of South Florida study, people who drank three or more 4-ounce glasses of fruit or vegetable juice each week were 76 percent less likely to develop Alzheimer's disease than those who drank less. The high levels of polyphenols—antioxidants found in fruits and vegetables—may protect brain cells from the damage that may be caused by the disease, says study author Amy Borenstein, PhD. Eating a diverse mix of fruits and vegetables also provides the greatest oxidative protection, according to a recent study in the *Journal of Nutrition* that compared people who ate 18 plant families with those who ate only five varieties.

Let Your Brain Kick Back

Don't feel too guilty about shootin' the bull at the watercooler. A recent University of Michigan, Ann Arbor, study found that people who chatted for 10 minutes before being tested for mental-processing speed performed better than those who didn't. "Social interaction seems to sharpen your memory and other brain functions because you have to process information and gauge re-

If you want to keep your wits about you as you age, start consuming omega-3s.

sponses, such as whether a person is being ironic or honest," says researcher Oscar Ybarra, PhD. Even if there's no office gang handy, make sure to give yourself a break anyway. Grinding away at your job may not give you the edge you think it will. Heck, it could blunt your brainpower. A 2009 study published in the *American Journal of Epidemiology* shows that clocking 55 or more hours on the job correlated with lower scores on vocabulary and reasoning tests, compared with working a 35- to 40-hour week. The researchers think stress from overwork can cause impaired sleep and other problems that can slow your CPU. "Reserve 20 minutes to lie down or sit quietly with your eyes closed, away from any stimulus," says Richard Best, PhD, an organizational psychologist in San Antonio, Texas. You aren't trying to fall asleep; you're simply giving your brain a breather from nonstop processing. Your recharged neurons will thank you.

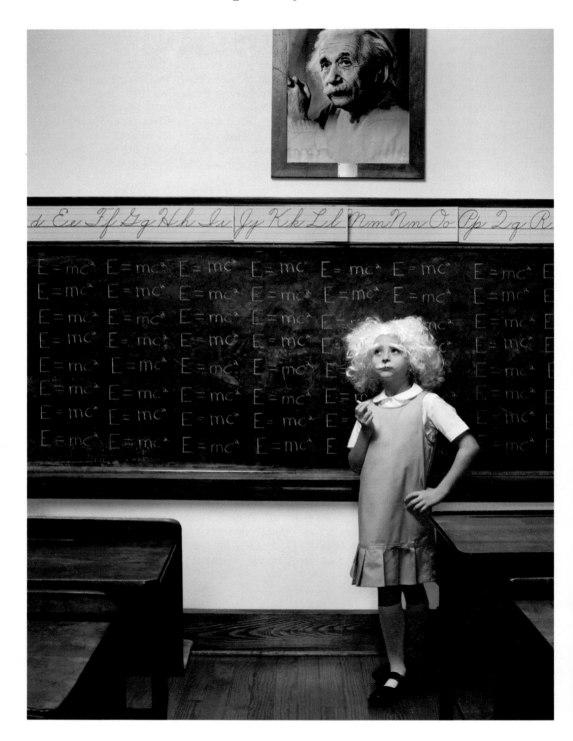

A Woman's Guide to Getting Einstein's Brain

THIS GENIUS HANDBOOK TO YOUR GRAY MATTER WILL HAVE YOUR NEURONS CRANKING LIKE LAB RATS.

By Valerie Reiss

Choose Kung Fu or Hip-Hop

Your gym membership benefits more than just your muscles and lungs. According to a 2007 Columbia University study, hitting the gym may help you sprout new cells in the dentate gyrus, an area of the brain vital to memory. Researchers measured blood volume in the brains of adults who worked out four times a week for 4 months and found that all that activity sparks the production of more neurons.

Genius move: Complexity is the key to a mind-growing workout, says John Ratey, MD, author of *Spark: The Revolutionary New Science of Exercise and the Brain*. His favorite activities: dance and martial arts. "Both require you to position different parts of your body simultaneously and in synchronicity—and with dance, you've got to move along to music," he says. "That's a lot of mental stimulation."

10 Parts of the brain simultaneously activated during orgasm

Crack Some Eggs

Woman cannot thrive on Pop-Tarts alone. Or even All-Bran. The best brain foods are those that would rot if the power went out, says Larry McCleary, MD, author of *The Brain Trust Program*. Pick fresh fruits, veggies, and lean proteins and avoid the dreaded duo, trans fats ("they diminish brain cells' ability to communicate with each other") and high-fructose corn syrup ("it can shrink the brain by damaging cells").

Genius move: An ideal breakfast, Dr. McCleary says, is an egg. The incredible edible contains B vitamins, which enable nerve cells to burn glucose, your brain's major energy source; antioxidants, which protect neurons against damage; and omega-3 fatty acids, which keep nerve cells firing at optimal speed. Wash it down with a cup of green tea, which supplies you with

163

theanine, an amino acid found almost exclusively in tea leaves. "Theanine is like the anti-speed," Dr. McCleary says. "It keeps brain cells from firing too fast and wearing out."

Keep On Moving On

Multitasking is like Kryptonite to gray matter. The key to remembering facts that dazzle is giving them your full attention when you first learn them. In a 2006 study at UCLA, participants were asked to memorize information, first while simultaneously counting beeping noises, then without the racket. Neural scans showed the distracted subjects utilized different systems in their brains, causing them to learn less efficiently. "The biggest reason we have trouble recalling information is that it never really gets into our memory stores to begin with," says Gary Small, MD, director of the UCLA Memory and Aging Research Center at the Semel Institute for Neuroscience and Human Behavior and the author of *The Longevity Bible*.
Genius move: When you have a crammed to-do list, rather than layering projects, take on one task at a time and change them up every hour. Can't finish something in 60 minutes? Schedule another slot for it later in the day. "Switching from one project to the next will engage different areas of the brain, keeping you mentally alert," Dr. Small says.

Breathe Like You Mean It

Sure, it might sound hippy-dippy, but meditation can expand your mind. In 2005 researchers at Harvard Medical School found that the brains of long-time meditators were bigger than those of nonmeditators. In particular, the frontal cortex, the part associated with attention, and the insula, which integrates thoughts and emotions, were thicker. By improving attention, "meditation may slow down or even reverse age-related memory decline," says Sara Lazar, PhD, who led the studies.
Genius move: Sit comfortably with your back straight. Close your eyes and take a few deep breaths. Then breathe naturally and direct your attention to the area where you feel your breath most—the nostrils, chest, or abdomen. When you notice your mind wandering to finishing a project, having sex, or eating cupcakes, refocus on your breath. Try to keep it up for 15 or 20 minutes.

Disconnect the Cable

After a deadline-filled day, it's tempting to zone out in front of a *Top Chef* marathon. But "too much TV may damage your memory," says Aric Sigman, PhD, psychologist, biologist, and author of *Remotely Controlled: How Television Is Damaging Our Lives*. "It's not a question of what's going on in your brain; it's what's not going on." Basically, your neurons can barely be bothered to fire when you're glued to the tube. A 2005 study published in *Brain and Cognition* found that for each additional hour per day a person spent watching TV between the ages of 40 and 59, the risk of developing Alzheimer's later in life rose by 1.3 percent. Yikes.
Genius move: Top out at 2 hours of TV a day, Sigman says. Instead of tuning in, consider brushing up on your Shakespeare or reading the latest David Sedaris book. A 2006 study published in *Neuropsychologia* found that reading sentences with metaphor or irony stimulates more brain activity than taking in straight-up facts.

Stroke Your Genius

Why they didn't mention this in science class we'll never know, but sex is brain food. In a 2004

Become a Chief Exercise Officer

Need a brilliant business plan? Hit the treadmill. Nearly 30 percent of entrepreneurs whose companies bring in at least $1 million a year exercise daily, according to an American Express survey. What's more, women respondents were five times more apt than the men to come up with their best ideas while sweating. "Women may be more likely to experience this [creative boost] if men are treating exercise as a competition, with themselves or others," says Kelly McGonigal, PhD. How to switch on that inner lightbulb? Vary your routine to keep your mind sharp, and crank up your iPod—it'll boost your mood and limit distractions.

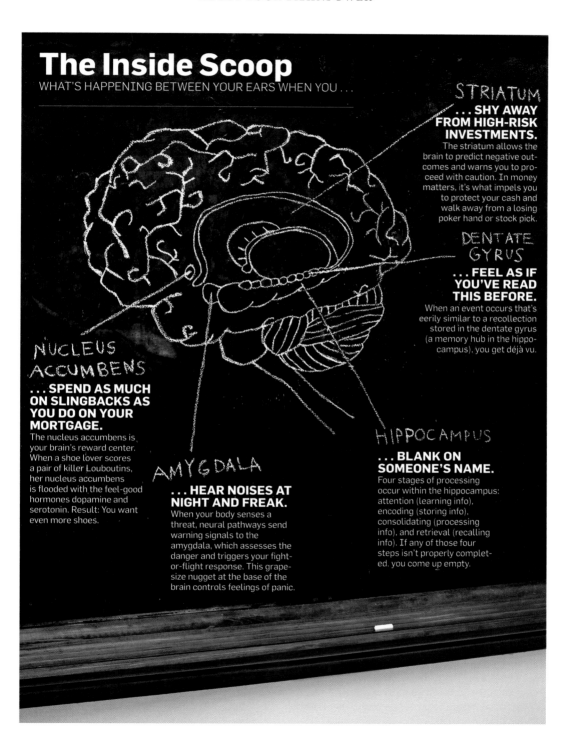

The Inside Scoop

WHAT'S HAPPENING BETWEEN YOUR EARS WHEN YOU . . .

STRIATUM
. . . SHY AWAY FROM HIGH-RISK INVESTMENTS.
The striatum allows the brain to predict negative out-comes and warns you to pro-ceed with caution. In money matters, it's what impels you to protect your cash and walk away from a losing poker hand or stock pick.

DENTATE GYRUS
. . . FEEL AS IF YOU'VE READ THIS BEFORE.
When an event occurs that's eerily similar to a recollection stored in the dentate gyrus (a memory hub in the hippo-campus), you get déjà vu.

NUCLEUS ACCUMBENS
. . . SPEND AS MUCH ON SLINGBACKS AS YOU DO ON YOUR MORTGAGE.
The nucleus accumbens is your brain's reward center. When a shoe lover scores a pair of killer Louboutins, her nucleus accumbens is flooded with the feel-good hormones dopamine and serotonin. Result: You want even more shoes.

AMYGDALA
. . . HEAR NOISES AT NIGHT AND FREAK.
When your body senses a threat, neural pathways send warning signals to the amygdala, which assesses the danger and triggers your fight-or-flight response. This grape-size nugget at the base of the brain controls feelings of panic.

HIPPOCAMPUS
. . . BLANK ON SOMEONE'S NAME.
Four stages of processing occur within the hippocampus: attention (learning info), encoding (storing info), consolidating (processing info), and retrieval (recalling info). If any of those four steps isn't properly complet-ed. you come up empty.

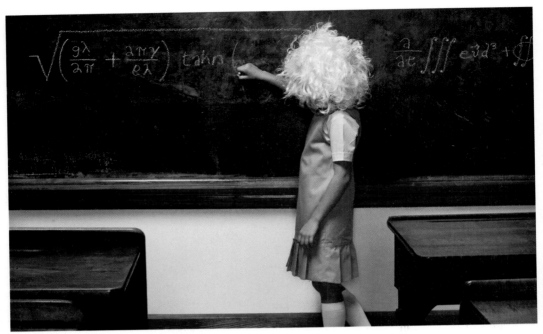

Rutgers University study, researchers found that orgasm simultaneously activates more than 10 parts of the brain, including the hippocampus, a memory hub; the amygdala, where emotion is processed; and the temporal lobe, an area associated with religious ecstasy ("Oh, God," indeed). "Sex is about stimulating everything at once," says Gina Ogden, PhD, a sex therapist and associate professor of sexology at the Institute for Advanced Study of Human Sexuality in San Francisco and the author of *Women Who Love Sex* and *The Heart and Soul of Sex*. "It's like a workout for your whole brain."

Give It a Rest

Getting plenty of snooze time is key to keeping your head on its toes. According to a 2007 study at Harvard Medical School, z's help memories lodge themselves in your brain (as anyone who has ever pulled an all-nighter and then tried to recall important details can attest). The study showed that the brain gathers disparate pieces of information and weaves them into a coherent whole while you're asleep.

Get Smart
3 GAMES TO SHARPEN YOUR WITS

Brain Age² for Nintendo DS
How it works: Your "baseline brain age" is assessed through three tests: Rock Paper Scissors, basic subtraction, and a few more-complicated equations. From there, you'll choose from 15 different puzzles and games. The program is based on the theories of a Japanese neuroscientist who maintains that the brain needs to be trained and toned just like any other muscle. His floating head acts as your virtual guide. (www.brainage.com)
Favorite challenge: Memory Sprint Training, in which you track a shaded runner in a race and determine what position he finished in (tougher than it sounds!)

Brain Games
How it works: Based on the research of Gary Small, MD, director of the UCLA Memory and Aging Research Center, this handheld device features five games—sequence, flash card, mind games, word hunt, and recall—and six levels of difficulty. (www.amazon.com)
Favorite challenge: In Word Hunt, a word is displayed and you use the letters to make as many new words as you can

FitBrains.com
How it works: Choose from beginner, intermediate, or advanced levels and then pick from three types of challenges: language, concentration, or memory. (Free)
Favorite challenge: Street of Dreams, a concentration game in which you have to place words in the appropriate category (like beer into beverage and television into appliances) as they cruise across the screen

Flex Your Mental Muscle

Mental exercise can reduce your risk of developing Alzheimer's disease and increase your brain's efficiency, says UCLA researcher Gary Small, MD, author of *The Longevity Bible*. Try the challenges below, adapted from Dr. Small's book, to give your brain its workout for the day.

1. *Triangles*
How many triangles (of any size) are in this diagram?

2. *Pac-Man fever*
Figure out which object does not match the others. This puzzle works the right side of your brain, specifically your visual and spatial skills.

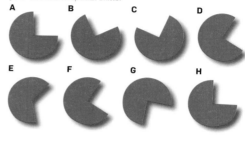

3. *Kind-of-like-Scrabble*
See how many words you can create from the letters below. Each word can't contain a repeated letter, but must contain the letter M. This puzzle exercises your language skills, which reside on the left side of your brain.

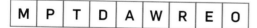

| M | P | T | D | A | W | R | E | O |

4. *Just plain hard*
Add two lines to any of the shapes below to complete the sequence. This whole-brain puzzle improves your ability to solve problems.

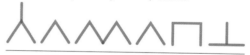

Answers: 1: 24; 2: E; 3: There are 43 words, including mowed, Warm, and Dream; 4: ⊤UvvⅤⅩYⅤ

Be the Square

PROVE YOUR MENTAL PROWESS BY GETTING ACROSS THE GRID

The rules: Moving one square at a time, either vertically or horizontally (not diagonally), find a path from the circle in the upper left corner to the circle in the lower right corner. One twist: You must switch shapes on every move—circle, triangle, circle, triangle, etc. There's only one solution.

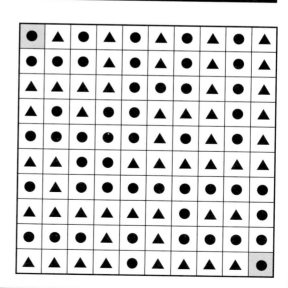

Part Two

Keep Your Memory Strong and Live Worry-Free

Total Recall

4 BRAIN BOOSTERS THAT CAN HELP YOU JUMP-START YOUR MEMORY.

Forgot about the water you started boiling for a cup of tea 20 minutes ago? D'oh! Can't remember the name of your sister's new boyfriend? Yikes! Having trouble recalling which password goes to which of your many online accounts? Ack! No worries. Even brainiacs forget this stuff. They just know how to kick-start their craniums, says *Memory Power* author Scott Hagwood, who memorized the order of nine decks of cards in an hour to become the first American Grandmaster of Memory. To limit future brain hiccups, try these tricks to remember . . .

1. Long Lists

Walk into a grocery store or a discount store without a list, and chances are you'll forget something you came for. Mental lists can dissolve when you're faced with many choices.

Brain booster: Visualize each option. "The more unusual the image, the more easily the information can be recalled," says Shane Bush, PhD, a neuropsychologist on Long Island, New York. Imagine Hugh Jackman holding the milk in one hand and a loaf of bread in the other, wearing nothing but boxer briefs made out of your favorite cereal. Bizarre? Sure. Effective? Definitely.

2. Phone Numbers

The brain can handle only so many numbers. So "combine them into units," says George W. Rebok, PhD, a professor in the department of mental health at Johns Hopkins University in Baltimore.

Brain booster: Divide a long string of numbers into sections that mean something to you. (Phone numbers are already grouped, so regroup them.) Look for three- and four-digit patterns and link them to your lucky number, your birthday, whatever. Once there's an association, the digits are less random and therefore easier to remember.

3. A Date's Details

Say you're back in the dating scene. Remembering little things—his mom's name, his March Madness pick—will always impress him. But that laundry list of information can be difficult to sort out, particularly when you're a few drinks into the night.

Brain booster: Use the room technique by picking a room that's familiar to you. As he's telling you things about his life, imagine him doing them (okay, mom was a bad example) in different parts of that room. Say, shooting hoops in a University of North Carolina jersey in the kitchen.

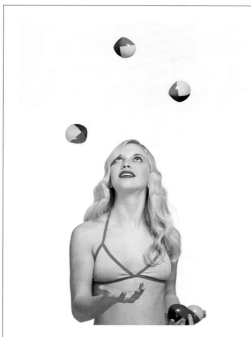

Increase Your Efficiency

Very few jobs can qualify as both physically *and* mentally challenging, but Air Force fighter pilot is certainly one of them. Not surprisingly, staying strong and calm while juggling life-or-death decisions at 10 Gs requires a good deal of training. Enter a word you probably know pretty well: multi-tasking.

Pilots prioritize a multitude of tasks and toggle back and forth between them rapidly . . . all while flying $130 million fighter jets at 1,500 mph. Here's how you can use their techniques to get more done in your daily life.

HABITUALIZE YOUR ROUTINES

Air Force: Novice pilots memorize the architecture of the cockpit and the aircraft's systems using mnemonics.

Civilians: To avoid what John Ratey, MD, an associate professor of psychiatry at Harvard, calls the "driveway pirouette," pack your gym bag the night before, and stash items you always carry (wallet, keys, BlackBerry, cell) in one spot. Recite your own shorthand phrase (e.g., "wa-key-Black-cell") before you leave.

KNOW THYSELF

Air Force: Pilots undergo a range of exercises (spinning in centrifuge machines, hypoxia tests, etc.) that teach them to recognize and operate within their own limits.

Civilians: Much less traumatic, but just as useful, is this concentration threshold test, devised by corporate productivity consultant Julie Morgenstern, author of *Never Check E-Mail in the Morning*. Throughout the day, create "concentration windows"—stretches of time when you're in a phone-and-e-mail blackout. Determine the length of your windows from a personal perspective (how long you can maintain peak mental performance?) and a practical one (how long you can stay silent before people think you've gone AWOL?).

HONE YOUR ATTENTIONAL FLEXIBILTY

Air Force: Grossly simplified, pilots learn various tasks and practice those tasks until their execution is almost automatic. Then, they practice switching back and forth between tasks until they can do it seamlessly.

Civilians: Recent research by Microsoft shows that multi-tasking can actually reduce productivity, because it takes most people 15 minutes to return to a serious mental task after responding to an incoming e-mail. So whenever possible, perform tasks sequentially, starting and finishing one before moving on to the next.

If you must multi-task, order your tasks from one to five and start at the top. If the list is too long, apply what Morgenstern calls the four Ds: Delay (schedule it for a more appropriate time when you can handle it properly), Diminish (do a down-and-dirty version), Delegate (assign the task to someone else), or Delete (omit a task that isn't worth doing).

ANALYZE YOUR PERFORMANCE

Air Force: After every mission comes the debriefing, sometimes hours long. These skull sessions identify mistakes and how to avoid making them again.

Civilians: Your debriefing takes only 10 minutes. Morgenstern calls it "tomorrow plus two." Take 10 minutes at the end of the day to assess—in your planner or in an online calendar—what got done and what didn't, and then plan out the next 3 days. Once you nail that, try a biweekly "next week plus two," and eventually "next month plus two." If a crisis hits, you'll have a long-term plan in place and be free to focus on the immediate issue.

4.

Names

"It doesn't matter how good you are at remembering things," Hagwood says. "Even the best experts can forget information if it's delivered too quickly."

Brain booster: Control the flow of information. If you're being introduced to a large group—at the wedding shower your future mother-in-law is throwing for you, for example—pause at the third person. Comment on her name, outfit, or resemblance to some celebrity. As others join in the banter, mentally review the names of the other two people you just met. Repeat with every third person you meet.

Research from the University of Richmond in Virginia found that the brain cell structures vital for communication double during pregnancy and that postdelivery the pathways to the hippocampus (where learning and memory are focused) are redefined and more efficient.

The Future of Alzheimer's

The chance of developing Alzheimer's before the age of 50 is less than 1 percent, says Thomas Crook, PhD, author of *The Memory Advantage* and former chairman of the National Institute of Mental Health's task force on age-associated memory impairment. About 10 to 15 percent of people in their seventies develop Alzheimer's, and the odds rise to about 50 percent by the time you hit your eighties, according to Bill Thies, PhD, vice president of medical and scientific relations for the Alzheimer's Association. But you can decrease your risk before you're in your golden years, even if the disease runs in your family. "Aerobic exercise appears to lower the risk of Alzheimer's by stimulating bloodflow and oxygenating the brain," Dr. Crook says. And, if we're lucky, someday it will become a manageable disease, like high blood pressure.

7 Everyday Tips for a Sharper Mind

IF YOU WANT TO JUMPSTART YOUR GRAY MATTER, "ACTIVELY START CARING FOR YOUR BRAIN AND ACTING FOR ITS BETTERMENT," SAYS DANIEL G. AMEN, MD, AUTHOR OF *MAGNIFICENT MIND AT ANY AGE*. HERE'S HOW.

1. Break Your Routine

Pursue anything that forces you to deviate from your daily patterns, such as brushing your teeth with your non-dominant hand and jogging backward. "In so doing, you'll stimulate new parts of your brain, encouraging it to make new connections," says Dr. Amen. Other ways to keep your brain agile: traveling to new places, learning to juggle, playing instruments, and dancing. "Few activities stimulate as wide a variety of brain systems as dancing does," says Dr. Amen. "Dancing requires everything from coordination and organization to planning and judgment."

2. Hydrate, Hydrate, Hyrdrate

"Your brain is 80 percent water, and if it's not hydrated, your neurons can't perform properly," says Dr. Amen.

3. Make Your Brain Purr

Achieve a calm, clear, stress-free brain through meditative belly breathing: Inhale slowly, allowing your stomach (not your chest) to rise, and then say the word "one" as you exhale. Repeat for 10 minutes.

4. Join a Reading Group

"Reading is good for your brain only when it involves storing and retrieving information," says Dr. Amen. That's why reading groups are beneficial. "And the social aspect of book groups adds another dynamic that bolsters cognitive functioning."

5. Kill the ANTs

"Automatic negative thoughts (ANTs) inflame the areas of the brain responsible for anxiety," says Dr. Amen. They also increase the production of stress hormones, which kill brain cells. Whenever an ANT enters your mind, write it down and devise a plan to correct it.

6. Pair Oats with OJ

Eat a power breakfast of oatmeal topped with chopped nuts, raisins, sesame seeds, and low-fat milk. The long-burning carbs and protein will fuel your body and brain for hours. Wash it down with two 8-ounce glasses of orange juice. A recent University of Alabama study found that 400 milligrams of vitamin C per day (the amount in a pint of OJ) significantly reduces the secretion of stress hormones.

7. Nap Like an Astronaut

In a NASA study, a 25-minute nap increased alertness by 54 percent and performance by 34 percent. Even catnaps of 5 or 10 minutes can help improve memory and learning.

Return to Glory

BELIEVE IT OR NOT, YOU CAN PREVENT BRAIN DAMAGE.
BUT TO ACHIEVE YOUR MAXIMUM POTENTIAL, YOU NEED TO KNOW
ABOUT THESE 6 MENTAL BOOSTS.

By Christina Goyanes

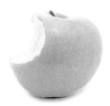

*O*f all the things you've got on your mind—work; bills; that weird, new stain on the kitchen floor—your mind probably isn't one of them. But now that you've started blanking on your own cell phone number and freezing when the ATM asks for your PIN, maybe it's time to start thinking about it. See, your brain tissue is steadily being chipped away—some of it by the natural aging process and some of it by brain shrinkers such as stress and cigarettes. Luckily, there are ways to strengthen your brain the way you build your abs. All it takes is a quick seven-step diet and exercise plan designed to boost your memory, attention span, and all the other things that will restore your skull-covered hard drive to its maximum power.

Brain Booster 1: Your Heart

The reason you misplace keys or can't remember what you ate 9 minutes ago? Normal aging shrinks neurons (brain cells) and drains neurotransmitters (the messengers that communicate between and among cells). But getting your

heart rate up can reverse this process by increasing bloodflow to the brain to improve memory and overall brain function, says Arthur Kramer, PhD, a professor of cognitive neuroscience at the University of Illinois at Urbana-Champaign. "We examined brain structure before and after fitness training and we found increases of brain volume in a number of areas," says Dr. Kramer, whose patients improved 10 to 15 percent on a variety of memory and attention tasks after exercise. The minimum: You can reap benefits from as little as walking 30 minutes three times a week.

Brain Booster 2: Your Back

Hauling your everyday (80-pound) shoulder bag can leave you tired. Carrying whiny kids can leave you frazzled. And both may injure your back—and your brain—in the process. A recent Northwestern University study found that people who suffered from chronic back pain lost up to $1\frac{1}{2}$ cubic centimeters (equivalent to 1 teaspoon) of gray matter per year. That's because the area of the brain that copes with the stress of the pain (the lateral prefrontal cortex, for those scoring at home) becomes depleted and dysfunctional enough to affect emotional decision making, says A. Vania Apkarian, PhD, whose previous work found that patients with chronic back pain were slower decision makers. The best way to beat back pain: Build muscle in your lower back and abdominals to support the spine. Try the reverse trunk curl: Lie flat on your belly and fold your hands under your chin. Lift your chin and chest off the floor about 3 to 6 inches. Aim for three sets of 10 to 15 repetitions three times a week.

Brain Booster 3: Your Waist

A body mass index (BMI) in the low twenties not only means you'll look great in a bikini, but also that you'll be more likely to remember that you do. A recent Swedish study found that women who had a BMI of 27 (25 to 30 is considered overweight) were more likely to experience loss of brain tissue in the temporal lobe (that's your brain's main hub for memory function and one of the first areas affected by Alzheimer's). This is because extra fat generates more chemicals that can be toxic to your brain, says Deborah Gustafson, PhD, the lead study author and assistant professor at the Institute of Clinical Neuroscience at the University of Göteborg in Sweden. One class of these chemicals—called free radicals—latches on to cells, disrupts the way they function, and can kill them. Aging naturally chews away at your memory, but excess fat may speed up the process. For each point your BMI increases, your risk increases 12 to 16 percent. "If you decrease your body weight, you're going to slow potential atrophy," says Dr. Gustafson, who recommends maintaining a BMI of below 25.

Brain Booster 4: Apples

Eat one a day and keep your neurologist away. Researchers from Cornell University in Ithaca, New York, recently discovered that animal brain cells treated with the antioxidant quercetin were able to resist damage from those brain-frying free radical cells (described above). "We know that quercetin, commonly found in apples, has a great potential to protect against chronic diseases, including Alzheimer's," says Chang Lee, PhD, the

principal study author and chair of the department of food science and technology at Cornell. Since fresh apples contain high levels of quercetin, Dr. Lee suggests that one a day may help combat neurodegenerative diseases. Pair your Red Delicious with a little cheese for an afternoon snack. Other foods high in quercetin include onions, plums, and berries.

Brain Booster 5: Your Desktop Wallpaper

Set up a Kandinsky painting as your desktop wallpaper, and it's like your brain doing 10 pushups every time you look at it. Researchers from the University of California at Davis found that the brain first detects recognizable patterns, such as shapes and lines, and then starts to break down new and different elements. Taking in an eyeful of complex images may ultimately help slow natural brain deterioration, says study author Scott Murray, PhD, a researcher at the University of Minnesota. Looking at a painting that actively engages your thoughts is far more challenging—and better—for your brain than staring out a window, which likely offers familiar views and much easier interpretation, Dr. Murray says.

1.5
Cubic centimeters of gray matter chronic back pain causes you to lose every year

Brain Booster 6: The Mall

In a recent study of 1,000 participants, researchers set out to find why 75-year-old women tend to maintain better brain function than 75-year-old men. The result: They shop. That's because shopping requires more physical and mental activity than sitting around and watching golf, says Guy McKhann, MD, study author and professor at the Center for Mind–Brain Research at Johns Hopkins University. "They're being physically active, mentally active, and tend to see themselves as having a role to play in life," says Dr. McKhan. Deciding what to buy, for whom, and how much to spend is one way to keep your brain—and your eye for a bargain—active on weekends. Watching sports does have a few benefits, but this is definitely one reason to hide the remote from your husband when you grow old together.

A Thinking Woman's Snack Plan

SNACKS TO KEEP YOU SANE ON THE MOST INSANE OF DAYS

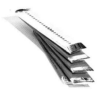 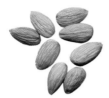 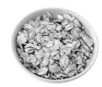

1. Gum A wad of Wrigley's can boost your attention and processing speed. Researchers in the United Kingdom had people complete four tests while chewing gum and found that it enhanced the delivery of glucose (aka blood sugar) to the brain, improving cognitive function. Another UK study had participants chew spearmint gum either before learning a word list or during the recall phase. Those who chewed during the learning phase were significantly more successful at recalling words than the latter group.

2. Nuts Most nuts are rich in choline, a nutrient that may improve memory. Researchers from the University of North Carolina at Chapel Hill found that the body uses choline to make neurotransmitters, which send signals across nerve endings. "Choline is also important for making the membranes around cells and nerve cells, [which will stop working] if these wrappers leak," says Steven Zeisel, MD, PhD, lead study author. Just 2 ounces of mixed nuts— especially pistachios, cashews, almonds, and peanuts—will help you meet the suggested daily intake of 425 mg for women. For an added boost, spread 2 tablespoons of peanut butter (20 mg of choline) on 2 wheat crackers (34 mg of choline).

3. Oatmeal Just ¼ cup of this carb-rich food supplies your brain with more of that great glucose stuff, which it needs to function. Iranian researchers recently found a clear correlation between blood glucose levels and memory: Of 20 participants who ate either a glucose-loaded breakfast (such as oatmeal), 50 grams of a protein drink, or a placebo, those who consumed glucose saw the most improvement in memory performance 60 minutes after ingestion.

4. Strawberries This sweet berry, as well as other dark-colored fruits and vegetables like blueberries and spinach, is loaded with vitamin C, which may ward off the development of Alzheimer's disease. Researchers working on the Cache County (Utah) Study on Memory, Health, and Aging recently found that women who consumed high amounts of vitamin C had a significantly lower risk of cognitive decline. A little less than a cup of strawberries is all you need to meet the USDA's daily dietary reference intake of 60 milligrams (mg) of vitamin C.

173

Focus, Dammit!

LIFE MAKING YOU CRAZY?
HERE'S HOW TO JUST DO WHAT YOU HAVE TO DO.

By Christina Goyanes

First of all, take a moment to freak out. "Everybody assumes that if we do everything right, everything will run smoothly," says Michael Carroll, author of *Awake at Work*. Wrong. Logging 50-hour weeks to get everything done can turn the job you love into a pothole of fear and frustration, Carroll says. Instead, think about doing your job properly, not perfectly. The next time you wig out, stop what you're doing. Sit up straight, eyes open, and try to calm your mind for 5 minutes. Let those first few thoughts of "This is ridiculous. I do not have time for this!" run their course, but don't give in to them. "If you can tame that restlessness, you'll be able to—in the midst of work's chaos—let go and find a sense of relief," Carroll says.

Set Your Agenda

"We think everything is urgent, and it's really not," says Fran Hewitt, coauthor of *The Power of Focus for Women*. "There are lots of reasons we do it— sometimes it's a personality thing where we like things completed for that sense of satisfaction. Sometimes we don't want to feel so overwhelmed, and other times we just don't prioritize." Determine what you must get done, set priorities, and then, suggests Hewitt, set up time blocks. "Make a conscious effort to cut back," she says, "otherwise your energy is going to be totally scattered." Turn off your cell phone, stop checking e-mail, and shut your door. Start by blocking out an hour each day. Once you reap the productive benefits of your

60-minute lockdown, set up time blocks throughout your day as needed.

Don't Be a Know-It-All

Acting like you know everything may be your way of dealing with job insecurities, Carroll says. This is stressful, especially when you overlook information that could make you more effective. Get to know the problem before you try to fix it. Drop your preconceptions and rely on your peers for information. "If we give ourselves enough room to not know everything," Carroll says, "we develop this ability to be open, alert, and inviting, rather than afraid of what we might not know."

Clear Off Your Desk

If your desk is cluttered, your gray matter is probably pretty scattered, too. "In an office, the environment is a reflection of the order of the person's mind," Hewitt says. Every random pile of papers is another brick in the wall blocking your clear train of thought. Instead of spending 3 hours looking for the misplaced file, "take the time to clean and reorganize your desk," Hewitt says. Once you know where everything is, you'll be able to focus on the task in front of you.

Don't Forget the H$_2$O

Next time you order a venti nonfat vanilla latte, grab a bottle of water—or two. "Our brain is only working at a third of its capacity when we're dehydrated," Hewitt says. For every cup of coffee, you need 2 cups of water to rehydrate. Tag-team

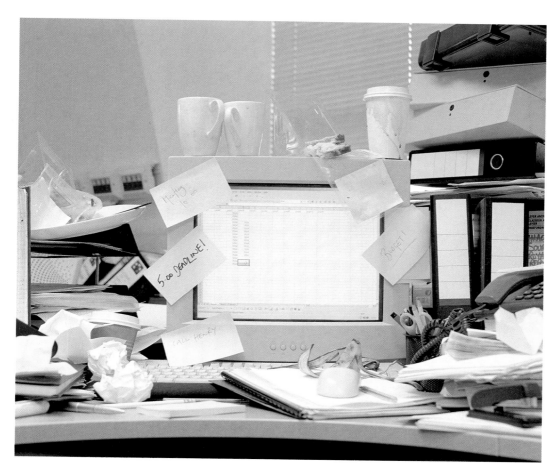

your 4 p.m. jolt of joe with at least 8 ounces of the clear stuff to help keep you fresh.

Ride the Elevator

Literally. But instead of skimming the latest memo, checking your watch, or averting eye contact, drop all your thoughts, stand still, and take a minute to, well, just be in the elevator. Embracing these small, personal moments, Carroll says, will help you relax so you're primed and ready to start working your little fanny off once you're back at the desk.

Let the Painter Paint

Get more from your job by zeroing in on your specialty. Take note of your low points during the day, Hewitt says, and watch for patterns that indicate you're not performing at your best: spending too much time in meetings, for example, or getting bogged down in computer tasks you haven't mastered yet. Ask your boss if other people in your department may be better at what's slowing you down, and suggest other areas where you can help. You'll win points for improving office efficiency, in addition to being able to focus on what you do best.

Look Back, Move Forward

Most of us don't take the time to appreciate what we've done, or how far we've come professionally. "We have this picture of what we want, and we create this discontent between where we are and where we want to go," Hewitt says. But looking back does push you to move forward. Instead of being frustrated by how far you have to go, think about times you were successful. Apply that sense of confidence and accomplishment to reaching your next goal.

The Importance of Turning It Off

ONCE YOU FIND WHAT SLEEP—AND THE LACK OF IT—DOES TO YOUR BODY, YOU'LL WANT TO GET THE MOST OUT OF ONE OF THE BEST THINGS YOU CAN DO BETWEEN THE SHEETS.

There's no such thing as a brain transplant, so taking care of this organ should be your top priority. "The best thing you can do is get enough sleep," says Rhonna Shatz, DO, associate professor of neurology at Wayne State University in Detroit. Yet as we struggle to allot enough time to the job, kids, family, friends, and *Lost,* sleep stands out as a suspiciously long block of idle hours. We set the alarm early, stay up late, and order a tall whatever-we-want to help us get by on the minimum. But the fact is: When you lose sleep, you lose your health.

Experts say most of us need about 8 hours of sleep a night, but half of us don't get it. And more than 80 percent of working women report exhaustion. According to the National Sleep Foundation's annual survey, US adults get, on average, just 6.7 hours of sleep a night. Now researchers are discovering that a decline in sleep time means a decline in your health. Some examples:

• Getting just an hour or two less sleep than needed per night can impair brain function. "You don't cycle enough through deep sleep, the stage when your body solidifies and stores memories," Dr. Shatz explains.

• Insufficient sleep is associated with cancer, heart disease, obesity, and diabetes—not to mention early death.

• It's also a risk factor for depression, infertility, miscarriage, and postpartum depression.

To top it off, sleeping less to do more doesn't even work: People who skimp on sleep may be devoting more hours to getting things done, but they work more slowly and accomplish less. "There really isn't a good substitute for sleep," says Donna Arand, PhD, a psychologist and the clinical director of the Sleep Disorders Center at Kettering Medical Center in Dayton, Ohio.

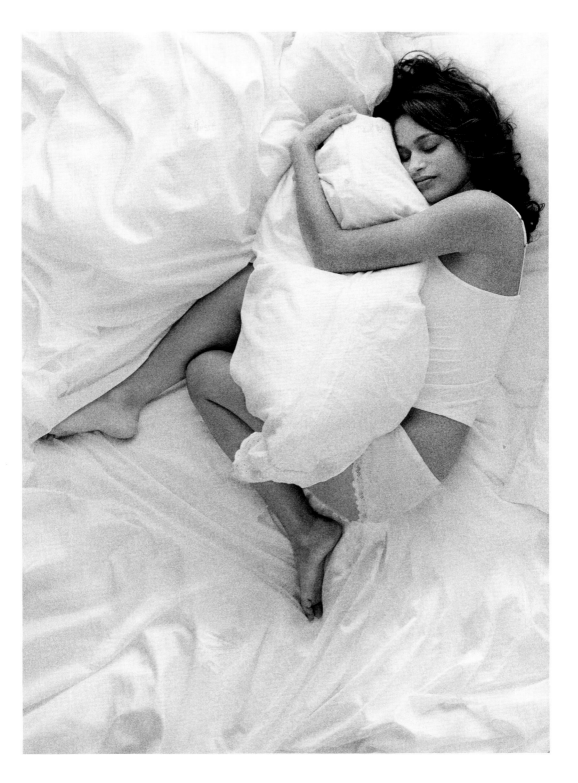

Scientists haven't yet grasped all the functions of sleep, but they know that sleep is needed every bit as intensely as food or water. It enables our bodies to regulate temperature and fight off infection. It may help our brains retain things we learned the previous day. If you take a peek inside your body and brain during a typical night's sleep, you'll find out how it rejuvenates you and why you should care. Let's start at the beginning, as your day is winding down . . .

9:34 p.m. It's been a crazy week, but with your 2-year-old daughter tucked in, tonight you found a much-needed hour to address invitations to your mom's retirement party. Now it's not even 10 o'clock and you're actually in bed, alone, with a mug full of peppermint tea and a new cookbook you've been dying to page through. When you start having trouble grasping the distinction between chiffon and meringue, you realize you're getting drowsy and reach for the light.

10:01 p.m. At this moment your bloodstream is full of a sleep-triggering chemical called adenosine. Adenosine is created whenever your body does work. So as you went about your day—thinking, talking, driving, digesting—adenosine was accumulating, gradually telling your brain that it was time to sleep. If you were to drink a cup of coffee right now, it would jolt you awake because caffeine wedges itself into the places in brain cells where adenosine would normally attach, preventing the fatigue signal from reaching your brain.

10:03 p.m. When you're awake, the electrical activity in your brain is varied—slow, fast, strong, faint. But when you fall asleep, your brain waves slow and synchronize. You initially enter a doze, known as Stage 1 sleep, from which you can be easily awakened. Falling asleep should take at least 5 minutes; tonight it took you 2. According to experts, that's a sign of a problem—it means you're overtired. "One of the major misconceptions is that it's a good thing if you fall asleep as soon as your head hits the pillow," says Kathryn Lee, PhD, a sleep specialist and nursing professor at the University of California at San Francisco. "Actually, it means you're a sleep-deprived person."

Over the next hour or so, you transition into increasingly intense slumber. Next comes Stage 2. This is "baseline" sleep—over the course of the night you'll spend half your time in this state, but not all at once. Right now you spend just 15 to 20 minutes here before entering Stages 3 and 4, known as slow-wave sleep, the deepest and most restorative kind. You're breathing evenly and slowly, the very picture of serenity. Then every-

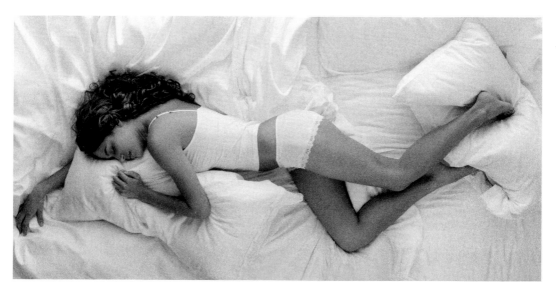

thing changes. You shift into REM (rapid eye movement) sleep. Your brain emits a cacophony of electrical signals—it's as active as when you are awake. But you're not awake, of course. REM sleep is the phase when most dreaming occurs. Your eyes dart back and forth, and the muscles in your arms and legs are paralyzed. Sleep researchers believe this inertia may have evolved to prevent us from acting out our dreams.

11:38 p.m. One 90- to 110-minute sleep cycle ends and the next begins. Each of the ensuing cycles will contain a different proportion of light, medium, deep, and REM sleep.

Although experts don't yet fully understand what sleep is for, they know it is crucial: Rats normally live 2 years or more, but when deprived of sleep they die within 3 weeks. If you stay awake for 24 hours straight, you will involuntarily begin undergoing regular bursts of "microsleep"—2- to 3-second intervals in which you essentially lose consciousness. An Australian study published in the journal *Nature* found that people kept awake for 28 hours did as poorly on a hand-eye coordination test as did people who were legally drunk (having a blood alcohol concentration of 1.0).

But you don't have to pull an all-nighter to feel the effects of sleep loss. The past few nights, you've stayed up late—to work, pay bills, help your husband pack for a business trip. You think you do fine on 6 hours' sleep, but you're actually accumulating a "sleep debt." Recent research shows that spending just a couple of hours less in bed each night for a week or two—basically your normal schedule—lowers your spirits. "Sleep deprivation has significant impacts on mood in healthy individuals," says J. Todd Arnedt, PhD, a University of Michigan, Ann Arbor, sleep specialist. "People get more depressed; they may get more anxious." Sleep loss also slows your reflexes and impairs your memory, judgment, and mental acuity. In a landmark 2003 University of Pennsylvania study, people who were limited to 6 hours of sleep per night for 2 weeks did significantly worse on tests of alertness and reasoning than people who got their full 8 hours.

But get this: The subjects in the Penn study had no idea how impaired they were. They reported an initial increase in sleepiness, but as time wore on they did not complain of additional exhaustion, though their test scores continued to decline. "One of the first things that goes in our

Some people inherit genes that make them early birds.

brains is our insight," says Joyce Walsleben, PhD, a psychologist at New York University's Sleep Disorders Center. "A sleepy person generally does not perceive how badly they are functioning."

Thankfully, your sleep debt can be paid, and you don't have to make up every lost hour. When you're overtired you slip more quickly into slow-wave sleep and stay there longer, which helps you recover faster. But don't make a practice of playing catch-up—repaying your sleep debt works only in small doses (and there's no set ratio for how much makeup time is needed). If the deprivation is chronic, catching up won't work. "When you stress the system, you can recover. Will it always recover 100 percent? Some of those problems are more likely to stay with you as time goes on," says Damon Salzman, MD, director of the Sleep-Wake Disorders Center at New York–Presbyterian Hospital in White Plains, New York.

3:21 a.m. You're awakened by your daughter calling for you. You grope for your slippers, go into her room, then sit with her as she sinks back to sleep. If only it were that easy for you. Back in bed, you can't stop your mental gears from grinding. Should you ask your sister to chip in for the party expenses? What will you say in your toast?

3:56 a.m. You glance at the clock for the third time—and feel the pressure. Recent research reveals that getting an hour or two less sleep than you need on a regular basis doesn't just slow your brain and make you irritable, it's a risk factor for illness, including heart disease and diabetes.

Sleep loss also hampers your immune system, making you more susceptible to colds and the flu. And it might make you fat. People who sleep less than 7 hours a night are more likely to be obese, and in 2004 researchers at the University of Chicago discovered one of the reasons why. In people who had slept just 4 hours for 2 consecutive nights, they found an 18 percent decrease in leptin, a hormone that tells your brain you're full, and a 28 percent increase in ghrelin, a hormone that triggers hunger.

4:03 a.m. You happen to be in the second half of your menstrual cycle. That means your body is producing lots of progesterone, a reproductive hormone that in animal experiments has been shown to induce sleep. So you fall back to sleep. If instead you were about to get your period, a time when progesterone levels drop, you might have had more trouble. If this is a monthly problem, experts suggest you take sleeping pills just for those couple of days.

4:25 a.m. The time between now and your alarm—the last few hours of sleep—may be especially important: Recent research suggests that this is when your brain rehearses what you learned the previous day. And "sleeping on it" does more than help you remember new things—it may make you better at them. In a 2002 study, scientists asked people to type a sequence of numbers over and over. The volunteers got faster with practice, then plateaued. Tested later in the day, they performed no better, but the next day, after the benefit of a good night's sleep, they sped up an additional 20 percent. Curtailed sleep eliminates those sorts of gains.

So as for that cake-decorating class you took yesterday: Right now, your brain is reviewing how to color the icing and choose the appropriate nib for the pastry bag. Thanks to tonight's sleep, when you bake a cake for your mom's party, you'll fashion sugary roses more expertly than you did in class. "It will feel sort of magical to you, but your performance will have improved," says Robert Stickgold, PhD, a Harvard Medical School neuroscientist who coauthored the typing study.

7:00 a.m. *Banh banh banh banh. . .* You fumble for the alarm. You've never been a morning person—now it turns out your preference for sleeping in is genetic. Coordinating basic daily needs to Earth's 24-hour light/dark cycle is so crucial to survival that even the most primitive creatures possess internal biological clocks. These clocks tell them when to forage for food, when to rest, when to mate, when to migrate. In humans the clock regulates sleep through the release of the hormone melatonin—that substance sold as a sleep aid at health food stores.

In recent years biologists have discovered at least 10 "clock" genes, and these genes, it turns out, occur in more than one variety. Some people

Turn Off Your Headaches

When neurologist Joel Saper, MD, began his career 35 years ago, experts argued that women suffered from migraines more often than men as a result of their "anxious natures." Dr. Saper rejected that idea, and new research linking women's higher headache rates to estrogen receptors in the brain backs him up. "These days, nearly everyone can find relief thanks to new therapies like neurostimulation, which may 'turn off' headaches by using electrical pulses to block the sensation of pain in the brain," says Dr. Saper, director of the head pain treatment unit at Chelsea Community Hospital in Ann Arbor, Michigan.

Lose the flab, stop the stab. "Eating a healthy diet and losing excess weight can actually help reduce the frequency of migraines," Dr. Saper says. "Evidence shows that the heavier a woman is, the more estrogen her body produces and the more headaches she tends to have."

Avoid pill pitfalls. "Many pain medications, if used too often, cause a rebound effect that leads to even more headaches," says David Buchholz, MD, associate professor of neurology at Johns Hopkins University. Instead, he suggests taking a preventive approach, which includes 8 hours or more of sleep each night and regular exercise. Also keep in mind: Other types of drugs—including birth control and antidepressants—often increase headaches, and may be best avoided.

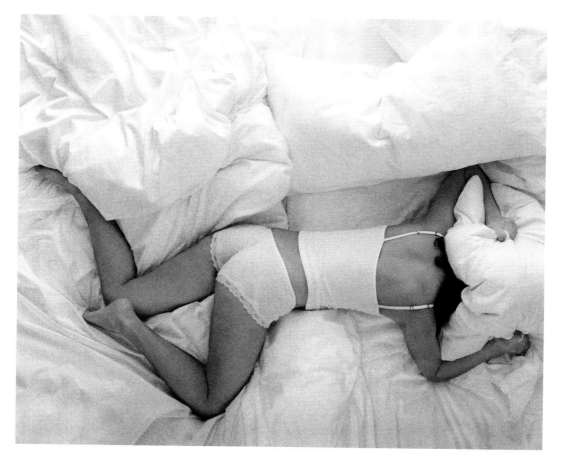

inherit genes that make them natural early birds; others are born to be late risers. It's biology that makes your inner morning person reassert itself after cramming for a deadline. "When the pressure to change goes away, you're likely to slip back," Dr. Salzman says.

Now that you've showered, though, you're feeling unusually chipper. It's been a while since you felt so rested. You actually have the energy to multitask, scanning the headlines as you pack your lunch. And when you snap your daughter into her car seat to drive her to day care and yourself to work, that extra sleep will make you both safer. The National Transportation Safety Board estimates that driver fatigue causes at least

100,000 auto accidents a year. Crashes are more likely in people sleeping less than 6 hours a night, and, according to the National Sleep Foundation's poll, 28 percent of adults drive drowsy at least once a month.

Maybe, you think, you should try harder to get enough sleep. You make an effort to accomplish so many other things. And what could be more important than your mood, your health, and your family's safety? "It's just a matter of prioritization," says Eric Olson, MD, codirector of the Mayo Sleep Disorders Center in Rochester, Minnesota. "People have to decide where sleep falls in how they're going to spend the 24 hours we're all limited to."

28
Percentage of adults who drive drowsy at least once a month

Secrets to a Good Night's Rest

WHAT WORKS—AND WHAT DOESN'T— IN THE FRUSTRATING QUEST FOR SLUMBER.

By Paige Greenfield

According to the 2009 results of the National Sleep Foundation's annual Sleep in America poll, 64 percent of adults in the US have trouble sleeping at least a few nights a week, and 41 percent say it's a nightly occurrence. What's more, the same survey found that women are 10 percent more likely than men to report insomnia.

Unless you live next door to a 24-hour car-alarm testing facility, the likely cause is stress. Chronic anxiety makes your adrenaline and cortisol spike, your heart race, and your blood pressure increase. The result: You feel as if you're hooked up to a nonstop caffeine drip. "Stress shifts the brain and body into fifth gear, but you need to be in neutral to fall asleep," says Donna Arand, PhD, of the Kettering Medical Center Sleep Disorders Center in Dayton, Ohio.

Experts say that if you find yourself suffering from acute insomnia—a week or two of very poor sleep quality—you need help. "For a lot of people, insomnia takes on a life of its own," says Wilfred Pigeon, PhD, a sleep specialist at the University of Rochester in New York. "The longer someone has insomnia, the more intractable it becomes." Why? Because when you spend night after night lying awake, you start to anticipate not falling asleep, and you develop habits that prolong the problem. Here, the nation's leading sleep experts help you put your anxieties to bed.

1. **Sleep Stopper:** Going directly from your desktop to your pillowtop **Solution:** Create a routine that sets you up for snoozing.

If you give your body cues that it's time for bed, you'll drift off faster once your head hits the pillow. "About 20 minutes before bedtime, step into a hot shower or bath," recommends Michael Breus, PhD, author of *Beauty Sleep: Look Younger, Lose Weight and Feel Great through Better Sleep*. Warm water relieves muscle tension, and when you step out, the cool air dials down your inner thermostat, mimicking the way your body naturally cools itself during sleep.

2. **Sleep Stopper:** Watching financial doom and gloom on the 10 o'clock news **Solution:** Laugh at funny reruns.

"Watching CNN before bed is like eating a spicy meal and then trying to nod off," says Rubin Naiman, PhD, a sleep specialist at Andrew Weil's Center for Integrative Medicine at the University of Arizona. Old-school advice calls for switching off the tube, but new research suggests that sitcoms may be a better antidote. A 2008 review of scientific literature confirms that laughter results in decreases in heart rate, respiratory rate, and blood pressure. (Just don't watch in bed, because the blue glow from the TV can keep you awake.)

3.

Sleep Stopper: Lying in bed planning tomorrow's to-do list
Solution: Do a data dump at dinner.
At least 2 hours before bedtime, write out tomorrow's to-do list and jot down a possible solution next to each item. "The only time most of us have a moment to ourselves is when we're trying to fall asleep," says Mark Mahowald, MD, a neurologist and director of the Minnesota Regional Sleep Disorders Center. And we typically don't spend it calmly recalling last summer's vacation; we use it to worry about unfinished business, he says. Cycling through your thoughts earlier in the evening will desensitize you to them later on. "If you start thinking about a task on the list when you're trying to fall asleep, remind yourself that you have a plan," Dr. Arand says.

4.

Sleep Stopper: Taking a trip down what-if way
Solution: Balance your perspective.
"People tend to catastrophize when they feel stressed," says Karen Reivich, PhD, a research associate at the University of Pennsylvania's Positive Psychology Center and coauthor of *The Resilience Factor*. Next time a problem has you in bed wrapped up in what-ifs, follow Reivich's Rx: Draw a line down the middle of a sheet of paper. On one side, list all your worst-case scenarios until you come up dry. On the other side, write the best possible outcome for the same situation. Balancing catastrophic scenarios against their best-case counterparts makes it clear that neither is likely to happen. So you can rest assured that the actual outcome will probably be somewhere in the middle and something you can handle.

5.

Sleep Stopper: Downing a pinot to take the edge off a rough day
Solution: Practice relaxation techniques that work.
Alcohol suppresses the central nervous system, so drinking can help you doze off. But 3 or 4 hours later, once your body has broken down that half bottle of vino, it acts as a stimulant—meaning you're wide awake at 3 a.m. and unable to fall back asleep, Dr. Arand says. Next time, try these techniques to keep you snoozing through the night.

- **Ease your breathing.** "Your respiratory rate slows about 20 percent during sleep," says Dr. Breus. Inhale all the way, then let it out. Repeat.
- **Picture yourself on a warm beach.** Visual imagery can replace stressful thoughts with soothing ones. Even mentally planning tomorrow's outfit may help you drift off faster (and cut down on morning prep time).
- **Flex, relax, repeat.** Tense the muscles in your right foot for 10 seconds, then release. Repeat on the left side, then work the rest of your body's muscles one by one. This exercise helps you relax and puts your focus back in the here and now.

6.

Sleep Stopper: Frequently checking your alarm clock
Solution: Organize your night table.
Turn your clock around so the numbers face the wall; the constant reminder that you're running out of sleep time adds stress. In a no-boss kind of world, the ideal is to go to bed early enough so that you wake up naturally—and don't need to be buzzed at 6:15 a.m. "If you absolutely need an alarm clock to get out of bed, you're not sleeping enough," says Meir Kryger, MD, author of *A Woman's Guide to Sleep Disorders*.

27
Percentage of people who are kept awake by money worries

7.

Sleep Stopper: You're tossing and turning.
Solution: Don't take it lying down.
If you can't sleep, get out of bed. Wrestling with pillows only conditions your brain to associate your bed with sleeping problems. Get up, get out, and do something else until you feel sleepy again. First stop: The fridge. Milk is rich in the amino acid tryptophan, which affects serotonin, a neurotransmitter that is key to sleep, according to Duke University's Andrew Krystal, MD. Just don't do anything too active. Exercising close to bedtime can keep you awake. Sex, fortunately, is an exception.

10 Instant Sighs of Relief

UNFORTUNATELY, A RESTFUL NIGHT'S SLEEP OR AN HOUR AT THE GYM ISN'T ALWAYS POSSIBLE. HERE ARE THE BEST WAYS TO BEAT STRESS IN 10 MINUTES OR LESS.

1 Second: Swear

Researchers at England's University of East Anglia Norwich looked into leadership styles and found that using swear words can reduce stress and can actually boost camaraderie among co-workers. Good luck, asshole!

5 Seconds: Pop Fish Oil

According to research from the University of Pittsburgh, people with the highest blood levels of EPA and DHA omega-3 fatty acids are happier, less impulsive, and more agreeable. Try a daily supplement of 400 milligrams each of EPA and DHA fish oils.

10 Seconds: Eat Dark Chocolate

A study published in *Proceedings of the National Academy of Sciences of the United States of America* showed that the flavonoids in cocoa relax your body's blood vessels. Look for low-fat dark chocolate, which has more stress-busting flavonoids than milk chocolate.

30 Seconds: Know Your Hoku

Acupressure is a quick tension releaser, according to researchers at Hong Kong Polytechnic University who found it can reduce stress by up to 39 percent. For fast relief, massage your *hoku* (the fleshy part between the thumb and index finger) for 20 to 30 seconds. "This is the universal pressure point for easing upper-body tension," says Patrice Winter, a spokeswoman for the American Physical Therapy Association.

30 Seconds: Sit Back

Forget what you've been told about sitting up straight to relieve tension in your back. Researchers at the University of Alberta Hospital in Edmonton found that leaning back at a 135-degree angle is the best sitting position for alleviating back pain.

1 Minute: Add Garlic

Researchers at the University of Alabama at Birmingham believe they've figured out why garlic is good for heart health, and their finding implies it's a powerful stress buster too. When you digest garlic's main ingredient, organosulfur allicin, your body produces hydrogen sulfide, which relaxes blood vessels and increases bloodflow.

5 Minutes: Take a YouTube Timeout

Just the anticipation of laughing decreases the stress hormones 3,4-dihydroxyphenylacetic acid, cortisol, and epinephrine by 38, 39, and 70 percent, respectively, according to researchers at Loma Linda University in California. And when researchers at the University of Maryland in College Park showed short movie clips to study participants, those who watched funny films experienced a 22 percent increase in bloodflow to their hearts.

10 Minutes: Just Do It

Kissing or hugging can reduce stress because it raises levels of oxytocin, the hormone associated with bonding and love, say researchers at the University of North Carolina at Chapel Hill. And a Scottish researcher found that having sex regularly lowers anxiety, stress, and blood pressure. No need to take our word for it, though—find out for yourself!

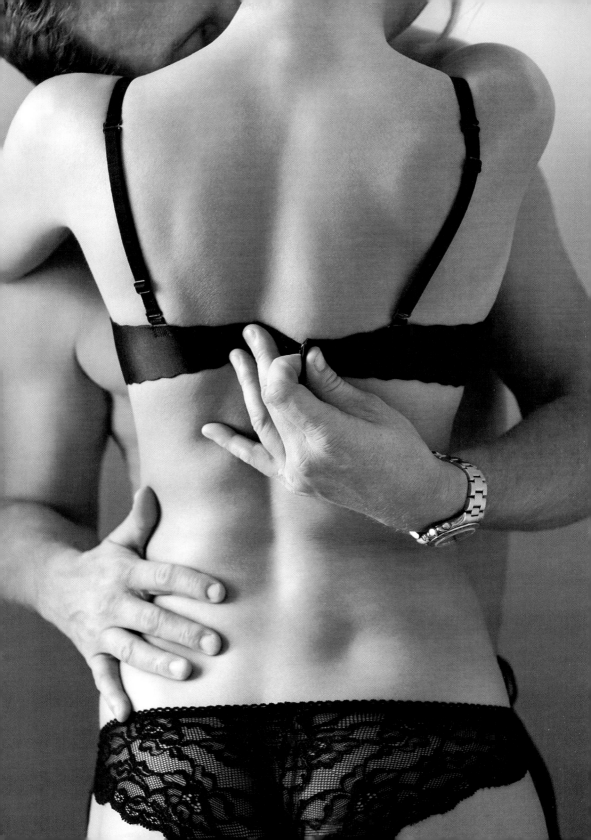

Go Ahead, Laugh Your A** Off!

NEW STUDIES ARE REVEALING THE SURPRISING HEALTH BENEFITS OF BUSTING A GUT.

By Dan Ferber

Let's say your boss pops into your office, and instead of that third-quarter report on your screen, she spies Sarah Silverman spewing one of her infamously off-color jokes: "When God gives you AIDS—and God does give you AIDS, by the way—make LemonAIDS." Mortification would be the typical go-to response. But if you both knew that cracking up makes you smarter, more creative, and more productive, you'd tilt the screen her way, turn up the volume, and get your giggles on.

Laughter, it turns out, nearly rivals exercise when it comes to health and brain-boosting powers. For starters, a Loma Linda University study found that it raised levels of disease-fighting immunoglobulins by 14 percent. Another at UCLA discovered that kids could endure having their hands submerged in ice water 40 percent longer while watching comedies. And a cardiologist at the University of Maryland Medical Center in Baltimore measured subjects' bloodflow as they watched *There's Something about Mary* and concluded that laughter increases circulation about as much as a treadmill session.

Beyond the physical perks, a few guffaws can sharpen your thinking. Ron Berk, PhD, a recently retired psychologist from Johns Hopkins Medical School, started using jokes and gags back in 1993 to combat his students' lecture-induced narcolepsy. He soon noticed that his one-liners did more than keep them awake; they caused a spike in their test scores. To prove it, he and a colleague divided 98 students in a graduate biostatistics class into two groups. Each took the same 57-item exam, but one group's test had funny instructions. As the two researchers reported in the scientific journal *Humor,* the students who got a dose of silliness scored significantly higher on the exam.

The results of that experiment probably didn't surprise one school of brainiacs: positive psychologists. Unlike traditional psychologists, who focus on negative emotions such as fear and anger, these guys research desirable feelings like happiness and satisfaction. Until the past decade or so, scientists knew astonishingly little about the benefits of feeling good. In the late 1990s, Barbara Fredrickson, PhD, a psychologist at the University of North Carolina, came up with a theory: A positive state of mind—whether caused by humor, love, or contentment—broadens people's thinking and ability to adapt to changing circumstances.

An experiment with penguins illustrates the

30
Times you're more likely to laugh in company of others than alone

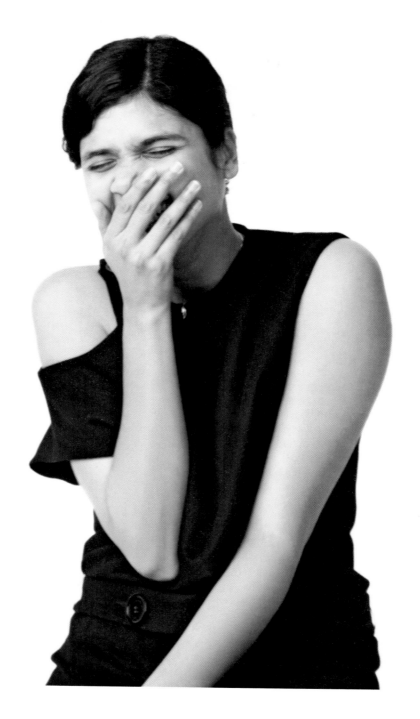

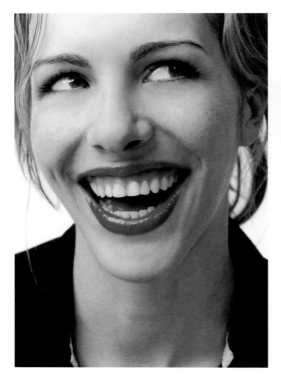

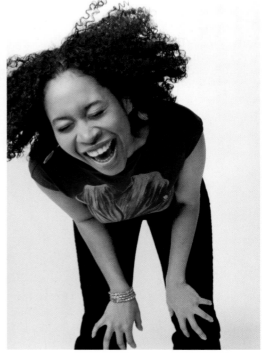

point. In a 2005 study, Fredrickson showed 104 undergraduates a 2-minute video of waddling penguins that only a major scrooge could fail to find funny. An equal number of students watched an abstract video of, er, colored lines, which left them predictably unmoved. Then Fredrickson tested the students for big-picture thinking by showing them four small triangles arranged as a square or three small squares arranged as a triangle. Amused subjects were significantly more likely to focus on the overall pattern rather than the component shapes: They were better able to see the big picture, literally.

In a separate experiment, students were asked to watch the penguins and list up to 20 things they'd like to do at that moment. The people who had watched the goofy film thought of more things to do, which indicates more flexible and creative thinking.

How does humor help us think? Scientists are

14

Percentage that laughing raises disease–fighting immunoglobulins

pretty sure it has to do with the way amusement stimulates the brain's reward center. In a landmark 2003 study at Stanford, researchers put subjects in MRI machines and showed them *Bizarro* cartoons. When they got a joke, a midbrain area known as the nucleus accumbens became active. The nucleus accumbens is part of a neural pathway that scientists call a reward circuit, the same one that's triggered when we eat chocolate or have sex. There's evidence that this circuit pumps out dopamine, a brain-signaling chemical that stimulates the frontal lobe—the place where we do most of our mental heavy lifting. So humor and other positive feelings effectively fuel our noodles.

It's amazing what a little kidding can do for your social life. Consider that jelly-bellied Jack Black scores leading roles opposite the likes of Cameron Diaz and Kate Winslet or that beady-eyed Vince Vaughn got a shot at Jennifer Aniston.

Making chicks laugh can transform so-so guys into studs—and we have more than celeb examples to back that up. Researchers at McMaster University in Ontario recently had more than 200 college students examine photos of members of the opposite sex accompanied by either funny or bland quotes. Women rated the funny men as more attractive. But while guys said they preferred a woman with a good sense of humor, they didn't actually find the funny females foxier. These egomaniacs did, however, rate women who found them funny as more attractive.

Off the meet market, goofing around can help you warm up to a new bud. In 2000, Arthur Aron, PhD, a social psychologist at the State University of New York at Stony Brook, separated 96 undergraduates into same-sex pairs and had one teach the other dance moves. In half of the pairs, the "teacher" held a straw in her teeth, which garbled her speech, and the "student" was blindfolded. The shenanigans elicited plenty of giggles, and the pairs who laughed together reported feeling closer afterward than those who took the exercise seriously.

According to Dr. Aron, humor softens us up by distracting us from the anxiety we feel when meeting someone new and by creating the sensation of something exciting, which makes the experience more pleasurable. Experts also believe that people who can see the funny side of a situation have a greater level of "emotional intelligence"—the ability to manage their own emotions and accurately read another person's. In a 2006 study, Rod Martin, PhD, professor of clinical psychology at the University of Western Ontario and past president of the International Society for Humor Studies, gave students questionnaires to measure their senses of humor, then had them analyze the emotions of faces on a computer screen. The upshot: People who joke around more often tend to read other people better. Not surprising when you consider that humor usually involves addressing touchy subjects in a way that's provocative but not upsetting, e.g., making LemonAIDS.

Silly skills score points at work too. Fabio Sala, PhD, an organizational psychologist at EMC Corporation, analyzed audiotapes of 20 male executives. The execs rated "outstanding" by their staff used humor—by either cracking jokes or cracking up—more than twice as often as those rated "average."

Whether at home, on a date, or in the office, humor works kind of like a couple of martinis—only better. It greases the social wheels by reducing stress and putting people at ease. And luckily, you don't have to be as funny as Sarah Silverman to reap the benefits. All you have to do is laugh.

What's So Funny?

THE SCIENCE BEHIND THE
THINGS THAT SPLIT YOUR SIDES

A falling anvil crushes a cuddly cartoon character; a grown man dresses like an elf; a dinner guest washes his face in the toilet. Why do we laugh at this stuff?

It's all about incongruity, scientists say. When we expect one thing and get another, the surprise triggers several different areas of the brain at once, causing our diaphragms to convulse and goofy sounds to come out of our mouths. But incongruities are funny only when no one gets hurt, says Paul McGhee, PhD, psychologist and author of Health, Healing and the Amuse System. The cartoon character feels no pain. The man in the elf costume isn't really insane. And the toilet has just been cleaned. (You hope.)

But what tickles your funny bone might not tickle his. Northwestern University's Jennifer Hay, PhD, taped adult friends as they hung out together. Women were eight times more likely than men to tell funny, revealing stories about themselves. Men went more for slapstick and canned jokes and used humor to impress others rather than to bond.

And sometimes we laugh when there's nothing remotely funny—to let off steam, to show we're friendly, to connect. According to Robert R. Provine, PhD, author of Laughter: A Scientific Investigation, people laugh 30 times more often with others than alone, even when they're watching the same comedy. "If you want more laughter in your life," Dr. Provine says, "spend more time with friends." Even if they're not particularly funny.

The Pursuit of Happiness

IT HAS A BAD RAP AS A COMPLICATED, ELUSIVE
GOAL THAT WE CAN SPEND OUR WHOLE LIVES CHASING. BUT
LIKE ANYTHING ELSE, IT GETS A HELL OF A LOT
EASIER WHEN YOU HAVE SOME REALLY GOOD ADVICE.

*T*he bottom line of any self-help book at Barnes and Noble is probably the same mantra you used to hear from your mother: "You have to make *yourself* happy." Great advice, yes. But what if you don't know how to make yourself happy? What if you're trying your damnedest, but your best days seem as much the result of blind luck as strategic planning? Could there be some secret formula out there for attaining happiness?

The answer to that question is yes—and, surprisingly, no prescription drugs are involved. A small but increasing number of psychologists have shifted the focus of their work from curing mental illness to discovering which character traits, attitudes, and habits make people deeply and lastingly happy. These "positive psychologists" figure that while alleviating conditions such as depression and anxiety are worthy goals, most people don't want to settle for feeling "not bad." They want to feel really, really good. Amen to that.

Of course, it's impossible to be happy all of the time. "We've found that even the top 10 percent of happy people, rigorously measured, have some unhappy moments every day," says Martin Seligman, PhD, author of *Authentic Happiness* and founder of the positive psychology movement. While adversity—whether in the form of a bitchy cashier, a failed relationship, or a natural disaster—is unavoidable, research shows that the positive feelings you have deep down about yourself, the people close to you, and the world at large can be profoundly and permanently improved.

Find Your Good Side

Between college psych classes, daytime talk shows, and those leading questions posed by pharmaceutical ads ("Have you been feeling bored, tired, or unmotivated?"), most people have already self-diagnosed their "mental weaknesses," not mention those of their friends, family members, and significant others: obsessive-compulsive disorder, social anxiety, fear of failure, attention–deficit/hyperactivity disorder . . . call it a postmodern hobby. But if happiness is really what you're after, you need to quit zeroing in on your pathologies and start pinpointing—and using—your strengths. "Countless therapies advocate focusing on your shortcomings, but doing so can often cause you to backslide and feel worse," Dr. Seligman says. "Identifying and burnishing your signature strengths, however, is fun and effective for increasing positive emotion, and there's no backsliding."

In this model of happiness building, everyone wins because everyone has built-in, signature strengths just waiting to be tapped. People who

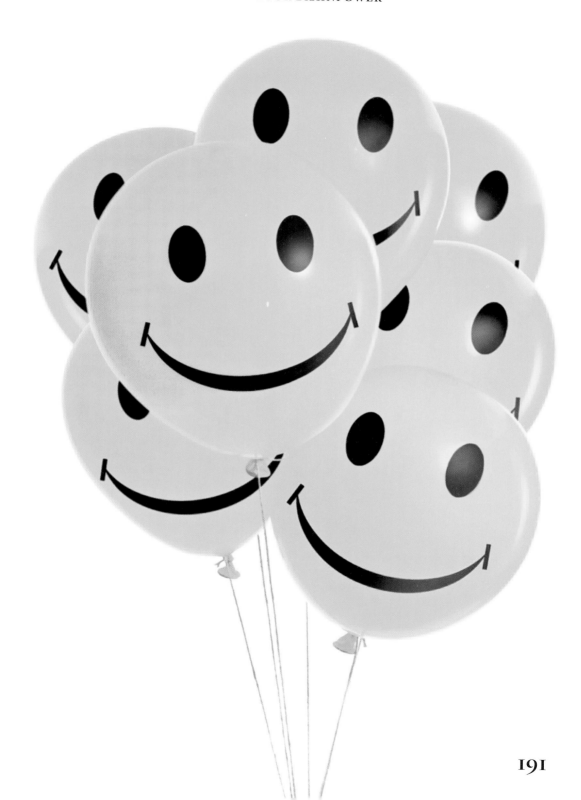

detest teamwork are advised to revel in their originality. The seldom cautious can take pride in their passion. It doesn't matter what your virtues happen to be, as long as you know what they are. (To reveal your top five strengths, take the "Satisfaction Guaranteed" quiz on page 195.) Citing dozens of psychological studies as backup, Dr. Seligman states that finding ways to use your character strengths on a daily basis will directly lead to feeling better about yourself and your life in general.

The reason it works is simple: Doing good makes you feel good. And since there's no struggle or massive transformation necessary, the warm, fuzzy effects start to kick in immediately. You increase your sense of self-worth. You're more confident and more fulfilled. Even if you have a bad day, a bad week, or a bad year, you rest more easily at night knowing that— at least in some ways—you're a fundamentally good person.

Fuel Your Resilience

Since adversity is inevitable, getting better at enduring and bouncing back from negative situations will do more for your overall happiness than trying to avoid them. "A common misconception about happy people is that few bad things have ever happened to them, or that they don't have their share of down days," says the University of Pennsylvania's Karen Reivich, PhD. "The truth is that happy people are just better at acknowledging that setbacks are only temporary." And while that translates to being more optimistic, it doesn't mean being unrealistic. A recent eye-opening study led by Harvard psychologist Daniel Gilbert, PhD, revealed that people almost always overestimate the damage negative events will have on their lives. According to Dr. Gilbert's research, "common events typically influence people's subjective well-being for little more than a few months, and even uncommon events—such as losing a child in a car accident or being diagnosed with cancer—seem to have less impact on long-term happiness than one might naively expect." Telling yourself that you're going to be okay, it turns out, isn't a white lie. It's a fact of life.

For those times when things go so wrong you can't even remember what right looks like, Dr. Reivich presents some simple techniques that will help you avoid getting sucked into a black hole.

• It may seem depressing, but thinking back to past events that you were convinced would crush you (okay, it is depressing) will ultimately reveal that you're tougher than you think. Whether it was a breakup, a botched interview, or a broken

To foster optimism, write down what you're thankful for.

ankle on the first day of a weeklong vacation in Vail, Colorado, you survived and managed to be happy again, right? Right.

• No one likes being the girl blubbering on her friend's shoulder at the end of the bar, but spilling your guts to the people who care about you is highly therapeutic. As your pile of wadded tissues grows, so does your sense of intimacy and connectedness with others, which scientists have found directly leads to greater happiness.

• Use good old corny gratitude like a drug. Richard Emmons, PhD, a psychologist at the University of California–Davis, found that simply writing down what you're thankful for helps alleviate depression and foster optimism. Before you go to bed, make a list of five ways other people have helped you during the day—whether it was a colleague who reminded you of a meeting or the guy who found your dry cleaning despite your lost ticket.

• Be your own defense attorney. Every time you catch yourself thinking in a melodramatically negative way, like "I can never do anything right" or "This relationship sucks," present yourself with cold, hard evidence to the contrary. Remember the time you solved a difficult problem and got tons of positive feedback. Flip through a photo album filled with visual proof of all the happy, romantic moments you've had with your significant other.

The more skillful you become at bouncing back, the less any kind of adversity will be able to shake your inner sense of well-being. Your new, high-resiliency motto: "Shit happens, but that doesn't mean I have to stand in it."

Engage in Mind-Bending Behavior

The discovery of antidepressants made it clear that changing your brain chemistry can have positive effects on your behavior. Studies now show that changes in behavior can also have positive effects on your brain chemistry. Take, for example, the work of Richard Davidson, PhD, professor of psychology and psychiatry at the University of Wisconsin in Madison. He monitored the brain activity of Tibetan Buddhist monks who had logged between 10,000 and 50,000 hours of meditation over the course of their lives. He found that while they were meditating, the area of their brains associated with happiness and positive thoughts—the left prefrontal cortex—lit up like the big screen at Yankee Stadium. And even when they weren't meditating, their happiness nodes were unusually active.

To find out if meditation could increase positive emotions in the average American, Dr. Davidson and Jon Kabat-Zinn, PhD, founder of the Stress Reduction Clinic at the University of Massachusetts Medical Center in Worcester, asked a group of employees at a biotech company to begin meditating just once a week for 8 weeks. Those who completed the study showed increased activity in their brains' pleasure centers and reported feeling more positive and at ease. Two months later, when they were tested again, the benefits were still noticeable. How do you start meditating? "You put aside a few minutes of your day to focus solely on the present moment," says Noah Levine, a Buddhist therapist, meditation instructor, and author of *Dharma Punx*. "The simplest way is to sit in a chair with your back straight, your hands resting on your knees, and your eyes closed. Concentrate on the sensation of your breath moving in and out of your body. When you notice your mind wandering away from your breath, gently refocus your attention."

You won't be surprised to hear that exercise has also been found to change your brain—and disposition—for the better. But the fact that exercise can be a more effective treatment for depression than drugs is pretty amazing news. Researchers at Duke University followed the progress of patients with major depressive disorders who were prescribed Zoloft, Zoloft combined with an exercise routine, or just plain exercise. Six months after the study ended, they found that the patients who had relied on exercise alone were more likely to be partly or fully recovered. In other words, whenever you decide that you're too tired, busy, or out of shape to move your body, you're basically asking for a bad mood.

Know That Some Big Things Matter Little . . .

Despite the fact that money can buy African safaris and hot young tennis instructors, it is nonetheless true that it doesn't have much impact on day-to-day happiness. Psychologists Daniel Kahneman, PhD, of Princeton University and David Schkade, PhD, of the University of California–San Diego conducted a survey of 909 working women that asked them to rate how much they had enjoyed the different activities they engaged in throughout the previous day. Wealthier women reported getting just about the same amount of pleasure as everyone else. Same goes for education. An advanced degree didn't result in greater satisfaction.

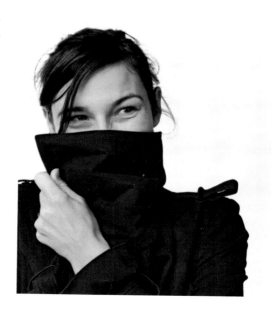

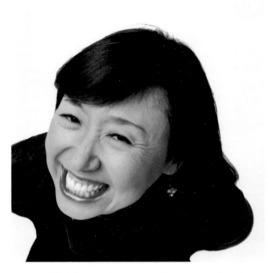

You'd think that in our youth-obsessed culture, young people would be happier and more optimistic than the old and wrinkled. Not the case. In a 2003 study of 144 participants, researchers at the University of California–Irvine found that while people in their twenties tend to dwell on negative images and memories, older people focus more on the positive. A different study conducted by psychologists at the University of California–Berkeley examined whether personality changes after the age of 30. It revealed that women become more warm, generous, and helpful in their thirties than they are in their twenties.

People who like to fantasize about how much happier they'd be if they moved to a sunnier location will have to find something else to daydream about. In 1999, Dr. Schkade and Dr. Kahneman discovered that college students from the West Coast didn't claim to be any more self-satisfied than students on the East Coast. And if you've always loved big families and are considering a minivan full of your own babies, you might want to take into consideration the results of a groundbreaking University of Pennsylvania study on parenthood and life satisfaction. Sociology professor Hans-Peter Kohler, PhD, found that while mothers with one child were at least 20 percent happier than childless women, having more than

one didn't increase happiness at all. In fact, two or more kids were shown to decrease satisfaction, due to increased stress.

…And That Some Little Things Matter Big

On the flip side, some small-scale, everyday stuff can produce disproportionate amounts of pleasure. Instead of the massive responsibility of raising a third child, for example, you'd be better off raising a little dog. According to the Mayo Clinic, caring for a cat or a dog will lower your blood pressure, help you deal better with stress, and add to your overall sense of well-being. In one study, AIDS patients with pets experienced less depression than those without. What does a pet offer that's so beneficial? Unconditional love.

Your nonfurry friends aren't anywhere near as forgiving, but insisting on squeezing them into your weekly schedule is another major harbinger of happiness. Study after study shows that extroverted people report feeling more fulfilled, and in that survey of 909 women, the activity enjoyed above all others was socializing with friends. Combining girlfriend time with a fun activity that requires skill and attention can be a veritable pleasure bomb, according to scientists who are studying the happiness-producing phenomenon known as "flow." The gist is that people enjoy themselves most when they're so fully engaged in what they're doing that they lose all sense of place, time, and even self. Theoretically, it's possible to achieve "flow" in just about any situation, but sports and hobbies are the most common.

Last but not least, you'll be much, much happier if you stop obsessively comparing yourself to people you think have better lives than you do. "To a certain degree, happiness is relative to others' attainments," says David G. Myers, PhD, author of *The Pursuit of Happiness*. "Whether we feel good or bad depends on who those others are." Go ahead and be inspired while watching gorgeous Scarlett Johansson stroll down the red carpet on Oscar night, just be sure to have a DVD of *Meet the Fockers* standing by. We're not saying that you should take pleasure in the sight of Ben Stiller being humiliated and embarrassed, but there's nothing wrong with reveling in the fact that you're you and not him.

Satisfaction Guaranteed

According to Martin Seligman, PhD, author of *Authentic Happiness*, feeling content with yourself and your life is as easy as recognizing the amazing personality strengths you already possess and using them as often as possible. To pinpoint your top virtues (most people find they have about five), take a quickie version of his quiz below.

Circle N (never), S (sometimes), or A (always), depending on how often you—honestly—feel that each statement is true about you.

1. This world is so damn fascinating that I could never be bored.................................**N S A**
2. No matter how things look, I don't jump to conclusions......................................**N S A**
3. I do what I think is right, even if it's difficult or unpopular.............................**N S A**
4. Taking time to help someone is a pleasure, not a chore................................**N S A**
5. Working as part of a team is fun and rewarding...**N S A**
6. People use the term "cutting edge" to describe me or my work...............................**N S A**
7. I am blown away by art, technology, or just looking at the sky.............................**N S A**
8. Every decision deserves careful consideration...**N S A**
9. I finish what I start..**N S A**
10. Compliments are embarrassing. I prefer to praise others...............................**N S A**
11. When I say "Count me in," I mean 100 percent in.....................................**N S A**
12. I seldom feel envious, because I'm already so lucky......................................**N S A**
13. I can do anything if I really set my mind to it..**N S A**
14. I don't easily get caught up in the details....**N S A**
15. Even if I can't stand someone, I treat him or her with respect.....................**N S A**
16. I believe I'm alive for an important reason..**N S A**
17. I say what I mean and mean what I say...**N S A**
18. There are people who would sacrifice everything for me and for whom I would sacrifice everything.........................**N S A**
19. I'm good at getting diverse people to work together......................................**N S A**
20. No matter where I am, I can connect with the people around me......................**N S A**
21. I jump at the chance to learn something—anything—new.........................**N S A**
22. I give people second and third chances....**N S A**
23. My emotions don't get the best of me........**N S A**
24. I crack myself up...**N S A**

Consider each statement for which you circled "A" to be one of the signature strengths you should show off regularly.

The Scorecard ....
 1. Curiosity..
 2. Good judgment..
 3. Courage...
 4. Kindness ....
 5. Teamwork..
 6. Originality ....
 7. Appreciation of beauty ....
 8. Caution ....
 9. Perseverance..
10. Modesty ....
11. Enthusiasm..
12. Gratitude ....
13. Optimism..
14. Perspective...
15. Fairness ....
16. Spirituality ....
17. Integrity and honest..
18. Capacity for love ....
19. Leadership ....
20. Social intelligence...
21. Passion for learning ....
22. Forgiveness ....
23. Self-control ....
24. Playfulness..

Chapter Eight

Build Lean Muscle

KEEP THAT TIGHT AND TONED LOOK FOR LIFE!

> INVESTMENT: 3 WEEKS
> AGE ERASED: 2 YEARS

Introduction

How does a woman's body grow stronger? Here's what happens when you engage in a weight-training program: Just before you, say, take a step to begin a lunge, your brain sends a message to your muscles—"We're about to lunge, folks!"—via your spinal cord. Muscles are made of bundles of fibers that contain two types of proteins, which slide across each other when given the green light, causing the fibers to contract. This motion moves the bones attached to the muscle, and off you go, bobbing across the gym floor.

As you move, the lunge causes microscopic tears in the muscle fibers involved. To repair them, your body rushes healing white blood cells, proteins, and other fix-its to the scene. This increases the size of the muscle fibers and strengthens them. *Ta da!*—next time at the gym, you can add two lunges to your set.

Resistance training will not turn you into the Hulk, however. It's just not in your blood. "Testosterone helps men gain bulk," says Suzanne Meth, MS, CSCS, a manager at Equinox Fitness in New York City. When men lift weights, the hormone causes their muscle fibers to grow. Since women have 20 to 30 percent less testosterone than guys do, we gain strength without the heft.

Unfortunately, some women think "resistance training" means walking past a shoe store and trying not to go inside. And that's bad: As you get older, your fast-twitch muscle fibers—the stringy part of your muscles responsible for generating power so you can jump to snag a shirt from the top shelf of your closet or sprint to your 10 o'clock appointment—get increasingly fickle. Maintaining muscle power requires fast, explosive movements, the kind you used to get playing soccer or hoops, but most of us stopped doing those once we graduated from middle school. But don't worry! So long as you're willing to sweat and feel a little burn in your muscles, you *can* keep your power levels high. Why wait? The only thing you need to transform your body into the one you've always wanted is the right direction, and that's what this chapter is all about.

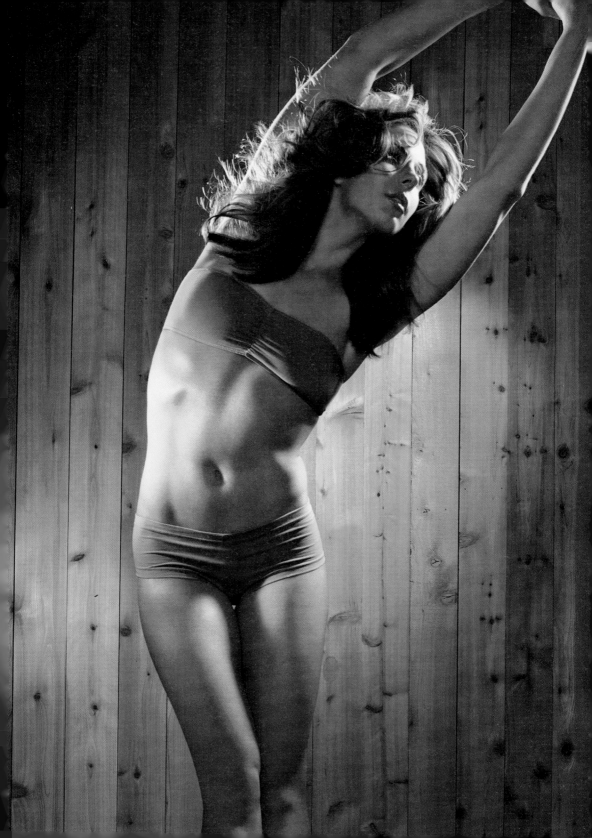

Part One

Create a Strong Fitness Strategy

Muscle, Defined

HOW TO MAKE THE MUSCLES RIPPLING UNDER YOUR SKIN
STRONG, SEXY, AND SO WORTH THE SWEAT.

By Allison Winn Scotch

When it comes to your body, knowledge is power. Literally. The better you understand your muscles and what they're capable of, the more you can do with them. But when there are about 650 muscles, and millions of individual fibers, to get intimate with, it's more than a little daunting. So we're going to keep it simple. Here's the least you need to know to get the most from your body.

Meet and Greet

You have three types of muscles: the cardiac muscle found in your ticker, the smooth muscle that lines such organs as your stomach and esophagus, and skeletal muscle, which attaches to your bones via tendons. You use these to suck in your belly at the beach or lift groceries onto your countertop. They make up 30 to 40 percent of your body mass and are largely voluntary, meaning that you make them move—except when someone scares the crap out of you.

Muscles Marinara

Grab a handful of dry spaghetti. This is what skeletal muscle looks like: Each strand of spaghetti represents a muscle fiber. These fibers are bundled together—larger muscles, such as your quads, pack up to 150 in one bunch—and huddle with other bundles to make up the entire muscle.

Grow What You've Got

How many muscle fibers you have was determined by the time you dumped your middle-school boyfriend. "The number may increase early in life, but it becomes set at puberty," says C. David Geier Jr., MD, director of sports medicine at the Medical University of South Carolina in Charleston. What you can control: how big the fibers get, which determines how tight and strong you look. The scientific word for muscle growth, by the way, is "hypertrophy."

We're Be-Twitched

All muscle fibers are not created equal. Slow-twitch fibers are perfect for endurance but don't pack a lot of power. Fast-twitch fibers do the opposite: They offer bursts of rapid-fire energy, but only for a short time. Your genes control how much of one type or the other you have. If you're looking to jack up your endurance for a marathon, hone your slow-twitchers by lifting two or three sets with lighter weights, eking out 12 to 15 reps in each set, suggests Jason Conviser, PhD,

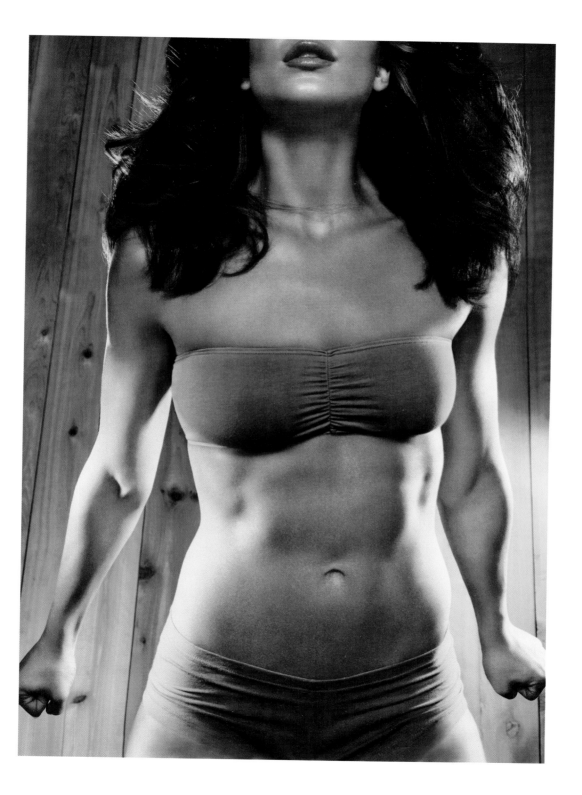

an exercise physiologist at Insight Psychological Center in Chicago. To improve your 5-K kick, do three sets of 8 reps using heavier weights.

Your Muscle Has an IQ

When you fire a power-punch in kickboxing class, your brain sends a signal down a nerve cell, telling certain muscle fibers in your arms, back, core, and legs to contract. After a series of microscopic chemical reactions—*bam!*—you deliver the KO blow. As you practice, your brain and muscles learn to communicate more efficiently and you become more coordinated.

Best. News. Ever.

If you can't fit "gym" on your to-do list, thinking about exercises may help bolster the pathways between your brain and your brawn. In 2007, researchers found that when healthy men and women spent 4 weeks visualizing themselves lifting weights, their actual strength went up 4 percent—without their hoisting a single dumbbell.

The Best Way to Safeguard Fast-Twitch Muscles

Add the jump squat to your gym routine. Stand with your feet shoulder-width apart, knees slightly bent, arms hanging at your sides. Keeping your torso as upright as possible, quickly bend your knees and lower your hips back and down until your thighs are parallel to the floor. Then immediately jump straight off the floor as high as you can. Land as softly as possible, sinking back down into a squat position—that's 1 rep. Repeat the jump. Do three to four sets of 6 reps, resting for 1 minute between sets.

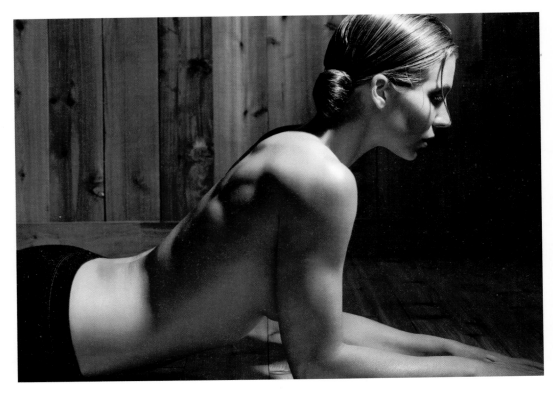

Step Into the Toned Zone

USE THESE 4 STRATEGIES TO DESIGN YOUR ULTIMATE WORKOUT.

By Liz Plosser

Designing your own workout can feel like an insurmountable challenge—which is why people hire personal trainers. You could do that . . . or you could learn from some of the nation's top trainers and fitness researchers, who have distilled their cumlative wisdom into this easy-to-understand, step-by-step system for customizing an exercise program. Follow these guidelines to create a personal fitness plan—and upgrade your body to the one you've always wanted.

1. Nail a Goal

And make it attainable and detailed. According to a American College of Sports Medicine study, women who set smaller, specific goals are 30 percent likelier to reach them than those who shoot for big, general ones. To keep things simple, pick one of these (the three most often heard by trainers): a toned upper body; flat, bikini-worthy abs; or a strong, lean lower body. Then write down a weekly plan or register at www.traineo.com. This site not only helps you track your workouts, it also lets you designate up to four motivators (co-worker, boyfriend, etc.) who will get weekly progress reports via e-mail. If you slack, it's their job to harass you.

2. Pick Six Moves

"Lifting weights two to three times a week is enough to get noticeable results without spending hours each day in the gym," says Tom Terwilliger, owner of Terwilliger Fitness in Denver. "But this means you need to hit every major muscle group whenever you work out." Aim for six moves per workout and be sure to target all of your key parts (abs, arms, back, chest, glutes, and legs). Use this chart to choose your moves. In all, the sequence shouldn't take longer than about five songs on your workout playlist.

YOUR GOAL	WORK YOUR	NUMBER OF MOVES
Toned Upper Body	Chest	1
	Back	1
	Arms	2
	Core	1
	Lower Body	1
Flat Abs	Core	3
	Chest	1
	Back	1
	Lower Body	1
Lean Lower Body	Glutes	2
	Quads	1
	Hamstrings	1
	Upper Body	1
	Core	1

Tackle the moves tied to your goal at the beginning of your workout when you have the most energy and focus.

3. Place Your Order

How many times have you saved your least favorite move for the end, only to rush through it while debating whether your post-gym beer counts as hydration? In a 2007 study published in the *Journal of Strength and Conditioning Research,* researchers found that women couldn't do as many reps toward the end of their workouts. "You lose mental focus, and your muscles fatigue during a strength session," says Jeffrey Willardson, PhD, an exercise physiologist at the University of Eastern Illinois in Charleston. Tackle the moves tied to your goal at the beginning of your workout when you have the most energy.

Some other general rules to lift by:

IF YOU WANT A TONED UPPER BODY Think big, then small. Do chest and upper-back exercises before targeting your smaller arm muscles. You'll work your biceps and triceps in most upper-body moves, and if you've already exhausted them with isolating moves, you won't get as much out of anything you do afterward.

IF YOU WANT FLAT ABS Squeeze them in. To get a firm, flat midsection even faster, insert a core exercise between your lower- and upper-body moves. "It will reactivate those muscles so they're constantly engaged during the workout," Terwilliger says. "It keeps them firing."

IF YOU WANT A LEAN LOWER BODY Start with your bum. Hit it first and hit it hard. Because your glutes are the biggest muscles of all, your rear end burns more calories than any other body part.

4. Get Your Numbers Straight

REPS The number of times you repeat a move is what strengthens your muscle fibers. How many reps do you need? That depends on your goal. If you want to . . .

Maximize strength: Do 4 to 6 reps with a weight heavy enough that you can barely get through the last one.

Maximize power (how fast the muscle can move): Do 8 to 12 reps.

Maximize endurance: Do 15 to 25 reps.

SETS Breaking up moves into groups of repetitions, or sets, allows you to get through more reps—because you can rest in between. Doing three sets is enough to challenge the muscle completely, Dr. Willardson says. If you're pressed for time, do one set of each move rather than skipping a move or two and doing all three sets. Studies show that you get 50 to 90 percent of your strength gains from your first set.

LOAD Generally, choose a weight that makes finishing your last set with good form barely doable. But once every four to six sessions, opt for a heft that leaves you totally spent after 4 to 6 reps (and, no, this doesn't get you out of the remaining two sets). This activates your fast-twitch muscles—needed for short bursts of strength. "In everyday life, they don't get called on as often as other muscle fibers," says Mike Godard, PhD, a professor of kinesiology at Western Illinois University in Macomb. "So they're especially important to pay attention to in the gym."

REST BETWEEN SETS Every time you work out you produce growth hormone—your ally in the fight for a halter-ready body. Growth hormone levels spike following an individual set of moves and help amino acids—what protein is made of—latch on to and feed the muscle so it can grow stronger. The key to gaining strength is to keep your recovery time to 30 to 60 seconds, Dr. Willardson says, so hormone levels are consistently amped and ready to help fuel your muscles.

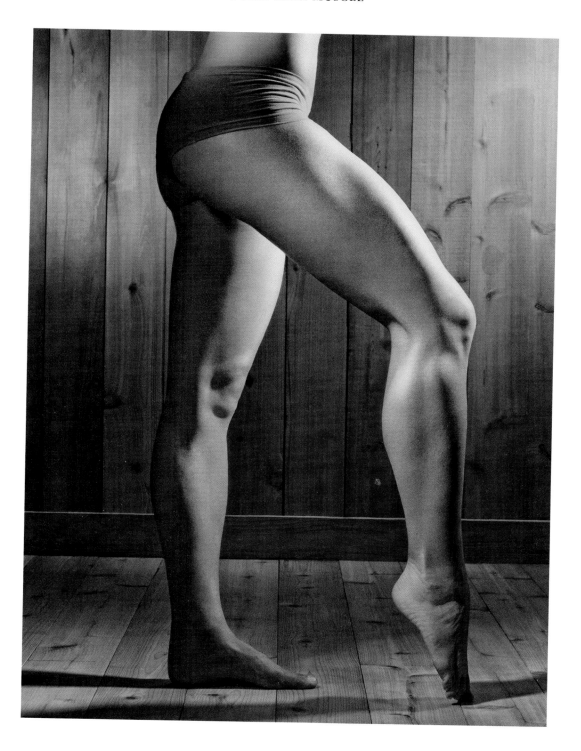

20 Ways to Stick to Your Workout

FOR THOSE DAYS WHEN YOU'D RATHER EAT NAILS THAN EXERCISE, THESE EXPERT TIPS WILL KEEP YOU MOTIVATED.

By Kelly Borgeson

There's no feeling like leaving the gym. It's getting there that's the problem. Like at the end of the workday, which suddenly becomes the perfect time to check the supply cabinet, IM about *Lost,* and—damn, look at the time; you'll get that workout in tomorrow. Why are we paying personal trainers after we get to the gym? What we really need them to do is carry us there. Your motivation needs motivating, so top trainers and athletes offered to help you firm up your resolve—and your glutes, thighs, and abs—with these stick-to-your-workout strategies.

1. Get In over Your Head

Sign up for a race and give yourself a reason to train. "After I retired, it was hard to motivate myself to work out, so I set a goal to run a marathon," says Olympian Nikki Stone, an aerial freestyle skiing gold medalist. "It gives you something to work toward." If you want help before you jump into a live race, most running clubs sponsor organized training runs, which match you with groups at your skill level and prepare you for specific races and distances. Visit the Road Runners Club of America at www.rrca.org/clubs to find a group near you.

2. Cut a Soundtrack

"Whenever I do cardio, I listen to something that gets me going," says Emily Copeland, a professional wakeboarder who's won gold at the X Games. Rip a playlist with music that gets you pumped up; leave off the slow tracks. Upbeat music makes a workout seem easier and go by faster, according to a study led by Ronald W. Deitrick, PhD, director of exercise science at the University of Scranton in Pennsylvania. That's because high-tempo music is a better distractor, Dr. Deitrick says. "It helps you block out the sensations you have regarding pain and effort."

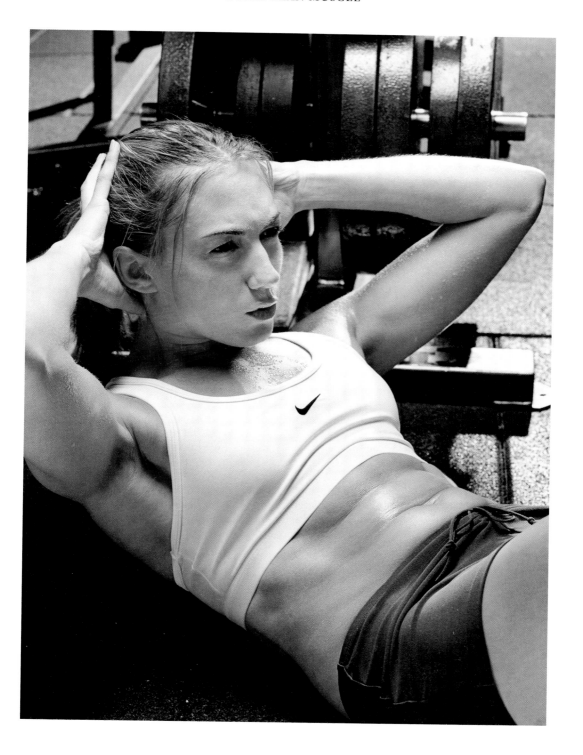

3. Book It

"You'll never find the time—you've got to make the time," says Chuck Wolf, MS, manager of sport science and human performance at the USA Triathlon National Training Center in Clermont, Florida. While that seems obvious, lack of planning continues to be the biggest reason people fail to work out, Wolf says. He suggests keeping a calendar and scheduling workouts—strength, cardio, yoga, new classes you want to try—at least a week in advance. Before you set foot in the locker room, have an agenda: which exercises you're going to do, what order, and how many sets and reps. Have a contingency plan, too—lifting dumbbells or jumping rope for 20 minutes at home—in case the unexpected cancels your workout. "You're 40 percent more likely to work out if you have strategies to help you overcome the obstacles," says Rod Dishman, PhD, an exercise scientist at the University of Georgia in Athens.

4. Get a Buy-In

Whether it's your husband, boyfriend, mother, father, or child, you're going to need support from anyone who has a claim on your time. Make an agreement with them: 4 or 5 days a week, you're entitled to 1 all-about-you hour to work out. "Since it's for your health, it's a contract they can't refuse," says Darren Steeves, a trainer in Nova Scotia. "That will allow you to exercise guilt-free." If you're in a relationship, make the deal a united effort and see if you can get him to work on his soft spots, too.

5. Start with Squats

Few people love this exercise. But the payoff in places where you're seeking results (glutes, hips, thighs) is unquestioned. It's simply one of the best full-body exercises you can do. If you don't have a specific goal or body part in mind when you enter the gym, consider beginning your workout with the squat. Starting with such a demanding move will help you finish strong. "You'll look forward to your favorite moves at the end of your workout, which will encourage you to complete the entire session," says John Williams, a trainer in Atlanta.

6. Ask a Friend

If you'd rather hit the snooze button than the treadmill, try some friendly intervention. Having a friend waiting for you at the gym three mornings a week will get you out of bed. "If you've made a commitment to someone, you have a tendency to keep it," says Tristan Gale, an Olympic gold medalist in women's skeleton (barreling head first down a bobsled track). But that doesn't necessarily mean your best friend is also your best workout partner. Look for someone who's at the same fitness level and has similar goals. "If there's too much of a disparity, no one will get a good workout," Wolf says.

7. Just Show Up

On really low-energy days, head to the gym with the promise that you can leave after you finish your warmup. "Tell yourself you'll just do some stretches and a few minutes of cardio," says Rachel Cosgrove, a personal trainer in Newhall, California. "Once you get to the gym and get your blood pumping, chances are you'll finish your full workout. Ninety percent of the time, our clients do."

8. Target Your Heart

High cholesterol isn't just a problem for men—heart disease is the No. 1 killer of women (more on that in Chapter 10). Make sure a cholesterol test is part of your annual checkup, and follow up with your doctor on the results to find out what your cholesterol levels are and what they should be. Then work toward meeting that target by exercising regularly. "You'll decrease your risk of heart disease while providing yourself with a very important, concrete goal," says John Thyfault, PhD, an assistant professor and health scientist in the department of internal medicine at the University of Missouri–Columbia.

9. Be Defensive

Need more inspiration than trimming your waistline? Consider enrolling in a self-defense class, which will increase your confidence and your heart rate. Learning practical defense skills—eye strikes, heel palms, knees to the groin—is a workout that will also bolster your

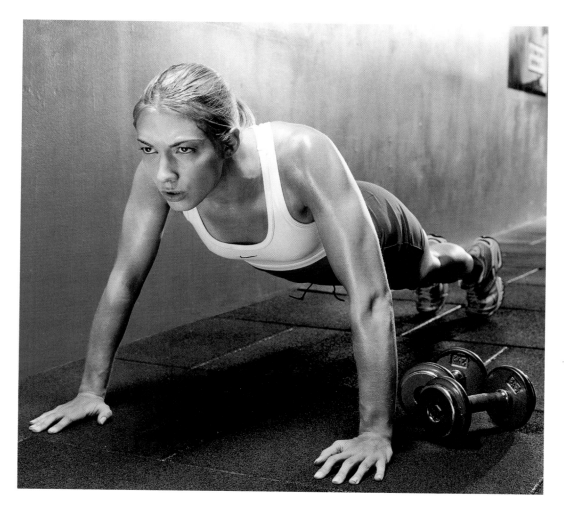

sense of control, says Dana Schwartz, who teaches self-defense at Prepare in New York City. "You get to fight every class, and every class you see improvement in yourself," Schwartz says. "I think people are surprised by how powerful they are."

10. Invest in a Trainer

If you don't know what you're doing when you get to the gym, it pays to hire someone who does. Beyond helping you plan your workout, a personal trainer will observe and correct your form to make sure you produce results and avoid injuries, and they'll provide constant motivation.

11. Don't Do It

"If I'm going to recommend exercise, I can say running is the best," Dr. Deitrick says. "But if a person doesn't like running, guess what? They're not going to do it. They don't care what the benefit is." The "perfect" exercise is the one you're happy doing, and you have plenty of options, indoors and out. So don't suffer through a less-than-stimulating routine. Find an exercise you like—cycling, yoga, hiking, that rowing machine in the corner of the gym that no one ever uses—and you'll find yourself wanting to exercise. That might require a little experimentation, but that's always the fun part.

12. Watch the Rut

You found the perfect routine—great. Just be sure not to make it as familiar as *Friends* reruns. What bores your mind also bores your body; you need variety to guarantee results like fat loss and muscle tone. If you do the same three-sets-of-8 circuit week after week, you'll stop challenging your body around Week 4 and your progress will quickly plateau. "When you impose a stress on your body, your body adapts to it," says Tom Holland, exercise physiologist and author of *The Truth about How to Get in Shape*. Switch your routine—do different strength or cardio moves, or take a new class—every 4 to 6 weeks to keep yourself fresh.

13. Write It Down

Write your fitness goals in a journal, and track your workouts. Include the usual stats, such as specific exercises, duration, weight, sets, and reps. Write down your perceptions, too. "Think: Am I having fun, or does it feel like work?" says Sara Ivanhoe, instructor of the *Yoga for Dummies* VHS/DVD series. Figure out which exercises make you feel good and produce results, and note the stressors that tend to derail workouts. "It's a good opportunity to explore what gets in the way of being consistent," Ivanhoe says, whether it's a traffic jam at the leg-press machine at the same time every night or too much time chatting with friends.

14. Work with Him

"Eighty percent of couples who divorce say they grew apart," says Pat Love, EdD, a relationship therapist and coauthor of *Hot Monogamy*. "Sharing activities is a surefire way to help keep you together. Especially activities where you both end up feeling good and energized." Nikki Stone is a believer. She regularly jogs with her husband, and they take their English sheepdog for long walks. "We get quality time together—and a workout," she says. Exercise releases neurohormones that make people feel happier, more motivated, and less anxious, Dr. Love says. "And anytime you have a pleasurable experience when you're with your partner, your brain associates him with pleasure."

15. Streak!

No, don't sprint out of the locker room naked. See how many days you can go without missing a workout, and then try to beat your record. "Every time your streak ends, strive to set a longer mark in your new attempt," Williams says.

16. Reward Yourself

After 2 months of training, you ran your first sub-8:30 mile. Celebrate by treating yourself to a deep-tissue massage. But don't let the moment pass. Because sometimes, that short-term reward might be the only evidence of your long-term success, says Jacqueline Wagner, a certified trainer in New York City. "Some of the things we see in exercise in terms of maintaining balance, of maintaining bone mass, of maintaining function, we're not going to see for years down the road," Wagner says. That massage, meanwhile, can make you feel good right now.

17. Play the Percentages

Have your body-fat level measured every few months to gauge your fit-

Learn to Love the Burn

For decades scientists thought the burning sensation was a result of your body's producing lactic acid to slow you down when you're going too hard. Seemed logical, until 2006, when researchers at the University of California–Berkeley discovered the real reason your muscles burn. Turns out that although the burning is caused by lactic acid, it's not your body putting the brakes on your workout. The acid actually is a main source of fuel for your muscles. When you push yourself, your muscles convert glucose from food into lactic acid, which is moved via proteins to the mitochondria, your muscles' energy factories. The more you work out, the more efficiently your body uses lactate as fuel—which means you can go longer and harder.

ness progress. "You'll actually have numbers that you can shoot for, and something that you can definitely measure, as opposed to 'I just want my abs to look better,'" says Tim Kuebler, a certified trainer in Kansas City, Missouri. A body-fat percentage from the high teens to the mid-twenties is considered healthy for most women (ranges vary by age), according to the American College of Sports Medicine. A trainer can estimate your percentage using calipers, and most gyms offer this service for a minimal charge; just have the same person do it each time, as measurement techniques can vary.

18. Take a Chance

Boost your adrenaline with a workout that challenges both your body and your fears—rock climbing, for example, or whitewater kayaking. Besides being great exercise, such adrenaline-spiked adventures will help you better manage stress in everyday life, according to a study from Texas A&M University. Adventure sports raise your levels of adrenaline and the stress hormone cortisol, and also provide you with an immediate way—exercise—to efficiently work that stress out. The fitter you are, the study found, the better you handle stress.

19. Run Away

Sign up for a race in another time zone. "Once you've paid for the airfare and a hotel room, you'll have extra incentive to follow your training plan," says Carolyn Ross-Toren, chairwoman of the Mayor's Fitness Council in San Antonio, Texas. Check www.theschedule.com for information on everything from 5-Ks to marathons, www.usatriathlon.org for triathlon events, and www.marathonguide.com for . . . well, marathons. Another great, all-purpose resource for runners: www.runnersworld.com.

20. Show Off

A boost to your appearance—be it a new haircut, a new sports bra, or fresh-out-of-the-box running shoes—can give you a lift in the gym. "Sometimes, those little things can be very uplifting and motivating," Wagner says. "And when you feel better about yourself, you're going to function better."

Build Your Basics— In 10 Minutes

A 10-minute workout is fitness's quickie. It's so fast it might not seem worth the effort, but you can still get satisfying results if you know what you're doing. While it's not enough time for a great fat-burning workout, 10 minutes will help you build a solid fitness foundation if you develop a strong core and sense of balance. "You can tone up key areas and work on stabilizing the spine, which will help you to avoid future injuries," says Chere Schoffstall, a trainer at the National Academy of Sports Medicine in Calabasas, California.

OPTION 1: STRETCH AND STRENGTHEN

Start your 10-spot with dynamic stretches, which are body-weight exercises that utilize your range of motion. They'll keep you flexible and work your core at the same time. Do two or three sets of 12 deep squats and walking lunges so you can warm your muscles as you stretch. Next, twist at the waist as you walk your lunges and do a set of 10 to each side. For a core work, do three sets of 8 full-range, slow situps to work the length of your core. "Keep your feet unanchored because it will force you to use your abs instead of relying solely on your hip flexors," says Mike Mejia, CSCS, a strength and conditioning specialist on Long Island, New York. "You'll have to focus and control your movement to pull yourself up and keep your feet on the ground."

OPTION 2: GET BALANCED

Balance work trains your small proprioceptive muscles to improve reaction time and strength and help prevent injuries. "It's also important to work your glutes, because that's where balance comes from. It's the bottom of your core," Schoffstall says. For core stability, do three sets of the plank (pushup position but this time with elbows on the floor, using the length of your abs to keep your body flat and still), 20 seconds each. Then do three sets of bridges. Finally, perform two sets of 10 to 12 repetitions of both single-leg squats and side lunges. When you press up from the side lunge, balance on your standing leg.

Part Two:
Work Less, Burn More Fat

Speed Up Your Metabolism

DON'T BEMOAN THE FACT THAT YOU WERE BORN WITH A
SLUGGISH CALORIE-BURNING SYSTEM. TURBOCHARGE IT WITH
THESE TIPS—SOME EVEN WORK IN YOUR SLEEP!

Here's a secret: Slaving away inside your body—right this minute—is your very own personal trainer, working tirelessly to help you burn calories and shed fat. It's called your metabolism, and it's the sum of everything that your body does. Each time you eat, enzymes in your body's cells break down the food and turn it into energy that keeps your heart beating, your mind thinking, and your legs churning during a grueling workout. The faster your metabolism runs, the more calories you burn. The more you burn, the easier it is to drop pounds.

As we've said, though, with each passing decade, a woman's metabolism slows by about 5 percent. Hormones play a role, but mostly it's because as you get older, you typically become less active. As a result, you lose muscle mass, a major consumer of all those calories you scarf down. So by the time you hit 35, you'll burn 75 fewer calories a day than you did at 25; by age 65, you'll burn 500 fewer, says Madelyn Fernstrom, PhD, director of the Weight Management Center at the University of Pittsburgh.

But get this—you can make your metabolism work harder, a lot harder, 24 hours a day, and there's still plenty of wiggle room to outsmart Mother Nature. "You have a huge amount of control over your metabolic rate," says John Berardi, PhD, CSCS, author of *The Metabolism Advantage*. "You can't affect how many calories it takes to keep your heart beating, but you can burn an extra 500 to 600 calories a day by exercising properly and eating right." And by making a few changes to your routine.

To make those changes simpler, we enlisted the help of leading experts and came up with a round-the-clock, turn-up-the-burn plan complete with new moves that will throw your metabolism into overdrive.

1: In the Morning
Eat (a Good) Breakfast

Every. Single. Day. If you don't, your body goes into starvation mode (it's paranoid like that), so your metabolism slows to a crawl to conserve energy, Dr. Berardi says. In one study published in

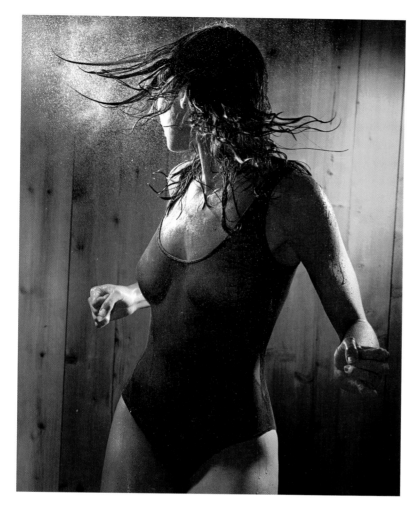

Race Against Time

MAPPING THE
DOWNSHIFT IN
METABOLISM THAT
COMES WITH AGING

Twenties:
Your muscle and bone mass
are at their peak.

Thirties:
Your mitochondria—cellular
powerhouses that fuel muscles
to use more oxygen and burn
more energy—become less
effective.

Forties:
A drop in estrogen production
further slows metabolism.

Fifties:
Sharp decreases in activity
reduce the levels of hormones
responsible for maintaining lean
muscle mass and bone density.

the *American Journal of Epidemiology,* volunteers who got 22 to 55 percent of their total calories at breakfast gained only 1.7 pounds on average over 4 years. Those who ate zero to 11 percent of their calories in the morning gained nearly 3 pounds. In another study published in the same journal, volunteers who reported regularly skipping breakfast had 4½ times the risk of obesity as those who took the time to eat. And the heartier your first meal is, the better—slow-digesting munchies leave you feeling fuller longer. Try a mix of lean protein with complex carbohydrates and healthy fats, like this power breakfast,

recommended by Dr. Berardi: an omelet made with 1 egg and 2 egg whites and ½ cup mixed bell peppers and onions, plus ½ cup cooked steel-cut oats mixed with ¼ cup frozen berries and 1 teaspoon omega-3–loaded fish oil.

Guzzle Your Water Cold

Chase your morning joe with an ice-cold glass of H_2O. Researchers at the University of Utah in Salt Lake City found that volunteers who drank eight to twelve 8-ounce glasses of water per day had higher metabolic rates than those who quaffed only four glasses. Your body may burn a

The best way to shorten your workout: Step up your intensity. You'll burn the same number of calories—or more—in less time.

few calories heating the cold water to your core temperature, says Madelyn Fernstrom, PhD, founder and director of the University of Pittsburgh Medical Center Weight Management Center. Though the extra calories you burn drinking a single glass don't amount to much, making it a habit can add up to pounds lost with essentially zero additional effort.

2. At the Office
Pick Protein for Lunch
Cramming protein into every meal helps build and maintain lean muscle mass. Muscle burns more calories than fat does, even at rest, says Donald Layman, PhD, professor of nutrition at the University of Illinois at Urbana-Champaign. Aim for about 30 grams of protein—the equivalent of about 1 cup of low-fat cottage cheese or a 4-ounce boneless chicken breast—at each meal.

Brew Up Some Green Tea
"It's the closest thing to a metabolism potion," says Tammy Lakatos Shames, RD, coauthor of *Fire Up Your Metabolism: 9 Proven Principles for Burning Fat and Losing Weight Forever*. The brew contains epigallocatechin-3-gallate (ECGC), a plant compound that promotes fat burning. In one study, people who consumed the equivalent of 3 to 5 cups a day for 12 weeks decreased their body weight by 4.6 percent. According to other studies, consuming 2 to 4 cups of green tea per day may torch an extra 50 calories. That translates into about 5 pounds per year. Not bad for a few bags of leaves, eh? For maximum effect, let your tea steep for 3 minutes and drink it while it's still hot.

Undo Damage with Dairy
Hey, it happens. There are days when no salad on earth can possibly overcome the seductive power

of French fries. But you can make up for it with a calcium-rich afternoon snack, like 8 ounces of milk or 6 ounces of low-fat yogurt. Calcium helps your body metabolize fat more efficiently by increasing the rate at which it gets rid of fat as waste (yes, that kind), reports a study from the University of Copenhagen. Sorry, supplements don't have the same effect.

3. In the Grocery Store
Choose Organic Produce
Researchers in Canada found that dieters with the most organochlorides (chemicals found in pesticides) stored in their fat cells were the most susceptible to disruptions in mitochondrial activity and thyroid function. Translation: Their metabolism stalled. Can't afford a full organic swap? Go to www.foodnews.org/fulllist for the most (and the least) contaminated produce, and then adjust your shopping list accordingly.

Seek Heat
It turns out that capsaicin, the compound that gives chile peppers their mouth-searing quality, can also fire up your metabolism. Eating about 1 tablespoon of chopped red or green chilies boosts your body's production of heat and the activity of your sympathetic nervous system (responsible for our fight-or-flight response), according to a study published in the *Journal of Nutritional Science and Vitaminology*. The result: a temporary metabolism spike of about 23 percent. Stock up on chilies to add to salsas, and keep a jar of red pepper flakes on hand for topping pizzas, pastas, and stir-fries.

Grab Some Metal
Women lose iron during their periods every month. That can throw a wrench into your metabolic machine, because iron helps carry oxygen

to your muscles. If your levels run low, your muscles don't get enough O_2, your energy tanks, and your metabolism sputters, Shames says. Stock up on iron-fortified cereals, beans, and dark leafy greens, such as spinach, bok choy, and broccoli.

4. At the Gym
Mix Things Up with Intervals

The best way to shorten your workout: Step up your intensity. You'll burn the same number of calories—or more—in less time. In one Australian study, female volunteers either rode a stationary bike for 40 minutes at a steady pace or for 20 minutes of intervals, alternating 8 seconds of sprints and 12 seconds of easy pedaling. After 15 weeks, those who incorporated the sprints into their cardio workouts had lost three times as much body fat—including thigh and core flab—compared with those who exercised at a steady pace. Bursts of speed may stimulate a fat-burning response within the muscles, says lead researcher Ethlyn Gail Trapp, PhD. Whether you ride, run, or row, try ramping things up to rev your burn: Start by doing three 8-second all-out, can't-talk sprints with 12 seconds at an easy pace between each effort. Work your way up until you can do 10 sprints over 20 minutes.

Take It Slow

This isn't easy, but when you strength train, count to 3 as you lower the weight back to the start position. Slowing things down increases the breakdown of muscle tissue; it sounds bad, but all that damage you're incurring is actually a good thing. The repair process pumps up your metabolism for as long as 72 hours after your session, according to researchers at Wayne State University in Detroit. But pass on those featherweight dumbbells—you need to use weights that are heavy enough that you struggle to complete the final few reps.

Pop Pills

Combining regular exercise with fish-oil supplements increases the activity of your fat-burning enzymes, reports a study published in the *American Journal of Clinical Nutrition*. Volunteers took 6 grams of fish oil daily and worked out three times a week. After 12 weeks, they'd lost an average of 3.4 pounds, while those who exercised exclusively saw minimal shrinkage. Look for brands containing at least 300 milligrams of the fatty acid eicosapentaenoic acid (EPA) and 200 milligrams of the fatty acid docosahexaenoic acid (DHA) per capsule. Pop 2 of these 2 hours before your workout.

5. At Home
Eat Nemo's Pals

Fatty fish like salmon, tuna, and sardines are loaded with hunger-quashing omega-3 fatty acids. These healthy fats help trigger the rapid transfer of "I'm full" signals to your brain, according to the National Institutes of Health. Bonus: A 3½-ounce serving of salmon nets you 90 percent of your recommended daily value of vitamin D, which will help you to preserve your precious calorie-craving, metabolism-stoking muscle tissue. And remember to always buy salmon labeled wild, not farmed.

Skip the Second Mojito

73

Percentage two alcoholic drinks puts the brakes on your body's fat-burning ability

Another reason not to overimbibe: Knocking back the equivalent of just two mixed drinks (or two glasses of wine or two bottles of beer) puts the brakes on fat burning by a whopping 73 percent. That's because your liver converts the alcohol into acetate and starts using that as fuel instead of your fat stores, report researchers from the University of California–Berkeley. To pace yourself, drink a glass of water between every alcoholic beverage.

Hit the Sack—Early

When you sleep less than you should, you throw off the amounts of leptin and ghrelin—hormones that help regulate energy use and appetite—that your body produces. Researchers at Stanford University found that people who snoozed fewer than 7½ hours per night experienced an increase in their body mass index. So make sure you get at least 8 hours of rest.

The 19 Best Fitness Foods for Women

STOCK YOUR FRIDGE AND PANTRY WITH THESE STAPLES
TO PERFORM AND FEEL YOUR ABSOLUTE BEST.

By Maureen Callahan, RD

Choosing a bagel over a peanut butter sandwich isn't the kind of life-altering decision that, say, changing your e-mail address is. But your pick could have heavy fitness repercussions. Just grab a lame prerun snack and you'll be dragging to the finish. Reach for the wrong food when you put down those weights and the next time you pump iron, you could be crashing harder than a disgraced beauty queen after an all-nighter. The simple truth is what you eat influences your performance in key ways. That's why we pored over a stack of scientific studies and picked the brains of a half-dozen experts—top-notch researchers, coaches, and sports nutritionists—to single out the top 19 foods for any activity, from yoga to running to rock climbing.

Avocados

The cholesterol-lowering monounsaturated fat in these green health bombs can help keep your body strong and pain-free. University of Buffalo researchers found that competitive women runners who ate less than 20 percent fat were more likely to suffer injuries than those who consumed at least 31 percent. Peter J. Horvath, PhD, a professor at the university, speculates that the problem is linked to extremely low-fat diets, which weaken muscles and joints. "A few slices of avo-cado a day are a great way to boost fat for women who are fat shy," says Leslie Bonci, RD, director of sports nutrition at the University of Pittsburgh Medical Center.

Whole Grain Bagels

Never mind Dr. Atkins—carbs are the optimal workout food. "You want complex carbohydrates in their natural package, aka whole grains," says Jackie Berning, PhD, RD, a nutrition professor at the University of Colorado at Colorado Springs and counselor to sports teams. "Not the simple ones, because they wind you up and drop you down." A whole-grain bagel is an ideal presweat-session pick: You'll digest it slowly because of all the fiber, which will deliver a steady flow of energy over time rather than one big burst.

Bananas

Thanks to bananas' high potassium content, peeling one is a speedy solution to that stitch in your side. While a lack of sodium is the main culprit behind muscle cramps, studies show potassium plays a supporting role: You need it to replace sweat losses and help with fluid absorption. Bananas are also packed with energizing carbohydrates. One medium-size fruit has 400 milligrams of potassium and as many carbs (29 grams) as 2 slices of whole wheat bread.

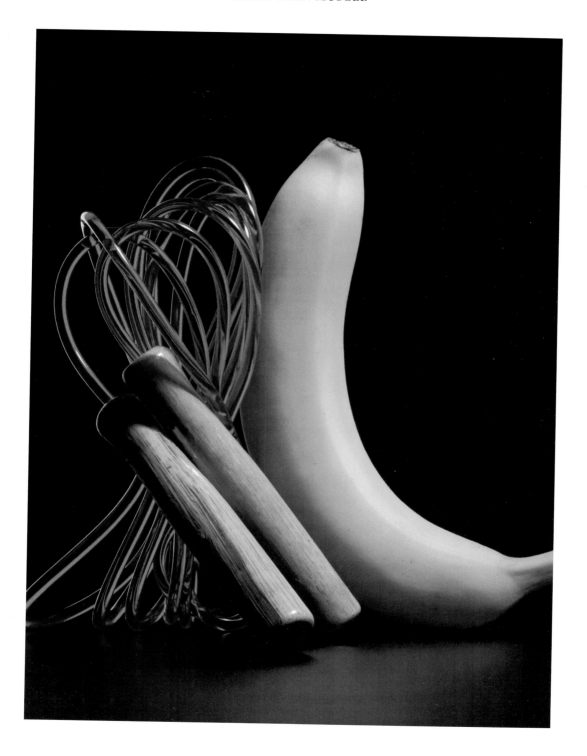

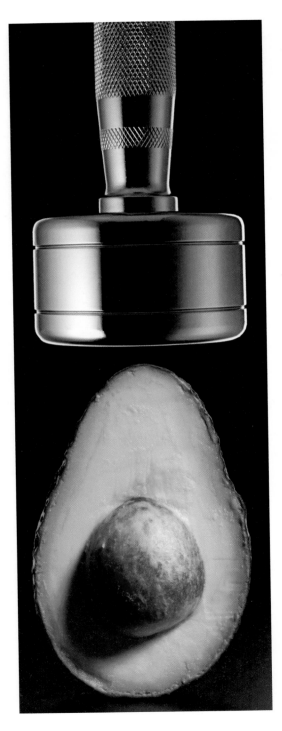

Berries

USDA researchers recently placed fresh berries on their list of the 20 foods richest in antioxidants. Just a handful of blueberries, raspberries, or blackberries is an excellent source of these potent nutrients, which protect muscles from free-radical damage that might be caused by exercise. Shop for berries by the shade of their skin: The deeper the color, the healthier the fruit.

Baby Carrots

Carrots pack complex carbs that provide energy to muscles and potassium to control blood pressure and muscle contractions, Bonci says. And $\frac{1}{2}$ cup has just 35 calories.

Whole-Grain Cereal

Looking for something to nosh before you hit the gym? Raid your cereal stash. The healthiest brands contain endurance-boosting complex carbs and muscle-building protein. Sixty minutes before a workout, fuel up with a 200-calorie snack: $\frac{3}{4}$ cup whole-grain cereal with 4 ounces fat-free milk. "When you eat something before exercising, you have more energy, so you can work out harder and perhaps longer. And you'll be less likely to overeat afterward," Bonci says.

Chicken Thighs

Skimp on iron and zinc and your energy will flag. Cooking up some juicy chicken thighs or turkey drumsticks is the best way to get more of both. "Dark-meat poultry is significantly lower in fat than red meat yet has all the iron, zinc, and B vitamins that women need in their diets," says Seattle sports nutritionist Susan Kleiner, PhD, author of *Power Eating*.

Low-Fat Chocolate Milk

There's way more to milk than just calcium. In fact, it's a damn near perfect food, giving you a lot of valuable energy while keeping your calorie count low, Dr. Kleiner says. The chocolate kind is loaded with calcium, vitamins, and minerals just like the plain stuff, but new studies confirm that milk with a touch of cocoa is as powerful as commercial recovery drinks at replenishing and repairing muscles.

Low-Fat Cottage Cheese

Despite its frumpy image, this diet staple packs 14 grams of protein per $1/2$-cup serving, along with 75 milligrams of calcium and 5 grams of carbohydrates. That protein is crucial to healing the microscopic muscle tears that occur during exercise, says Amy Jamieson-Petonic, RD, health education manager at Cleveland's Fairview Hospital.

Dried Cranberries

This packable fruit delivers a generous pre- or postworkout blast of carbohydrates (25 grams per $1/4$ cup). Plus, cranberries have proanthocyanins, compounds that help prevent and fight urinary tract infections. (Running to the bathroom every 5 minutes is an kind of annoying workout.)

Eggs

Don't skip the yolk. One egg a day supplies about 215 milligrams of cholesterol—not enough to push you over the 300-milligram daily cholesterol limit recommended by the American Heart Association. Plus, the yolk is a good source of iron, and it's loaded with lecithin, which is critical for brain health, Dr. Kleiner says. What does brainpower have to do with exercise? Try doing a sun salutation without it.

Ground Flaxseed

"Flaxseed is full of fibers called lignans that promote gut health," Dr. Kleiner says. Since flax lignans contain both soluble and insoluble fiber, they keep you regular. "When you're trying to do an endurance sport, it can be disruptive to have digestive problems," she notes. A daily dose of 1 to 2 tablespoons of ground flaxseed tossed in your cereal nets you fiber without fuss.

Hummus

Complex carbohydrates, protein, and unsaturated fats—all the right elements to fuel activity—meet in one healthy little 70-calorie, 3-tablespoon package. Plus, hummus is often made with olive oil, which contains oleic acid—a fat that helps cripple the gene responsible for 20 to 30 percent of breast cancers, according to Northwestern University researchers.

Oranges

"They're a rich source of vitamin C," Bonci says, "which helps repair muscle tissue." One orange has all the C a woman needs each day—close to 75 milligrams. Vitamin C is also key for making collagen, a tissue that helps keep bones strong.

Peanuts

No wonder Mr. Peanut never stops tap-dancing. Female soccer players kicked and sprinted just as well in the final minutes of a game as they did at the start when they added 2 ounces of peanuts a day to their regular diets, Dr. Horvath says. The extra fat may help improve endurance by giving muscles energy to burn up front so they can spare muscle glycogen stores later.

Baked Potatoes

Sweat like a pig? Four shakes of salt (about 1,100 milligrams of sodium) and a small baked potato is the perfect recipe for electrolyte replacement. "The electrolytes, sodium, and potassium help maintain fluid balance in and around cells and make sure muscles contract as they need to," Bonci says.

Salmon

Great for heart health, but here's an added twist: New studies are suggesting that monounsaturated fats and omega-3 fats might help lessen abdominal fat. It's too soon to understand the link, but "this could be particularly good for women working to tone their cores," Dr. Kleiner says.

Whey Protein

"Whey protein contains the ideal assortment of amino acids to repair and build muscle," Kleiner says. Plus, it's digested fast, so it gets to muscles quickly. Stir a scoop into a smoothie for a delicious boost before or after your next workout.

Yogurt

Immune-strengthening probiotics are a fabulous feature, but the best thing about yogurt is that it will spike your energy without making your stomach gurgle in yoga class. "It's liquidy in consistency and because you can digest it quickly, it's easy on the gut," Bonci says.

When a Ball Meets a Wall

HEAD–TO–TOE TONING IS EASIER THAN YOU THINK.

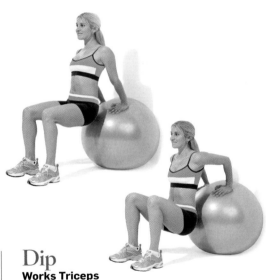

S omething flat and something squat should make for an awkward pair— think middle-school dances. But a wall and a Swiss ball are a power couple. The wall adds support for moves that would otherwise be dicey on a giant, roll-prone ball, so you have more muscle-working options. (And that will prove especially helpful if you're not yet the hard body of your dreams.) Try these moves from Shannon O'Regan, a certified group fitness instructor at the Evanston Athletic Club in Illinois. Work up to three sets three times a week, resting for 30 to 60 seconds between sets.

Dip
Works Triceps

Place the ball against the wall. Sit on the ball with your butt on its edge. Place your palms on the ball hip-width apart behind you, fingertips pointing toward your back. Push out from the ball so your hips are in front of it and your knees are at 90-degree angles (walk out a few steps if necessary). Plant your feet and contract your abs. Lifting your chest and pressing your shoulders down, bend your arms until your elbows are at right angles, keeping them pointing back. Straighten your arms, then repeat for 8 to 15 reps.

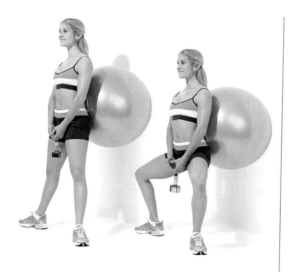

Plié Squat

Works Glutes, Hamstrings, Quads

With the ball between your lower back and the wall, hold a 10- to 20-pound dumbbell with both hands between your legs. Stand with your feet wider than your hips and turn your toes out. Contract your abs and lower for 4 counts until your knees are at 90 degrees. Hold for 4 seconds, then stand up for 4 counts. Repeat 8 to 15 times.

Wall Crunch and Twist

Works Center of Abs, Obliques

Sit on the ball facing the wall, then lie back so the middle to small of your back is resting on the ball. Place your feet hip-width apart on the wall with your knees bent to 90 degrees; cross your hands over your chest. Curl up and twist through the waist to the right, return to center, and curl down. Alternate to twist left. That's 1 rep; do 8 to 15.

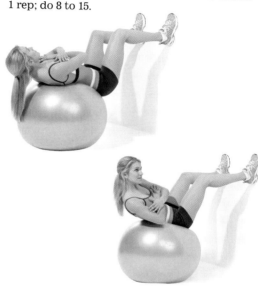

Static Squat with Front Raise

Works Shoulders, Hamstrings, Quads

With the ball between your lower back and the wall, hold a 3- to 8-pound dumbbell in each hand. Step forward with your feet hip-width apart. Lean back into the ball. Contract your abs and glutes, then lower your hips until your knees are at 90 degrees. In this position, slowly raise your arms in front of your body to shoulder height. Lower them to your sides and repeat 8 times. Rise to the starting position. That's one set.

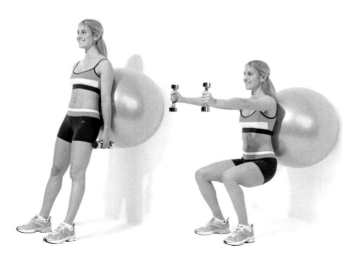

221

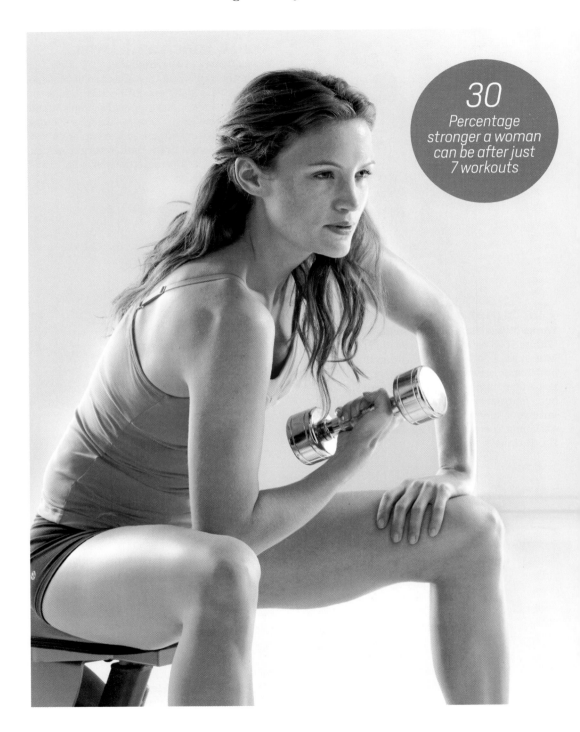

30
Percentage
stronger a woman
can be after just
7 workouts

A Total-Body Dumbbell Workout

TONE UP AND TRIM DOWN WITH THIS DO-ANYWHERE FITNESS PLAN.

Why wait in line at the gym when you can get the same results at home? This total-body dumbbell workout from Mike Mejia, CSCS, a personal trainer from Long Island, New York, hits several major muscle groups, and if you do one move after the other without rest, you'll torch serious calories.

Do 6 to 10 reps of each move, then go on to the next. After doing all four moves, rest for 60 seconds, then repeat. Choose a weight that lets you complete 6 to 10 reps of a bent-over row. To see results in about a month, do the workout two or three times a week.

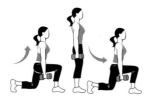

Lunge Works lower body
Grab the dumbbells and stand with your feet together, arms at your sides. Lunge forward with your right foot until your right thigh is almost parallel to the floor. Return to the start. Next, step backward with your left foot and sink into a lunge. Return to the start, then do a forward lunge with your left foot, then a back lunge with your right foot. That's 1 rep.

Bent-Over Row Works upper back and biceps
Grab the dumbbells and stand with your feet shoulder-width apart, knees slightly bent. With your arms at your sides, bend over from the hips until your back is almost parallel to the floor. Pull the dumbbells up, squeezing your shoulder blades together. Pause, then lower the weights. That's 1 rep. Complete all reps without standing up.

Romanian Deadlift Works glutes and hamstrings
Grab the dumbbells and stand with your feet hip-width apart, knees slightly bent. Position the dumbbells in front of your thighs, palms facing your body. Keeping your knees slightly bent, press your hips back as you bend at the waist and lower the weights toward the floor. Squeeze your glutes to return to standing. That's 1 rep. Up for a bigger challenge? Try this move on one leg.

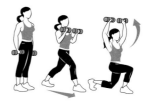

Curl and Press Works shoulders, biceps, and triceps
Grab the dumbbells and stand with your feet hip-width apart, arms at your sides. Step forward with your right leg as you curl both dumbbells up to your shoulders. Sink into a lunge and press the dumbbells directly overhead, rotating your arms so that your palms face forward at the top of the move. Pause for 2 seconds, then return to start. That's 1 rep.

Tone Your Arms

"When people say they dislike their arms, they're talking about their triceps," says J. J. Flizanes, director of Invisible Fitness in Los Angeles. If yours keep waving long after you've said good-bye, head straight to the dumbbell rack. Grab a 7- to 10-pound dumbbell, hoisting it behind your shoulder with your elbows bent. Lift the weight overhead by extending your elbow. Do three sets of 10 repetitions. Stand and burn more calories, says Douglas Lentz, CSCS, director of fitness for Summit Health in Chambersburg, Pennsylvania.

Strong Medicine

WHITTLE YOUR WAIST AND TORCH HUNDREDS OF CALORIES

If you liked pelting your crush with a rubber ball in phys ed class, you'll love these medicine ball moves designed by Steve Feinberg, an instructor at Equinox Fitness in New York City and founder of Speedball Fitness. This workout (based on a class Feinberg created called Speedball) combines high-intensity footwork with upper-body rotation—all while holding a 2- to 4-pound ball. Continue each move until you can't do another rep with perfect form. Rest for up to 3 minutes, then repeat. Do the routine 3 nonconsecutive days a week.

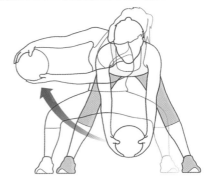

Monkey Swing

Grab a medicine ball and stand with your feet wider than your hips and your toes turned out slightly. Lower the ball so it's between your legs. Lean forward until your torso is parallel to the floor and bend your knees deeply. Swing your upper body to the right, raising the ball to shoulder level and rotating your spine to the right. Pause, then swing the ball to the left, allowing the spine to rotate. Pause. Continue alternating.

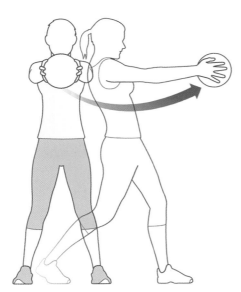

Lighthouse

Grab a medicine ball with both hands and stand with your feet wider than your hips. Raise the ball to shoulder height with your arms straight but not locked. Bend your knees slightly, then rotate your arms and torso 90 degrees to the left, pivoting on the ball of your right foot and turning from your hips. Repeat to the opposite side.

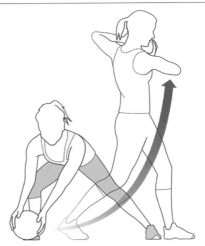

Side Touch

Grab a medicine ball with both hands and stand with your feet hip-width apart, your knees slightly bent. Hold the ball against your chest. Step to your right, turning your foot outward 45 degrees, and bend your right knee to 90 degrees. Rotate from your waist and touch the ball to the floor in front of your right toe. Lift the ball up, then quickly push off your right foot and rotate from your waist to the left while raising your left elbow up and behind you. Let your hips turn naturally and allow your right foot to slide in toward your body. Return to the start and repeat the entire sequence with your left foot forward.

Tip: Twisting is the best way to work your obliques.

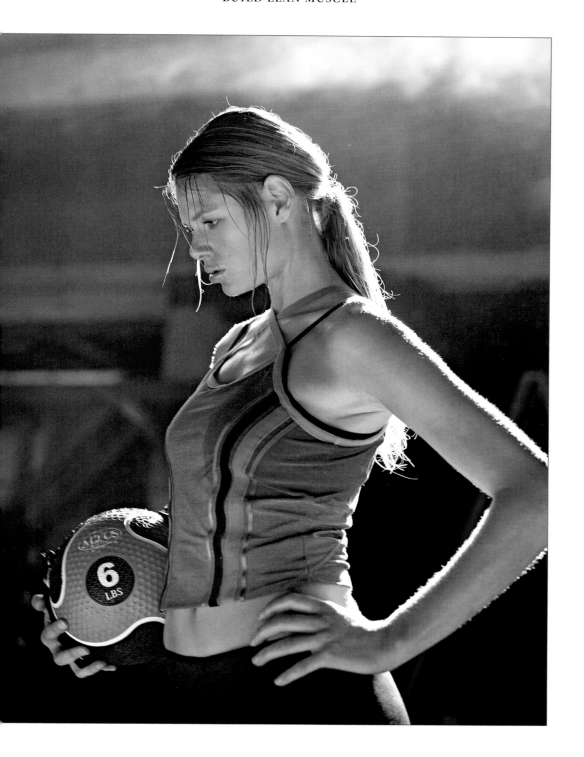

Pass the (Body) Bar

A WEIGHTED STICK WILL WORK YOUR WHOLE BODY IN WHOLE NEW WAYS.

Those black sticks in the corner of the gym are versatile pieces of equipment that give you a total-body workout while also delivering more stability than dumbbells. Claes Passalacqua, a senior trainer at Crunch in New York City, created these moves using the Body Bar (www.bodybars.com). Try them with a 9- or 12-pound bar.

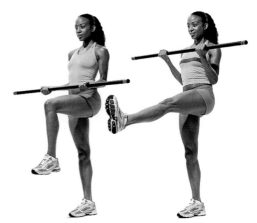

Stork Curl and Leg Extension

Stand holding the bar at your hips with a shoulder-width grip, palms forward. Draw your left knee up, bending it to 90 degrees, and curl the bar to your shoulders as you straighten your left leg. Bend the leg back to 90 degrees and lower. Repeat with the right leg. Alternate for 12 total reps.

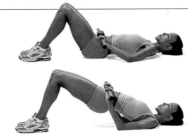

Bar Bridge

Lie on your back with your feet 1 foot from your butt. Using an overhand grip, hold the bar on your hips. Press up with your glutes so that your torso forms a straight line. Hold for a count of 10. Return to the start, and repeat for 5 reps.

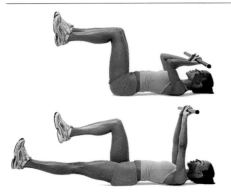

Lying Triceps-Abs Combo

Lie on your back with your knees bent to 90 degrees. Hold the bar just above your forehead, palms facing the ceiling. Press the bar up and extend your left leg to 6 inches off the floor. Lower the bar and return your leg to the start. Repeat with the right leg, then alternate for 12 total reps.

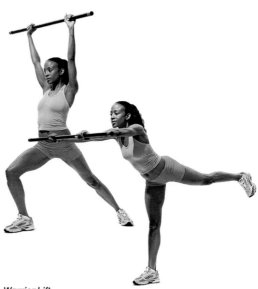

Warrior Lift

Hold the bar overhead with your hands shoulder-width apart, your palms facing forward. Then step into a wide lunge (right knee bent, left leg straight, and left foot turned outward). Lower the bar while straightening your right leg, and then lift your left leg straight out behind you while you simultaneously lift the bar in front of you. Return to the lunge stance and do 5 reps on each side.

Put Four on the Floor

BUILD A BETTER PUSHUP ROUTINE.

While the pushup—that age-old military classic—focuses on your chest, you can tweak it to strengthen your shoulders, arms, back, and whole core. These versions from Cliff Boyce, owner of Hollywood Fitness in Atlanta, will challenge your whole body. Do them all for a 15-minute workout, or sub them in during your regular routine.

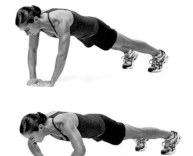

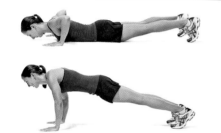

Flat Pushup Works your shoulders
Lie flat on the floor with your palms just outside your shoulders, toes on the floor, feet hip-width apart. Squeeze your core tight and push your entire body up. Pause for 2 seconds at the top, then lower to the floor and pause for another 2 seconds. Push up again and repeat. Start with three sets of 8 to 10 reps, working up to 15 to 20 reps per set. (If it's too difficult, put your knees on the ground.)

Pyramid Pushup Works your triceps
From a regular pushup position, place your hands on the floor to form a triangle (with thumbs and forefingers touching) and center them between your shoulders and your nose. Next, lower yourself until you're a few inches above your hands and pause for 2 seconds. Return to the start and repeat. Do three sets of 5 reps, working up to 20 reps per set. (Do it on your knees for an easier version.)

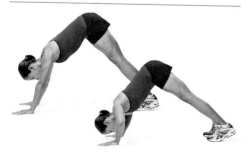

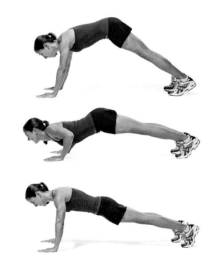

Decline Pushup Works your lower chest and abs
Start in a regular pushup position and walk your feet forward until your hips reach 90 degrees (pike position). Next, lower your upper body down and push up again, making sure to use only your upper body strength and not your legs for assistance. Start with three sets of 5 reps and work up to 15 reps per set.

Cobra Pushup Works your total body
With your hands on the floor just wider than your shoulders and your legs slightly wider than your hips, walk your feet forward into the pike position. Dip down with your chest, belly, hips, and then legs until your body is flat. When you dip down, your belly should almost touch the floor. Reverse to return to the pike position. Do three sets of 5 reps, working up to 10 to 15 reps. Too difficult? Walk your feet back a few steps before starting.

Chapter Nine

Tone Your Tummy

HOW TO WHITTLE YOUR WAISTLINE—AND THEN MAINTAIN YOUR IDEAL WEIGHT

INVESTMENT: 6 WEEKS
AGE ERASED: 2 YEARS

Introduction

Part One:
How to Get a Flat, Sexy Stomach
• The 8 Rules of Flat Abs
• Center of Attention
• Your Perfect Weight—Get There, Stay There

Part Two:
An All-Play, No-Work Guide to a Tighter Midsection
• Take a Firm Approach
• 8 Moves for Your Core—No Crunches Required
• One Good Turn
• A 20-Minute, Twice-a-Week Abs Workout

Part Three:
Watch Your Mouth
• Control Your Cravings
• 13 Flat Belly Food Tricks

Introduction

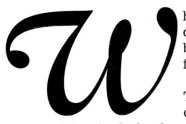

hen a family constructs its dream house, it doesn't begin with the landscaping. First, builders must pour footers and lay a sturdy foundation.

The same principle applies to your body. The foundation of the human body is the core, a web of muscles that spans the hips, abdominals, back, and shoulders. Every move you make—from lifting a package to picking up a crying toddler to acing that tennis serve—calls this support system into play. If you don't have a solid core, you don't have a strong body. And nothing—not your back, not your arms, and certainly not your abs—is going to grow strong and lean unless your foundation is powerful enough to support it.

"Your middle third must be integrated, because it's the hub," says physiologist Mark Verstegen, president of Athletes' Performance in Arizona and author of *Core Performance*. "If it's not dialed in, things will break down."

Your core network is made up of the muscles that keep you balanced and centered. They allow you to reach for a book without folding over at the waist, open a door without flipping backward, and make it through the last mile of a long run without doing a face plant.

And the core is also where all movement begins. Whenever your arms leave your sides or your legs bend at the knees, the transverse abdominis muscle—which wraps around your midsection—fires into action. Once activated, it works in concert with the rest of your core muscles to stabilize your hips, anchor the movements of your extremities, and transfer energy efficiently throughout the body. So the stronger your core, the more effectively you'll build muscle elsewhere—and the more you'll protect your body from injury, especially your back. Get your abs working today and you'll start building the foundation for a sleeker, stronger, sexier middle in no time.

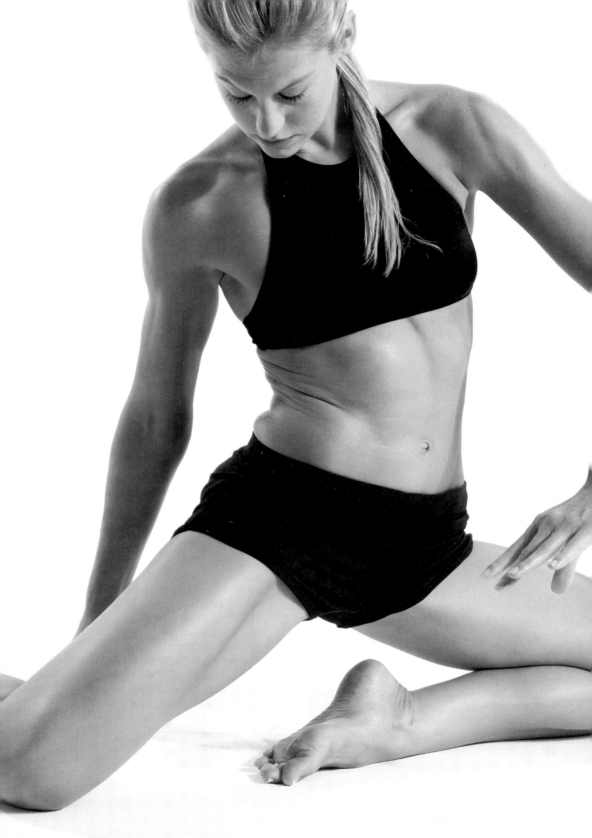

Part One:
How to Get a Flat, Sexy Stomach

The 8 Rules of Flat Abs

USE THESE SECRET STRATEGIES TO FINALLY REVEAL YOUR ABS.

By Bill Hartman, PT, CSCS, and Jen Ator

*I*f you've been doing crunches religiously for years and still have belly flab, don't blame your genes—blame your approach. The frustrating reality is that the midsection is one of the trickiest areas to tone. That's why even women dedicated to regular exercise often can't iron out their abs.

But if you take the right steps every single day, you'll ultimately get the toned tummy you've always dreamed of. Here's the solution: nine simple habits that will help you strip away extra belly fat for good. Think of these habits as daily goals designed to keep you on the fast track to a fit-looking physique. Individually they're not all that surprising, but together they become a powerful tool.

The effectiveness of this tool is supported by science. At the University of Iowa in Iowa City, researchers determined that people are more likely to stick with their fat-loss plans when they concentrate on specific actions instead of the desired result. So rather than focusing on abs that show, follow this daily list of nutrition, exercise, and lifestyle strategies for achieving that bare-worthy midsection. The result: automatic abs.

1. Follow These Easy Dietary Guidelines for a Flat Belly

Wake Up to Water. Imagine not drinking all day at work—no coffee, no water, no diet soda. At the end of an 8-hour shift, you'd be pretty parched. Which is precisely why you should start rehydrating immediately after a full night's slumber. From now on, drink at least 16 ounces of chilled H_2O as soon as you rise in the morning. German scientists recently found that doing this boosts metabolism by 24 percent for 90 minutes afterward. What's more, a previous study determined that muscle cells grow faster when they're well hydrated. A general rule of thumb: Drink at least a gallon of water a day.

Pump Up Your Protein Intake. Substituting meat, fish, dairy, and nuts for carbs can reduce the amount of fat around your middle. Researchers at McMaster University in Hamilton, Ontario, assessed the diets of 617 people and discovered that when they exchanged carbohydrates in favor of an equal amount of protein, they reduced overall belly fat.

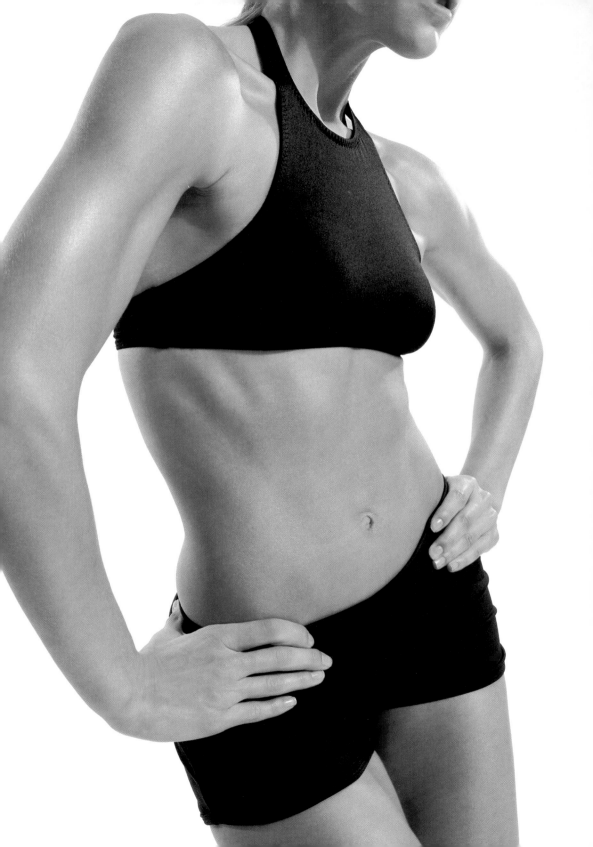

Eliminate Added Sugar. The average American eats about 20 teaspoons of sugar daily in the form of processed foods like soda, baked goods, cereals, and fruit drinks. That's about 325 empty calories every day. All that sugar increases insulin production, which slows your metabolism.

Don't Fear Fat. Research shows that diets containing more than 50 percent fat are just as effective for weight loss as those that are low in fat. "Fat is filling and adds flavor to your meals—both of which help you avoid feeling deprived, so you can stick to your diet," says Alan Aragon, MS, a nutritionist in the Los Angeles area. Eat foods rich in monounsaturated fats, such as olives, nuts, and avocados; research has even found that it's okay to enjoy whole foods that contain saturated fat (including milk, cheese, and butter) in moderation.

Beat the Bloat. No matter how much ab fat you lose or muscle you tone, if you're bloated, you won't look (or feel!) your best in a bikini. Carbonated beverages, and even good-for-you foods such as beans and broccoli, can make your stomach swell. The best guideline is really to keep your sodium intake in check: Nutritionists suggest you stay under 2,000 milligrams to avoid retaining excess water. (Most of us get closer to 5,000 milligrams a day.)

Eat Breakfast Every Day. A University of Massachusetts study showed that people who skip their morning meals are $4\frac{1}{2}$ times more likely to have larger waistlines than those who don't. So within an hour of waking, have a meal of at least 250 calories. British researchers found that breakfast size was inversely related to waist size (the larger the morning meal, the leaner the midsection). But keep the meal's size within reason: A 1,480-calorie smoked-sausage scramble at Denny's is really three breakfasts, so cap your intake at 500 calories. For a quick way to fuel up first thing, prepare a bowl of oatmeal and mix in a scoop of whey protein powder and $\frac{1}{2}$ cup blueberries.

Pack Your Lunch. If you don't have an insulated lunch bag already, get one. Take its contents seriously. In fact, packing your lunch should be as much a part of your morning ritual as showering. You don't need to overthink this habit, either. Here's a starting point:

* An apple (to eat as a morning snack)
* Two slices of cheese (to eat with the apple)
* A 500- to 600-calorie portion of leftovers (for your lunch)
* A premixed smoothie or a pint of milk (for your afternoon snack)

By using this approach, you'll keep your body well fed and satisfied throughout the day without overeating. You'll also provide your body with the nutrients it needs for your workout, no matter what time you exercise. Just as important, you'll be much less likely to be tempted by the office candy bowl. On that note, one simple rule to consider codifying into law: Don't eat anything that's not in your bag.

2. Review Your Fitness Goals Daily

Stay aware of your mission. University of Iowa scientists found that the people who monitored their diet and exercise goals the most frequently were more likely to achieve them than were goal setters who rarely reviewed their objectives.

Within an hour of waking, have a meal of at least 250 calories. Research shows people who skip breakfast have larger waistlines.

3. Exercise the Right Way

Everyone has abs, even if not everyone can see them because they're hidden under a layer of flab. So don't worry about "working your abs." Instead, you should spend most of your gym time torching fat.

The most effective strategy is a one-two approach of weight lifting and high-intensity interval training. According to a recent study at University of Southern Maine, Portland, half an hour of strength training burns as many calories as running at a 6-minute-per-mile pace for the same duration. (And it has the added benefit of helping you build muscle.) What's more, unlike aerobic exercise, weight lifting has been shown to boost metabolism for as long as 39 hours after the last repetition. Similar findings have been noted for intervals, which are short, all-out sprints interspersed with periods of rest.

For the best results, do a total-body weight-training workout 3 days a week, resting at least a day between sessions. Do an interval-training session on the days in between.

4. Attack Your Hidden Core Muscles

Crunches target only superficial muscles, so they aren't the most efficient way to work your abs. Hard fact: To burn just 1 pound of fat, you have to do 250,000 crunches, according to researchers at the University of Virginia. That's 100 crunches a day for 7 years. Uh, no thanks.

Instead, you really need to target the muscles that lie beneath the superficial ones: your transverse abdominis, multifidus, and internal obliques. Strengthening them pulls in your middle like a corset, keeping the area looking flat and toned. "Not only are these muscles weak in many women, but most of us don't have a clue about how to engage them," says celebrity trainer Valerie Waters.

To engage these "hidden" muscles, try this drill: Lie on your back and place your palms on your abdomen just below your navel. Exhale and allow your tummy to expand as far as you can, then focus on pulling your belly button toward your spine, drawing your abdomen toward the floor. Hold for 5 seconds. Repeat 8 to 10 times.

5. Ditch Your Daily Ab Workouts

You need only three sessions a week to see maximum results. Training every day with endless crunches won't flatten your belly faster; you'll see benefits quicker if you give your muscles a day to fully recover between workouts. That's because stressing your muscles during a workout breaks down the tissues, and they need recovery days to rebuild and get stronger. What's more, you should stick to only 15 to 20 reps of each move. "If you can easily do that many, it's time for harder moves," says Rachel Cosgrove, CSCS, owner of Results Fitness in Newhall, California.

And if flat abs are important to you, promote them to the top of your fitness to-do list. "A lot of people exercise their abdominal muscles at the end of their workout, and that's when you get sloppy or run out of time," Cosgrove says. "You should do them first, and then move on to your cardio. To get them looking great, you need to make them a priority." You'll be glad you did.

6. Move Your Butt

Your booty and your belly are unlikely partners in crime. Here's why: Over time, sitting around too much renders your glutes practically useless and causes your hip flexors—the muscles that connect your hipbones to your legs—to stiffen. This couch-potato combo tilts your pelvis forward, which increases the arch in your back and puts stress on your spine. From a cosmetic standpoint, it pushes your abdomen

Core Benefits

A TIGHT TUMMY DOES MORE THAN JUST TURN HEADS. CHECK OUT THESE OTHER SURPRISING BELLY BONUSES.

Steamier Sex

Strong abs and lower-back muscles give you the stamina and strength required to make the most of positions like Reverse Cowgirl and Wheelbarrow. But even more important: A smaller waistline means better bloodflow. When you're overweight, you tend to have significantly more artery-clogging plaque, which decreases bloodflow throughout the body. Researchers have found that increased bloodflow in the pelvic region improves vaginal lubrication, sensitivity, arousal, and sensation.

Fewer Injuries

Researchers for the US Army tracked the injuries of male and female soldiers during a year of field training in which they periodically performed the standard Army fitness test of situps, pushups, and a 2-mile run. Those who could crank out the most situps were less likely to suffer from injuries.

Better Health

Having a great belly doesn't guarantee you'll never call in sick, but studies show that people with flat abs are . . .

More than 25 percent less likely to develop heart disease
More than 35 percent less likely to have a heart attack
More than 41 percent less likely to develop high blood pressure
More than 40 percent less likely to develop kidney cancer
More than 60 percent less likely to develop gallstones
More than 14 percent less likely to develop osteoarthritis

A Longer Life

A Canadian study of more than 8,000 people over 13 years found that those with the weakest abdominal muscles had more than double the death rate of the people with the strongest midsections. No surprise when you consider all the health conditions associated with belly fat.

out, making even a relatively flat belly bulge. That means that to lose your gut, you've got to work your butt.

Two moves—the glute bridge march and hip-thigh raise (see pages 250–251)—will help you get a stronger behind. Combat tight hip flexors with this stretch: In a lunge position, lower yourself so your back knee is resting on the floor. Push your hips forward, keeping your back upright, until you feel a stretch in the front of the hip. Hold for 10 seconds, relax, and repeat. Switch legs. You can increase the stretch by reaching your arms over your head.

7. Stop Stressing

Anxiety can produce extra cortisol, a hormone that encourages the body to store fat, particularly in your belly. According to researchers at Yale University, your midsection is four times as likely as the rest of your body to store stress-induced fat. Keep anxiety in check by taking little breaks from work every 90 minutes to breathe and relax. "It's almost like recalibrating your body," Waters says.

Another way stress sabotages your abs: When tension runs high, we reach for fattening foods. So keep the office candy jar out of reach. In one study, participants who had to walk 6 feet to reach candy ate up to seven fewer chocolates per day than when the jars were conveniently located at their desks.

8. Skip the Late Shows

You need sleep to unveil a sexy stomach. That's because lack of shut-eye may disrupt the hormones that control your ability to burn fat. For instance, University of Chicago scientists recently found that just three nights of poor sleep may cause your muscle cells to become resistant to the hormone insulin. Over time, this leads to fat storage around your belly.

To achieve a better night's sleep, review your goals again 15 minutes before bedtime. And while you're at it, write down your plans for the next day's work schedule, as well as any personal chores you need to accomplish. This can help prevent you from lying awake worrying about tomorrow ("I have to remember to call Mom"), which can cut into quality snooze time.

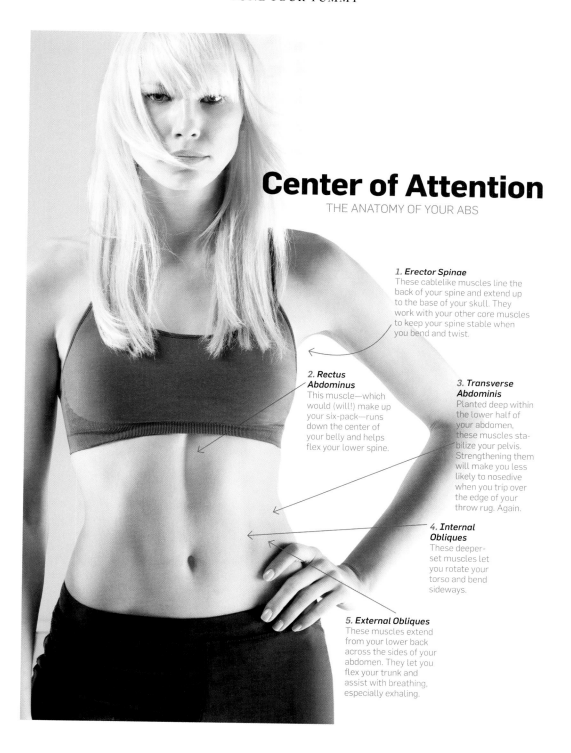

Center of Attention
THE ANATOMY OF YOUR ABS

1. Erector Spinae
These cablelike muscles line the back of your spine and extend up to the base of your skull. They work with your other core muscles to keep your spine stable when you bend and twist.

2. Rectus Abdominus
This muscle—which would (will!) make up your six-pack—runs down the center of your belly and helps flex your lower spine.

3. Transverse Abdominis
Planted deep within the lower half of your abdomen, these muscles stabilize your pelvis. Strengthening them will make you less likely to nosedive when you trip over the edge of your throw rug. Again.

4. Internal Obliques
These deeper-set muscles let you rotate your torso and bend sideways.

5. External Obliques
These muscles extend from your lower back across the sides of your abdomen. They let you flex your trunk and assist with breathing, especially exhaling.

237

Your Perfect Weight—Get There, Stay There

DETERMINE YOUR IDEAL SIZE WITH OUR BODY–ANALYSIS
GUIDE, THEN MAKE IT A REALITY WITH
OUR THREE–STEP SYSTEM TAILOR-MADE FOR YOU.

By Julie Upton, RD

Of all the numbers you carry around in your head, there's one series of digits that probably drives you crazy. Not because it's hard to remember—in fact, you could never forget it, no matter how hard you tried. This number represents your ever-elusive perfect weight. If you could only achieve it, and stay there, you're certain you'd be better in bed, more confident in meetings, sexier and sassier in jeans, and in every way 10 times happier than you are right this minute. But what is this magical number, and how do you arrive at it?

Is it a reasonable weight that falls within the ranges provided on doctor-approved charts? Or is it a weight you dipped to once, 4 years ago, after living through a painful breakup and that killer intestinal thing? The first key to hitting your number—and we promise you, you can do it—is to make it a realistic one, based on your bone structure and body type. The good news is that once you determine the right number and set your mind to reach it, your body will help you get there, despite late-night cravings and sluggish treadmill sessions.

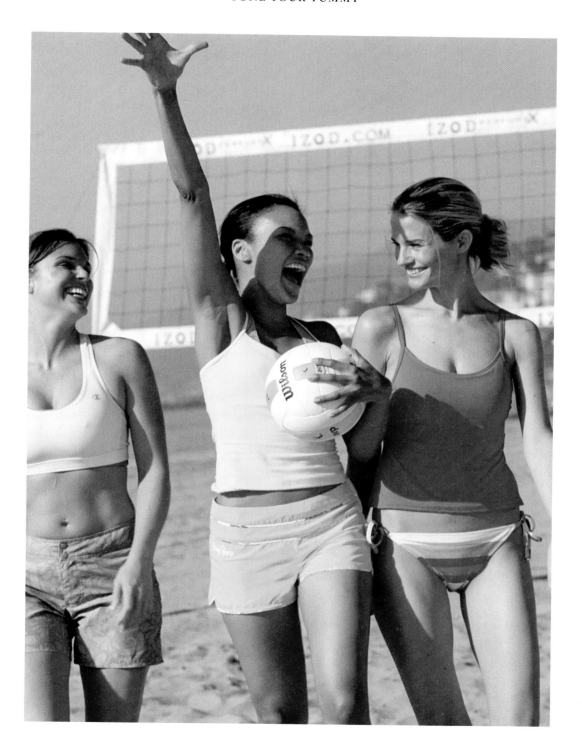

Step 1: Do the Math

There's no single formula for predicting an exact, down-to-the-decimal weight for every woman alive, but there are certain guidelines you can use to set a realistic weight-loss goal. Here are four that can help you find your magic number.

A. Your Baseline Figure

To start, let's go back to Health 101. Take the number of inches you are over 5 feet and multiply that number by five. Add this to 100 for a rough initial estimate of what someone of your height should weigh. So if you're 5 feet 7 inches, multiply 7 by 5 and add 100. Your target weight is 135. But wait! You're not done yet. You still need to assess—and factor in—the other elements that contribute to your perfect weight.

B. Your Bone Structure

Remember that phrase "you're just big-boned"? It seems like a euphemism for "fat" (see also "husky," "chunky," "pleasantly plump"), but the truth is that your frame—in effect, your bone structure—can run large or small, no matter how tall you are. Researchers now recognize that having a large frame can add up to 10 pounds of healthy, unavoidable weight to your body.

Okay, now take that baseline figure you calculated in Step A and adjust it accordingly—5 to 10 pounds more for a bigger frame, 5 to 10 pounds less for a smaller frame (see the chart below). Now you've got one number, but there are still two other important considerations, both having to do with your current body composition.

C. Your Overall Body Fat

One of the best indicators of whether you're at a healthy weight is how much of your bulk is fat. While between 20 and 31 percent is considered a "normal" range for women, an ideal level for fitness (and looking fit) is around 21 percent. The best way to measure body fat is with calibration tools—either old-fashioned skin-pinching calipers or more sensitive bioelectric impedance analysis machines, which use electrical currents to measure body mass. Is your bioelectric impedance machine in the shop? You can get a good estimation of your fat and how much of it you need to lose by using the chart on the opposite page.

21
Ideal body-fat percentage for women

D. Your Belly Fat

Now you want to figure out whether you are packing on too much belly fat—dangerous stuff because the same fat that gathers around your abdomen, called adipose fat, is also likely to be collecting around vital organs and preventing healthy bloodflow. And researchers at the New York Obesity Research Center at St. Luke's–Roosevelt Hospital found that waist size correlates better than overall body mass to risk factors for heart disease, such as high blood pressure, blood sugar, and cholesterol.

To calculate your waist size, wrap the tape measure around the tops of your hip bones. Take

Bone Structure Chart

Match your wrist measurements to your height	To determine your bone structure, measure the circumference of your wrist.		
	IF YOU'RE UNDER 5'2"	IF YOU'RE BETWEEN 5'2" AND 5'5"	IF YOU'RE OVER 5'5"
small frame	• *wrist size under 5.5"*	• *wrist size under 6"*	• *wrist size under 6.25"*
medium frame	• *wrist size 5.5" to 5.75"*	• *wrist size 6" to 6.25"*	• *wrist size 6.25" to 6.5"*
large frame	• *wrist size over 5.75"*	• *wrist size over 6.25"*	• *wrist size over 6.5"*

To Find Your Overall Body Fat . . .

1. First, find your body mass index (BMI), a ratio of weight to height. Say you're a 145-pound, 36-year-old woman who's 5 feet 10 inches (70 inches) tall. Multiply your height in inches by your height in inches.
Example: 70 x 70 = 4,900
Next, divide your weight by that number.
Example:
145 / 4,900 = 0.029
Now multiply that by 703 to find your BMI.
Example:
BMI = 0.029 x 703 = 20.39
Your BMI:　＿＿＿＿＿＿

2. To determine your body-fat percentage, multiply your BMI by 1.20.
Example:
1.20 x 20.39 = 24.47
Multiply your age by 0.23.
Example:
0.23 x 36 = 8.28
Add those two numbers.
Example:
24.47 + 8.28 = 32.75
Subtract 5.4 from that sum to find your body-fat percentage.
Example:
32.75 – 5.4 = 27.35
Your Body-Fat
Percentage:　＿＿＿＿＿＿

3. Use the body-fat percentage chart (below, right) to determine how far over the goal you are (or aren't!). At 27 percent body fat, our sample woman is carrying 21 percent more fat than the ideal of 21 percent.

4. Translate your body-fat percentage into how much sheer fat you're carrying by multiplying your body fat by your current weight.
Example:
27% x 145 = 39.15

In other words, almost 40 pounds of our 145-pound woman comes from her friend, fat.
Your Weight
from Fat:　＿＿＿＿＿＿

5. Finally, multiply your percentage over goal from Step 3 by your total body fat in answer 4. That's how many pounds of fat you should try to lose.
Example:
39 x 21% = 8.19 pounds
Your Weight-
Loss Goal:　＿＿＿＿＿＿

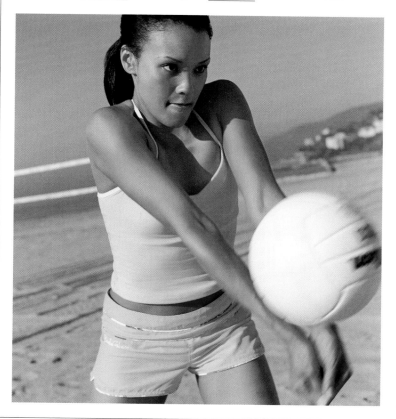

Body-Fat Percentage	
Body Fat	Percentage over Goal
22	4
23	7
24	11
25	14
26	18
27	21
28	25
29	29
30	32
31	36
32	39
33	43
34	46
35	50
36	54
37	57
38	61
39	64
40	68
41	71
42	75
43	79
44	82

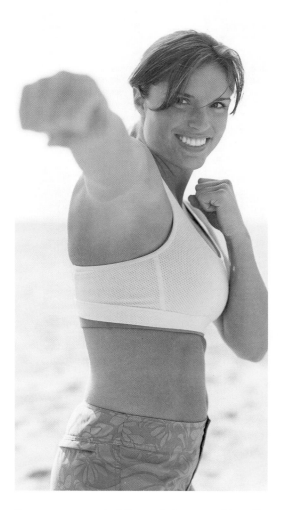

termined by the results of Steps C and D. You have the best understanding of what's realistic for you and how much your body can change, so don't let an overly ambitious goal ruin your day—or your healthy habits. Read ahead for our plan designed to burn off excess fat, build muscle, and get you to your perfect weight—and keep you there for good.

Step 2: Get There

You know the drill: To lose weight, you have to consume fewer calories than you burn. And to do that, you need to know your metabolic rate—the amount of calories you burn throughout the day. Most women have a metabolic rate of just under 1 calorie per minute, or about 1,440 calories per day, says David Nieman, PhD, a nutrition and exercise professor at Appalachian State University in Boone, North Carolina. Use this chart to determine your metabolic rate and daily calorie needs.

Your Vitals	Your Exercise	Your Calorie Needs
A. Your weight in pounds _____	D. **Aerobic Training** Multiply the number of minutes per week that you run, cycle, or play sports by 8 _____	G. Add C and F to get your daily calorie needs _____
B. Multiply A by 11 to get your basic calorie needs (how much your body burns just by existing) _____		H. If you're happy with your weight, stop here. Otherwise, subtract 500 from G _____
	E. **Strength Training** If you're doing two sets of an exercise plan similar to the ones in Chapter 3, add 600 to your answer from D.	
C. Multiply B by 1.6 to estimate your resting metabolic rate (rate of calorie burn when you factor in your daily activities) _____		This is your estimated daily calorie budget if you want to lose 1 pound per week. Subtract 1,000 to lose 2 pounds a week. Anything more and you'll lose more muscle than fat. You're on your way to your perfect weight!
	If you're doing three sets, add 840 to your answer from D.	
	F. Divide that by 7 _____	

the measurement at the end of a normal breath. Then place your index finger next to your belly button and, standing up straight, see how many inches of belly fat you can grasp between your index finger and thumb.

If your waist is over 33 inches and you can pinch 2 inches of fat, you need to lose at least 10 pounds from your current weight, no matter how you've scored in other tests. If you can pinch 1 inch, you need to lose at least 5 pounds.

Okay, so your "perfect weight," then, is between the figure you arrived at in Steps A and B and the amount of weight you need to lose as de-

On a healthy weight-loss diet, about three-quarters of every pound you lose is fat and one-quarter is lean body mass.

Step 3: Stay There

Losing weight is the easy part. But we all know that. Somehow, as soon as you've closed in on your magic number, it becomes harder and harder to stay there. And in fact, the wrong dieting habits can slow your metabolism, canceling out all your hard work. Well, no worries. Here's how to retool your eating behaviors and exercise routine to maintain your new, svelter self.

On a healthy weight-loss diet, about three-quarters of every pound you lose is fat and one-quarter is lean body mass. Lose too much too fast and you're more likely to have trouble keeping it off. "Depending on how rapidly you lose weight and on your diet and exercise patterns, your resting metabolic rate can decrease significantly during weight loss," says Chris Melby, DrPH, head of the department of food science and human nutrition at Colorado State University in Fort Collins. But even if you go at a safe, slow pound a week, your body still adapts to the loss—and makes it hard to stay slim. For every pound you lose, your total daily calories need to be reduced by about 10. Lose 10 pounds, and your body needs 100 fewer calories a day, on average, to sustain itself.

Getting more daily exercise is one way to help offset this drop in metabolic rate, but it still doesn't mean you can ignore what you eat. And beware of postworkout snacking: A study from the School of Human Kinetics at the University of Ottawa in Ontario found that a woman's appetite postexercise may drive her to eat as many calories as she burned during exercise. "Even if you exercise for an hour or more a day, our body is so fuel efficient that you'll still have to watch what you eat. Exercise because it's good for your health, but watch your diet because it ultimately controls how lean you are," Dr. Nieman says.

Slim Your Stomach Instantly

WHEN YOU WANT YOUR BELLY TO LOOK TRIM ON A DEADLINE—SAY, FOR THAT UPCOMING BEACH VACATION OR YOUR BEST FRIEND'S WEDDING—USE THESE THREE TRICKS TO LOOK EVEN SVELTER.

---

3 days before: Cut the carbs (except fruits and nonstarchy veggies). You'll shed any extra water you may have been holding on to, which can knock the scale down a notch or two. Skip excess salt too (it has the same water-retaining effect). Limit your daily sodium intake to 2,300 milligrams. Also, steer clear of cruciferous vegetables like broccoli, cabbage, and brussels sprouts—they're high in fiber and hard to digest, which means they make you bloated and, well, flatulent. They also contain sulfur, so when you let one rip, it's stinkier than a port-o-potty at Lollapalooza.

2 days before: Hit snooze. The amount of sleep you get affects the function of ghrelin and leptin— hormones that regulate your appetite and metabolism. Skimping on shut-eye can cause the hormone levels to fluctuate, which makes you hungry (especially for sugary, carb-heavy foods) and less able to tell when you're full. Aim for at least 7 hours of sleep a night and you won't be as likely to give in to that hot-dog hankering.

1 day before: Say *sayonara* to soda. When you drink carbonated beverages, you consume extra air, which makes your paunch puff up right after you've finished that Diet Dr. Pepper. So ditch the soda and seltzer and down water instead.

Part Two

An All-Play, No-Work Guide to a Tighter Midsection

Take a Firm Approach

FOCUS MORE ON YOUR CORE WITH 6 ACTIVITIES THAT WILL SHAPE YOUR MIDDLE—AND HAVE FUN WHILE YOU'RE DOING THEM!

By Alexa Joy Sherman

*W*aist flab is like a bad makeup job: Underneath it all there's something really attractive that you just can't see. Yet. And don't think you need to crunch yourself silly to morph your waist from drainpipe to hourglass either. The key is to burn off fat with cardio and work your core from every angle, so you'll have toned your whole waist—the front, the sides, and the back. We tapped top experts to show you how to get the most core-shaping benefits out of six popular activities, so you can do double duty during cardio and whittle while you work.

Tennis

Another reason to book lessons with the local Federer-wannabe: "You recruit your core muscles—stretching, twisting, and contracting your abs with every shot," says Bill Mountford, director of tennis for the US Tennis Association National Tennis Center in Flushing, Queens. And when you run for shots, you also burn calories and fat.

Waist Rx: To really kick your core and strengthen your obliques (the muscles on the sides of your waist), turn completely through the ball, fully

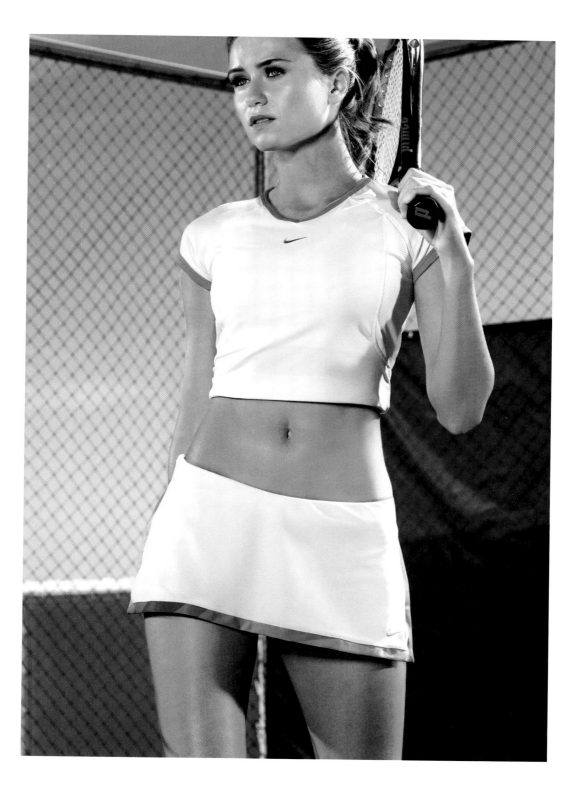

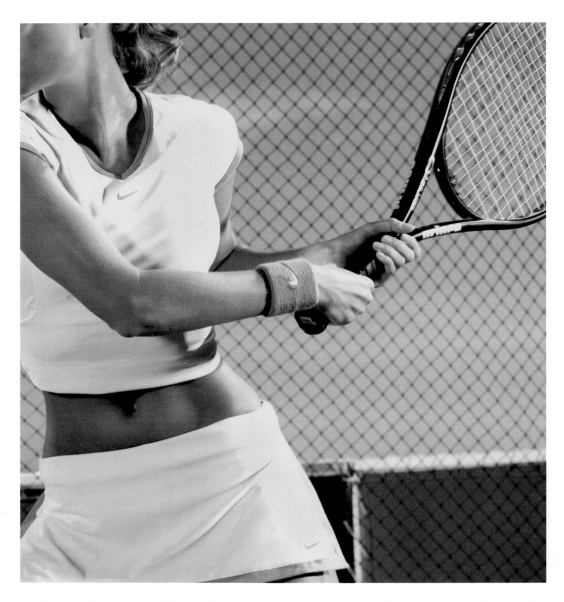

rotating your hips and shoulders in the direction of the shot—especially during forehands and two-handed backhands. "You'll hit the ball harder without compromising consistency, and you'll tax your core muscles," Mountford says. To emphasize your core, do the circuit below against a backboard or using a ball machine. Twist your torso completely through every hit to work your muscles through the entire range of motion. Do the circuit, rest for a minute, then repeat.

20 forehands
20 two-handed backhands
20 alternating forehands and two-handed backhands
10 serves (much of the power will come as you stretch, then contract, your core)

Bounding, especially on uneven terrain, forces your core to keep you balanced.

Trail Running

Running can burn more fat than a McDonald's franchise, but for a bigger calorie burn mixed with core stability work, head for rough ground. "Trail running offers more of a core challenge because you're constantly stabilizing on the uneven terrain," says Rebecca Rusch, a Red Bull adventure racer from Ketchum, Idaho. "You're forced to use your obliques to balance yourself with every step. The more uneven the terrain, the better your core workout."

Waist Rx: Find a trail with a variety of terrain, such as rocks, dips, and different degrees of steepness. For a 30-minute trail run that burns calories and will engage your core with every step, try this off-road workout.

Jog for 8 minutes at a relaxed pace. Then do 1 minute of running at a pace where you're not sprinting, but you're huffing hard. At the end of the minute, stop and do a series of 10 bounds—alternating one-legged leaps (pretend you're leaping over a small stream). Your bounds should be much longer than your average stride and much slower. Bounding—especially on uneven terrain—forces your core to keep you balanced, so you'll engage all of the muscles in your waist. For more of a twist, alternate between leaping forward and leaping laterally to work your obliques and the sides of your legs. Follow this with an easy 1-minute jog. Repeat the cycle of hard running, bounding, and jogging twice to complete the workout.

Hiking

A steep hike makes a fitness trifecta: You'll strengthen your legs, glutes, and abs. "Hiking downhill also strengthens your lower back because that part of your core works to compensate for the changing angle of the trail," Rusch says.

Waist Rx: To amplify your hike, Rusch recommends using poles (check www.leki.com for options) to add more total-body resistance. The poles allow you to pull and push your weight up the hill, so you burn more fat. Also, if you twist your middle to face the side of the pole you're pulling back, you can add a more focused resistance challenge that strengthens your obliques and the back of your waist. "Be aggressive, planting them at the same

The Best Move to Do at Work

STRENGTHEN YOUR BELLY IN LESS TIME THAN IT TAKES TO SEND AN E-MAIL.

This move from trainer Nick Tumminello, owner of Performance University in Baltimore, lets you activate those deep core muscles without leaving your desk. Do it anytime you need a break at work. For the best results, use a stable chair that doesn't swivel.

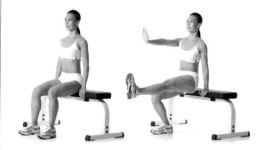

Upright Bird Dog

Sit at the edge of your chair with your feet flat on the floor, resting your hands on the seat next to your hips. Keep your hips, knees, and ankles bent at 90 degrees. Shift your weight forward off the seat so that all your weight rests on your hands and feet. Bracing your abs and keeping your torso stable, lift your left foot off the floor and your right arm straight in front of you. Hold for 10 seconds, then repeat the move with the opposite arm and leg. That's 1 rep; do 3 to 10 reps. Do this simple move three times a week and you'll be one step closer to a sexy core.

time as the opposite foot," Rusch says. "Your arm should be fully extended behind your body at the finish of each pole plant." Hike for at least 30 minutes to dip into your fat stores.

Swimming

Water provides natural muscle-toning resistance, but most of us overlook it as a waist workout. "While most people think of swimming with their arms, the best swimmers in the world rotate their hips to generate power," says Eric Harr, author of *Triathlon Training in Four Hours a Week*. "It not only builds your whole core, it helps you move efficiently in the water."

Waist Rx: When swimming freestyle, rotate your hips by rolling your body side to side as far as you can with every stroke. Focus on keeping your midsection tight, so it's aligned as one unit with your shoulders and hips. "Backstroke is also terrific for waist whittling because your whole core is constantly working to keep your body flat and stable on top of the water," Harr says. For more of a workout, warm up with 5 minutes of easy swimming and then grab a pair of fins. Float on your back with your arms stretched beyond your head and do dolphin kicks—kicking powerfully with both feet together—to propel yourself. Rest at the other end for 30 seconds and do 8 to 12 more laps before cooling down with a few minutes of easy swimming, fin free. "The fins increase resistance to work your core harder," Harr says.

Melt Your Middle

THIS TURBO-BOOSTED PLAN WILL SPEED UP YOUR SLIM-DOWN.

Follow this interval-training program to fire up your metabolism and burn off the fat that's hiding your abs. Intervals are short bursts of maximum-intensity effort—you're doing it right if you can't carry on a conversation—separated by periods of easy-pace recovery. In an Australian study, women who cranked out high-intensity interval training 3 days a week for 15 weeks dropped significantly more weight than those who exercised for the same period of time at a lower intensity.

	Max Effort	Easy Pace	Reps
WEEK 1	1 minute	2 minutes	5
WEEK 2	1 minute	90 seconds	6
WEEK 3	1 minute	1 minute	8
WEEK 4	1 minute	1 minute	10
WEEK 5	75 seconds	1 minute	10
WEEK 6	90 seconds	1 minute	10

Do the above routine three times a week after you work your core—and always remember to include an easy, 3- to 5-minute warmup and cooldown. You can run, bike, or use the cardio machine of your choice.

Mountain Biking

Cycling can burn your glutes, thighs, and usually your lungs, but if you want to recruit more ab and back muscles, get off the road. "The balance required to roll over undulating terrain builds core strength while burning massive amounts of calories," Harr says. And when you rise out of the saddle, you wind up using your core muscles to power your pedal strokes. (You can get similar benefits from rising out of your seat in spin class, sans rolling terrain.)

Waist Rx: Get up. "Include anywhere from four to eight standing intervals, ranging in length from 20 seconds to 2 minutes at a time, when you ride," Harr says. If you're a beginner, stick to the short intervals; if you're more advanced, stand for the full 2-minute sprints. If you're inside on a stationary bike or in spin class, getting out of the saddle will still force you to stabilize.

You can burn your core even more with this move: Turn the tension on your spinning cycle up high (so it feels like you're going up a steep incline), get out of the saddle, and pedal uphill. After 10 or 20 seconds, remove your firm grip

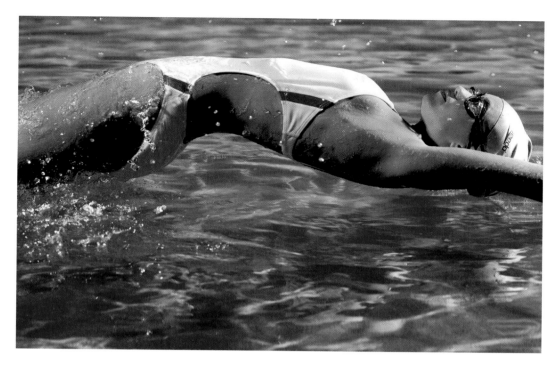

from the handles and stand up as straight as you can out of the saddle; now just lightly touch a few fingers on top of the handlebars (so you won't fall over). Without relying on your upper body so much for balance, you will force your core to keep you straight and keep you up. Alternate between 20 seconds on the handles and 40 seconds off for 2 to 3 minutes. Then sit back, spin for 3 minutes, and repeat the up-hill interval.

Rowing

That lonely piece of equipment in your gym is actually one of the most useful. It works your whole body, burning major calories, and it zeroes in on your back. "As you push with your legs, you pull with and really engage your lower back and lats," Rusch says.

Waist Rx: Most people round their backs while rowing, missing out on the back-flab toning benefits. The key is to keep your back straight and

80

Percentage more effort required from your shoulder muscles to slam a tennis ball when you have an unstable core

use it. Rusch's formula for good form: Start with knees bent and arms straight, and lean slightly forward with a straight back. "Lean from your waist," she says. Next, push with and extend your legs, and then tighten your core and slightly pull with your lower back, keeping your back straight. Finally, bring your fists to your chest and reverse the order to straighten arms, lean, and then bend legs. As the technique gets more comfortable, you can make each phase explosive. The return back to start is your rest time, so use that second to relax before exploding again. Row for at least 30 minutes for the best burn.

When you're finished with your workout, keep your legs stationary and for 5 minutes, do the last two phases of the stroke for an extra back burn and to emphasize the forgotten yet just as essential part of your core: your lower back. Sit and lean back (pull with your back muscles, keeping your back straight) and then snap your arms to your chest.

8 Moves for Your Core— No Crunches Required

GET A TIGHT STOMACH IN JUST 6 WEEKS WITH THIS QUICK, EASY, AND EFFICIENT WORKOUT.

This exercise plan, created by Rachel Cosgrove, CSCS, owner of Results Fitness in Newhall, California, combines fat-burning cardio with moves that target your entire core rather than individual muscles, so you'll burn more fat while toning up.

Directions

Do these moves on 3 nonconsecutive days a week. Start with the Basic Workout to prime your muscles. After 3 weeks, you'll be ready to graduate to the Advanced Workout. For maximum fat burning, perform the exercises as a circuit: Do one set of each move in the order shown, resting for 30 seconds between exercises. Then rest for a minute and repeat the circuit from the beginning.

Basic Workout

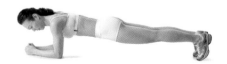

1. Plank Starting at the top of a pushup position, bend your elbows and lower yourself down until you can shift your weight from your hands to your forearms. Your body should form a straight line. Brace your abs (imagine someone is about to punch you in the gut) and hold for 60 seconds. If you can't make it to 60 seconds, hold for 5 to 10 seconds and rest for 5 seconds, continuing for 1 minute.

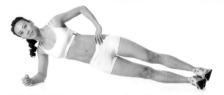

2. Side Plank Lie on your right side with your legs straight. Prop yourself up with your right forearm so your body forms a diagonal line. Rest your left hand on your hip. Brace your abs and hold for 60 seconds. If that's too long, hold for 5 to 10 seconds and rest for 5; continue for 1 minute.

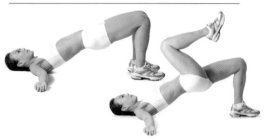

3. Glute Bridge March Lie on your back with your knees bent and your feet flat on the floor. Rest your arms on the floor, palms up, at shoulder level. Raise your hips so your body forms a straight line from your shoulders to your knees. Brace your abs and lift your right knee toward your chest. Hold for 2 counts, then lower your right foot. Repeat with the other leg. That's 1 rep. Do three sets of 10 reps.

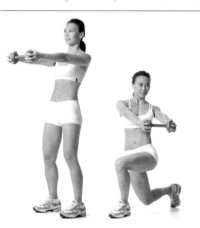

4. Lunge with Rotation Grab a light dumbbell with both hands. Stand with your feet hip-width apart and your arms straight out. Take a big step forward with your left foot and, bracing your abs, twist your torso to the left as you bend your knees and lower your body until both of your legs form 90-degree angles. Twist back to center, push off your left foot, and stand back up. Repeat on the other leg. That's 1 rep. Do two or three sets of 10 to 15 reps.

Advanced Workout

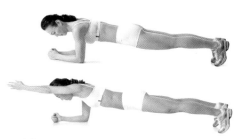

1. *Plank with Arm Lift* Get into the plank position (toes and forearms on the floor, body lifted). Your body should form a straight line. Brace your abs and carefully shift your weight to your right forearm. Extend your left arm in front of you and hold for 3 to 10 seconds. Slowly bring your arm back in. Repeat with the right arm. That's 1 rep. Do two or three sets of 5 to 10 reps, resting for 1 minute between sets.

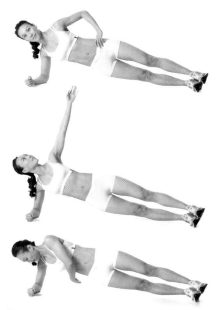

2. *Side Plank with Rotation* In the right-side plank position, brace your abs and reach your left hand toward the ceiling. Slowly tuck your left arm under your body and twist forward until your torso is almost parallel to the floor. Return to the side plank. That's 1 rep. Do two or three sets of 5 to 10 reps on each side, resting for 1 minute between sets.

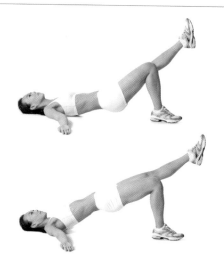

3. *Hip-Thigh Raise* Lie on your back with your right knee bent and your left leg extended. Rest your arms on the floor, palms up, at shoulder level with your hips about 2 inches off the floor. Raise your hips to form a straight line from your shoulders to your left foot. Hold for 2 counts, then return to start. That's 1 rep. Do 10 to 15 reps on each side. To make it harder, cross your arms over your chest.

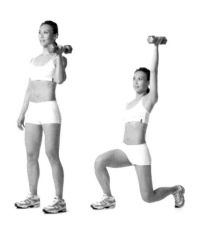

4. *Reverse Lunge with Single-Arm Press* Grab a 5- to 15-pound dumbbell in your left hand and hold it up next to your left shoulder, palm facing in. Step backward with your left foot and lower your body until your knees are bent to 90 degrees (your left knee should nearly touch the floor) while pressing the dumbbell directly over your shoulder without bending or leaning at the waist. Lower the weight back to the starting position as you push quickly back to standing. That's 1 rep. Do 10 to 15, then switch sides.

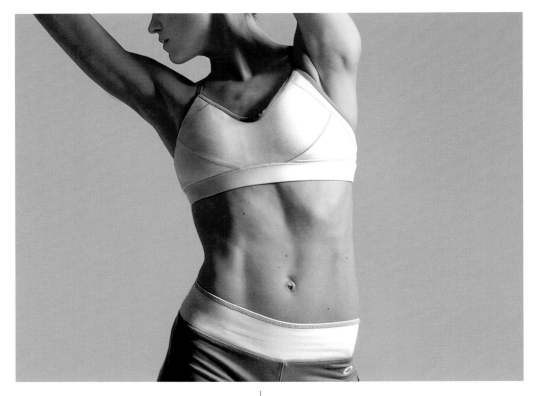

One Good Turn

IF THE ONLY THINGS YOU TWIST ARE
JAR LIDS, THEN YOU'RE MISSING
A GREAT CHANCE TO TONE YOUR BELLY.

Like martinis, updos, and the dance floor at that wedding last summer, your abs would be so much better with a twist. "Muscle fibers in the abdominals run diagonally," says Tom Holland, MS, CSCS, a trainer and exercise physiologist in Darien, Connecticut. "Working them in the way they were designed to move gets you the best results in both strength and tone." Twisting abdominal moves focus on your deepest core muscles, which will both strengthen and narrow your waist. Do either set of these four exercises three to five times a week.

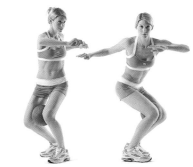

1. _Twister_
Works: Quads and obliques
Stand with your knees slightly bent and squeeze a small medicine ball between them. Take a small jump, rotating your knees to the right. Then jump to the left. Do two sets of about 20 jumps (or until tired). When 20 gets too easy, sink lower with each twist to a squat, and rotate back up. Repeat to your other side. Do 6 to 10 reps.

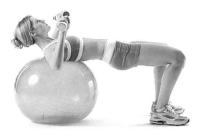

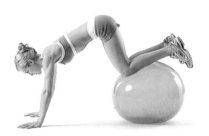

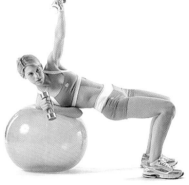

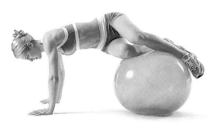

2. *One-Arm Rotational Press*
Works: Deltoids, glutes, and spinal stabilizers
Lie with your shoulders on a Swiss ball and hold a 2-
to 5-pound dumbbell in each hand. Keeping your hips
stable, press your left arm up and roll to your right
until you're on your right shoulder. Return to the start
and repeat to the other side. Aim for 12 reps.

3. *Swiss-Ball Twist*
Works: Hips, obliques, and spinal stabilizers
From the pushup position, place your shins on a
Swiss ball so you're straddling the ball from your
knees to your ankles. With your abs held tight,
slowly roll your knees to the left, then use your
obliques to roll your knees back to the start. Repeat
to the other side. Do 6 to 10 total reps (3 to 5 to
each side).

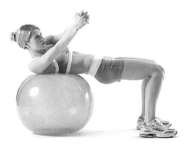

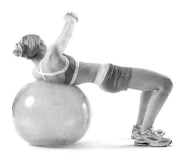

4. *Swiss-Ball Russian Twist*
Works: Obliques, glutes, and spinal stabilizers
Lie with your shoulders on a Swiss ball. Extend your
arms in front of you with your hands clasped together.

Press your tongue against the roof of your mouth to
stabilize your neck. Pull in your belly and rotate your
torso from side to side, keeping your feet on the
floor and your hips up. Do 10 reps to each side.

253

A 20-Minute, Twice-a-Week Abs Workout

GET A SLEEK STOMACH FAST—EVEN IF YOU ONLY HAVE MINUTES TO SPARE.

Challenge your core with these moves designed by Amy Dixon, exercise physiologist and group fitness manager at Equinox Fitness in Santa Monica, California. Do the recommended sets and reps, and use a weight that lets you barely complete the last rep of the final set with perfect form.

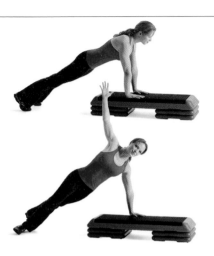

2. *Walk the Plank and Rotate*
Works: Entire core, shoulders, chest, back, and hips
Get in the plank position with your hands on a 12- to 18-inch step. With your weight on your left arm, rotate your body while raising your right arm toward the ceiling. Return to the plank position and step your right arm down to the right of the bench, then your left arm down to the left of the bench. Step back up, leading with your left arm. That's 1 rep. Do 8 to 10 reps, rest for 30 seconds, then repeat, twisting to the opposite side.

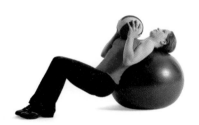

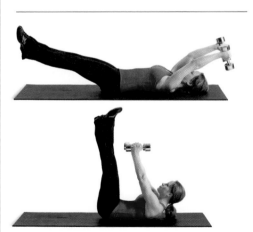

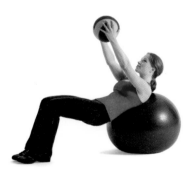

1. *Swiss-Ball Pelvic Tilt Crunch*
Works: Chest, abs, hips, and glutes
Grab a 5- to 10-pound medicine ball. Lie faceup on a Swiss ball with your back and head pressed into the ball, your feet together on the floor, and the medicine ball positioned against your chest. Brace your abs and crunch up until your shoulders are off the ball. Then reach the ball toward the ceiling. That's 1 rep. Do three sets of 12 to 15 reps, resting for 30 seconds between each set.

3. *Stiff-Leg Pullover Crunch*
Works: Upper back, abs, and hips
Grab a pair of 10- to 12-pound dumbbells and lie on your back with your arms extended beyond your head. Extend your legs at a 45-degree angle. Bring your arms up over your chest and lift your shoulders off the mat while raising your legs until they're perpendicular to the floor. Return to start (don't let your legs touch the floor). That's 1 rep. Do three sets of 15 reps, resting for 30 seconds between sets.

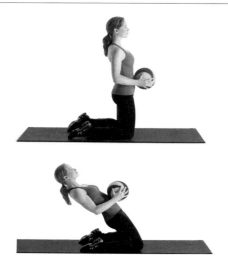

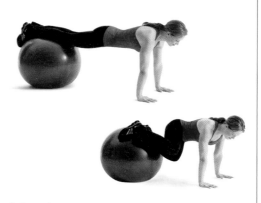

4. *The Matrix*
Works: Abs, back, glutes, and quads
Grab a 5- to 10-pound medicine ball and kneel on the floor with your knees hip-width apart. Lengthen your spine and press the ball against your abs. Slowly lean back as far as possible, keeping your knees planted. Hold the reclined position for 3 seconds, then use your core to slowly come up to the starting position. That's 1 rep. Do three sets of 15 reps, resting for 30 seconds between sets.

6. *Prone Oblique Roll*
Works: Shoulders, chest, obliques, back, and glutes
Get in the plank position with your shins about hip-width apart on a Swiss ball and your hands shoulder-width apart on the floor. Keeping your feet on the ball, draw your right knee toward your right shoulder (the left just comes along for the ride). Return to center. Do 12 to 15 reps, rest for 30 seconds, then repeat on the other side.
Trainer tip: As you draw your knees across your body, focus on rotating your core and activating your obliques. To help with balance, pick one spot on the floor and stare at it.

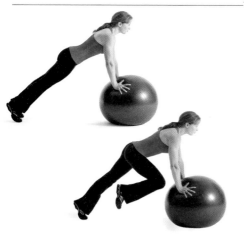

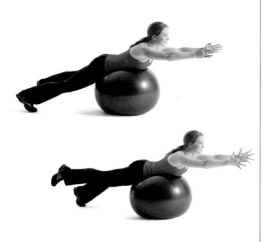

5. *Knee-to-Chest Crunch*
Works: Entire core, shoulders, chest, hips, and glutes
Get in the plank position with your hands shoulder-width apart on a Swiss ball. Draw your right knee toward your chest. Hold for 1 second, then return to the plank position. That's 1 rep. Do 12 to 15 reps. Rest for 30 seconds, then repeat with the other leg.

7. *Rear Leg Raise*
Works: Lower back and glutes
Rest your hips and belly on a Swiss ball. Straighten your legs and position your toes hip-width apart on the floor. Extend your arms in line with your shoulders. Lift your right leg about 6 inches off the floor while reaching out your arms as far as possible. That's 1 rep. Do 15 reps, then repeat to the other side without resting between sides.

Control Your Cravings

DON'T SABOTAGE YOUR HARD-EARNED ABS
WITH A MOMENT OF WEAKNESS! USE THESE TIPS BEFORE
GIVING IN TO YOUR SWEET TOOTH.

By Adam Campbell

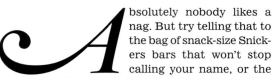

Absolutely nobody likes a nag. But try telling that to the bag of snack-size Snickers bars that won't stop calling your name, or the oh-so-salty French fries that keep pummeling your willpower.

A craving is like a little devil, constantly encouraging you to indulge. And dieting only turns up the pressure: A study published in the *International Journal of Obesity* found that 91 percent of women experienced food cravings when they weren't on a diet; once they started restricting calories, that figure went up to 94 percent. And we all know that giving in to urges is a ticket to nothing-in-my-closet-fits hell.

The good news is that, unlike, say, your mom's constant probing about future grandkids, these unhealthy tormentors can be fended off. The reason: Cravings are all about blood sugar. If your levels stay consistent throughout the day, your eating patterns will too. It's when you starve yourself for hours that cravings call.

"Your blood sugar can fall too low after just 4 hours of not eating," says Valerie Berkowitz, MS, RD, director of nutrition at the Center for Balanced Health in New York City. So you search the fridge, the food court, even the seat cushions for simple carbohydrates that will give you a quick boost.

Trouble is, the resulting blood-sugar spike triggers your pancreas to release insulin, a hormone that not only lowers blood sugar, but also signals your body to run through the craving cycle over

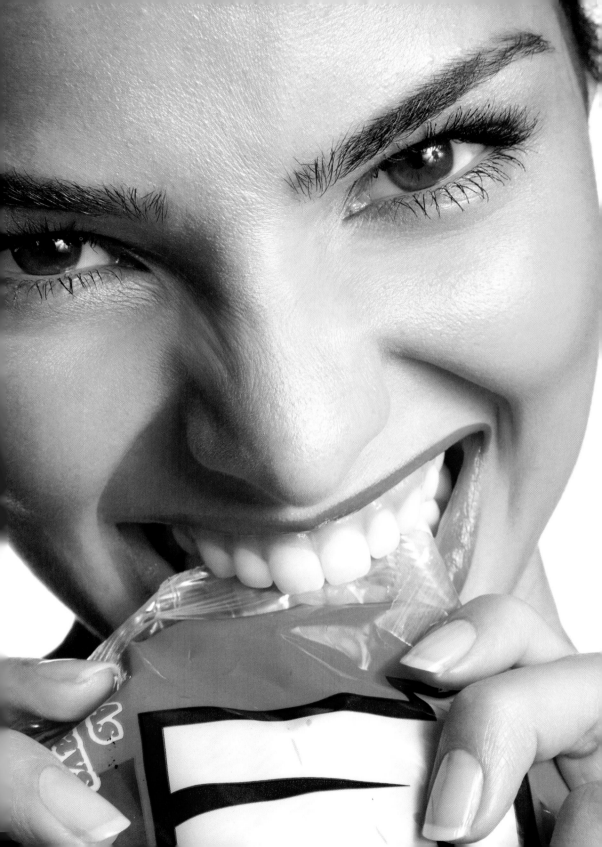

You're more likely to succumb to a craving when the object you desire is close at hand. So defy temptation by making sure it's not.

and over. In about half of us, insulin tends to overshoot—that's what sends blood sugar crashing. "This reinforces the binge because it makes you crave sugar and starch again," Berkowitz says. In other words, giving in to a carb craving only leaves you wanting more.

So how do you stop yourself from reaching for that Snickers? By following these seven steps designed to stop 99 percent of cravings before they start—and help you muzzle the 1 percent that never seem to shut up.

1. Ramp Up Your Resolve

One reason most diets fail is that long-term goals can be deceptively difficult: When the plan is to watch what you eat for the next 6 months, chugging one caramel latte with whipped cream seems like a minor slip. To avoid that kind of thinking, commit to eating well for a fixed amount of time that you're 100 percent confident you can manage, even if it's just a few days. "Once you make it to your goal date, start over," says Mary Vernon, MD, chairperson of the board of the American Society of Bariatric Physicians. "This establishes the notion that you can be successful and gives you a chance to notice that eating better makes you feel better, reinforcing your desire to continue."

2. Find Meaningful Motivation

If the main purpose of your diet is cosmetic—i.e., to look amazing in that body-hugging little black dress—you're unlikely to stick with it for the long haul. The solution: "Arm yourself with additional motivators," says Jeff Volek, PhD, RD, associate professor of kinesiology at the University of Connecticut in Storrs. He suggests keeping a daily journal in which you monitor migraines, heartburn, acne, canker sores, and sleep quality in addition to body measurements and the number on the

scale. "Discovering that your new diet improves the quality of your life and health is powerful motivation," Dr. Volek says.

3. Move On after a Mistake

Okay, you overindulged. What's the next step? "Forget about it," says James Newman, a nutritionist at Tahlequah City Hospital in Oklahoma, who followed his own advice to shed 300 pounds. (That's right, 300.) "One meal doesn't define your diet, so don't assume that you've failed or fallen off the wagon," he says. Institute a simple rule: Follow any "cheat" meal with at least five healthy meals and snacks. That ensures that you'll be eating right more than 80 percent of the time.

4. Roll Out of Bed and into the Kitchen

Sure, you've heard this advice multiple times already. But consider that if you sleep for 6 to 8 hours and then skip breakfast, your body is essentially running on fumes by the time you get to work. And that sends you desperately seeking sugar, which is usually pretty easy to find. The most convenient foods are typically packed with sugar (doughnuts, lattes) or other quickly digested carbohydrates (McMuffins, cinnamon buns). Which brings us to our next strategy.

5. Restock Your Shelves

How many times have you driven to the store in the middle of the night to satisfy a craving? Probably not nearly as often as you've raided the fridge. You're more likely to give in to a craving when the object you desire is close at hand. So make sure it's not: Toss the junk food and restock your cupboard and fridge with almonds and other nuts, low-fat cheeses, fruits and vegetables, and canned tuna and salmon. And do the same at work. "By eliminating snacks that

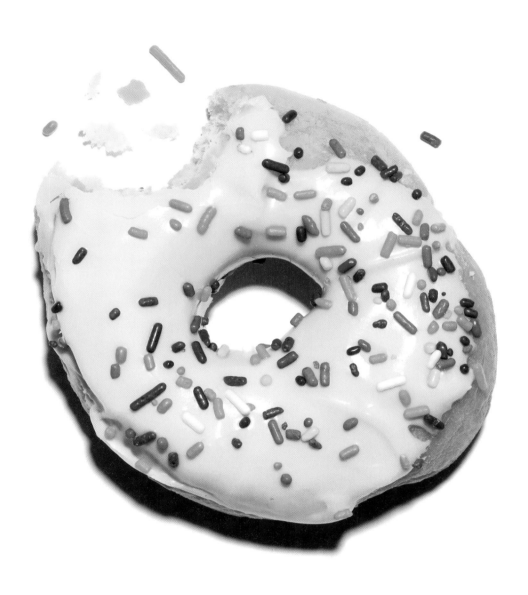

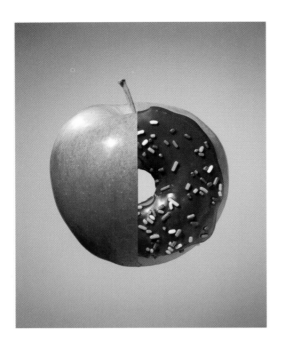

sound good, and you should eat," says Richard Feinman, PhD, a professor of biochemistry at the State University of New York Downstate Medical Center in Brooklyn. "If it doesn't sound good, your brain is playing tricks on you." His advice: Change your environment, which can be as easy as stretching at your desk or turning your attention to a different task.

Smart Swaps
YOU CAN GIVE IN AND STILL GET TRIM— IF YOU EAT THE RIGHT STUFF.

You feel like a salty snack
Glenny's Soy Crisps, lightly salted
Per half-bag: 158 calories, 2 g total fat, 0 g saturated fat, 20 g carbohydrates, 2 g sugar, 383 mg sodium, 3 g dietary fiber, 11 g protein

You want a sweet end to a meal
Fage Total 2% strawberry yogurt
Per 5.3 ounce container: 130 calories, 2.5 g total fat, 1.5 g saturated fat, 18 g carbohydrates, 17 g sugar, 40 mg sodium, 0 g dietary fiber, 11 g protein

You need chocolate
Sweetriot chocolate-covered cacao nibs (flavor 50)
Per ounce: 140 calories, 11 g total fat, 6 g saturated fat, 14 g carbohydrates, 10 g sugar, 0 mg sodium, 3 g dietary fiber, 2 g protein

You lust after something chewy
Dried mango
Per 6 pieces: 110 calories, 0 g total fat, 28 g carbohydrates, 20 g sugar, 1 mg sodium, 2 g dietary fiber, 2 g protein

You're dying for a decadent dessert
Dreamy Drizzle Chocolate Supreme VitaCake
Per 2-ounce slice: 100 calories, 2.5 g total fat, 0.5 g saturated fat, 24 g carbohydrates, 8 g sugar, 150 mg sodium, 6 g dietary fiber, 4 g protein

You long for a cool treat
Julie's Organic blackberry sorbet bar
Per 54 g bar: 60 calories, 0 g total fat, 16 g carbohydrates, 14 g sugar, 20 mg sodium, < 1 g dietary fiber, 0 g protein

don't match your diet and providing plenty that do, you're far less likely to find yourself at the doughnut-shop drive-thru or the vending machine," says Christopher Mohr, PhD, RD, president of Mohr Results, a fitness and nutrition consulting firm in Louisville, Kentucky.

6. Think like a Biochemist
Cookies made with organic cane juice might sound like something your yoga teacher would eat, but they won't help her fit into her Lycra pants. Junk food by any other name is still junk. Ditto for lots of "health foods" in the granola aisle. "Natural" sweeteners like honey raise blood sugar just like the white stuff. "If you're going to eat cookies, accept that you're deviating from your plan, and then revert to your diet afterward," Berkowitz says. Kidding yourself will only get you into trouble.

7. Spot Hunger Impostors
Have a craving for sweets even though you ate just an hour ago? Imagine sitting down to a delicious meal such as a sizzling steak, instead. "If you're truly hungry, the steak will

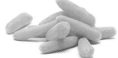

13 Flat Belly Food Tricks

THESE SIMPLE SHORTCUTS WILL HELP YOU SLIM DOWN.

1. Eat Dessert
Yes, always. "A small amount can signal that the meal is over," says Barbara Rolls, PhD, author of *The Volumetrics Eating Plan*. She ends her meals with a piece of high-quality chocolate—and she's a doctor.

2. Get a Mustache
Consuming 1,800 milligrams of calcium a day could block the absorption of about 80 calories, according to a University of Tennessee study. Jump-start your calcium intake by filling your coffee mug with skim or 1 percent milk, drinking it down to the level you want in your coffee, then pouring in your caffeine fix. That's 300 milligrams down, 1,500 to go.

3. Spice Things Up
Capsaicin, the substance that puts the hot in hot pepper, temporarily boosts your metabolism. Dairy blocks capsaicin's sweat-inducing signals better than water, though, so pair that searing-hot chicken vindaloo with yogurt lassi.

4. Go Organic
That's where you're likely to find bread and cereal with fiber counts that put the conventional choices to shame. Thought you were doing well with your 3-grams-per-serving Cheerios? Nature's Path Optimum Slim blows it away with 9 g.

5. Keep the Skin On
Speaking of fiber, a lot of it's in the peel, whether it's potatoes, apples, or pears. Even oranges—don't eat the whole peel, but keep the pith, that white, stringy stuff; it's packed with flavonoids.

6. Buy Precut Vegetables
Sure, they cost more, but you're more likely to eat them. "Make low-energy snacks as easy as possible," Dr. Rolls says. "Keep vegetables as near to hand as you can. Make it so you have no excuse."

7. Use Zagat's
Pick restaurants where you'll actually want to linger. "When the meals are not hurried, you can regulate your attitude," says Roberta Anding, a spokeswoman for the American Dietetic Association. That means your body—not the empty plate—will tell you when to stop.

8. Always Snack at 3:00 p.m.
"Have a 150-calorie snack [now], and it can save you 400 calories later," Anding says. An ounce of nuts or two sticks of string cheese weigh in at about 170 calories.

9. Drink with Your Dominant Hand
If you're circulating at a party, Dr. Rolls suggests keeping your glass in the hand you eat with. If you're drinking with it, you can't eat with it.

10. Plate It
Whatever it is, don't eat it out of the container and don't bring the container to the couch. "Part of satiety is visual," Anding says. "Your brain actually has to see the food on the plate, and when you reach into the jar, or the box, or the bag, you don't see it." If it's worth eating, put it on a plate. Eat what's there, then stop.

11. Start with Salad
It's the holy grail of dieting—eat less by eating more. Dr. Rolls's research has found that eating a salad as a first course decreased total lunch calories by 12 percent. Avoid the croutons and creamy dressings, which have the opposite effect.

12. Go Public
Enlist the help of friends, family, and co-workers—and know they're watching. "The power of embarrassment is greater than willpower," says Stephen Gullo, PhD, author of *The Thin Commandments*.

13. Use Your Fingers
Find a way other than food to work off your nervous energy. "It's behavior modification," Anding says. "Instead of grabbing chips, you pick up your knitting—or anything else that occupies your hands."

Chapter Ten

Strengthen Your Heart

KEEP YOUR TICKER STRONG AND DEFEAT A SILENT KILLER

INVESTMENT: 4 WEEKS
AGE ERASED: 2 YEARS

Introduction

Introduction

*I*n Hollywood, only men have heart attacks. Whether it's Jack Nicholson collapsing in *As Good As It Gets,* or Steve Buscemi dropping like a fly in *The Big Lebowski,* or Marlon Brando meeting his fate in *The Godfather,* you get the impression that every man over 40 is a walking time bomb, ready to implode at any moment. Yet heart attacks rarely strike men dead where they stand. In most cases, they're quiet killers, sneaking up and stealing heart tissue over the course of hours or even days.

Oh, and something else about heart attacks that Hollywood gets wrong: Their victims are just as likely to be women. Indeed, heart disease is the No. 1 killer of American women.

There are many risk factors for heart disease, and almost all of them—with the exception of your age and your family history—are factors you can significantly impact or, in many cases, eliminate entirely. Take smoking. "It's the most powerful risk factor for heart disease," says Sharonne N. Hayes, MD, director of the Women's Heart Clinic at the Mayo Clinic. In fact, your risk for having a heart attack drops just 24 hours after quitting.

But the first step toward preventing heart disease, says Barbara H. Roberts, MD, director of the Women's Cardiac Center at the Miriam Hospital in Providence, Rhode Island, is to alter your daily activities. "A healthy lifestyle goes a long way, but most Americans live on fast food and the most strenuous thing they do all day is pushing a computer key," she says. Exercising for just half an hour, 5 days a week, cuts your risk by 30 percent.

To make sure your ticker is in good shape, ask your doctor—or even your ob-gyn—to check your blood pressure, blood sugar, and cholesterol. "These are problems that often go undetected in young adults," says Dr. Roberts, "and by the time you've figured out that your numbers are high, they could already have caused severe damage." Read on to learn about more ways to protect your body's most important muscle.

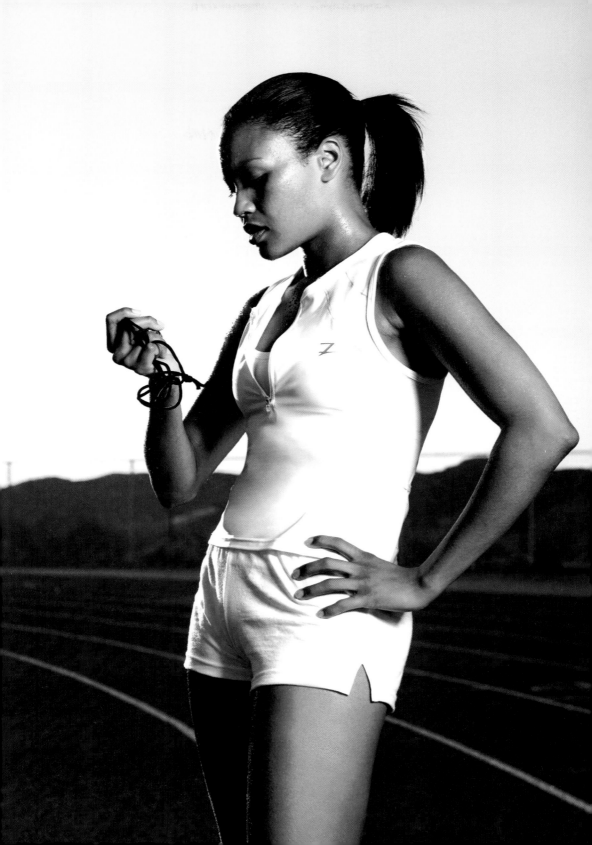

How Your Most Important Muscle Ages

CUTTING-EDGE, LIVE-LONG STRATEGIES FROM LEADING CARDIOLOGISTS.

You may have noticed a few of the outward signs already: slight lines around your eyes, a momentary memory lapse, longer recovery times. These indicators also signal that your body's key systems (your heart ranks as a fairly important one) are beginning to feel the effects of aging. The good news: Making simple, specific changes to your diet, exercise routine, and stress level will keep your heart healthy now, in 10 years, and for the rest of your life.

How Age Affects Your Heart:
1. Cholesterol Levels Shift
HDL (good) cholesterol sweeps up LDL (bad) cholesterol and shunts it to the liver for removal. Without enough HDL, the bad stuff builds up within your arteries and, over time, causes plaque to accumulate.

2. Plaque Causes Clots
Plaque is a mix of fatty substances, including cholesterol, which burrows into and inflames artery walls. When a plaque deposit bursts, the body's healing mechanism produces a clot. This can obstruct the artery and cause a heart attack.

3. Arteries Become Weak and Stiff
High blood pressure hardens flexible arteries, which strains the heart, rips open plaque deposits, and promotes blood vessel leaks that can cause an aneurysm or stroke. Blood vessels are lined with the same kind of tissue as your skin. "It's just as important to keep your inner skin as beautiful as the visible skin," says Lori Mosca, MD, PhD, an associate professor of medicine at Columbia University in New York City. "Instead of protecting it from the sun, you need to prevent damage from a poor diet or lack of exercise."

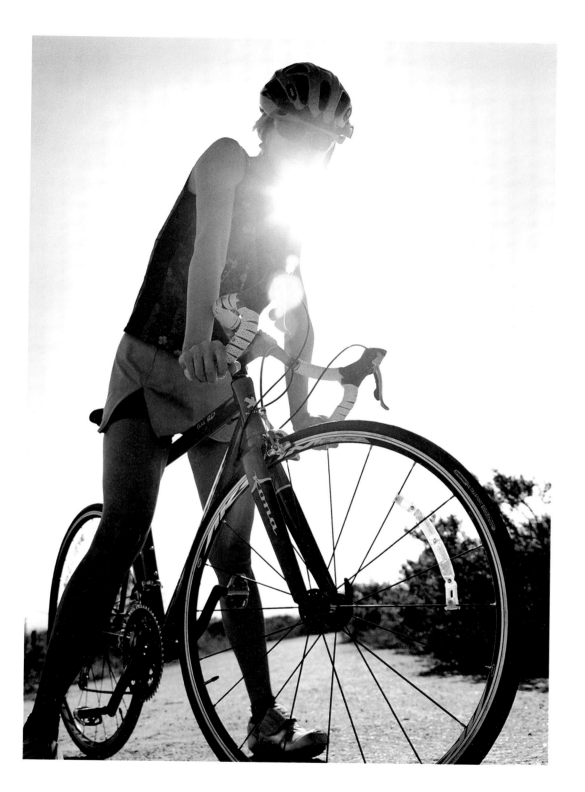

Anatomy of a Heart Attack

THE CLOT THICKENS.

Since the late 1990s, scientists have increasingly studied arterial inflammation to understand heart attacks. They now believe that 85 percent of heart attacks occur when excess cholesterol inside an artery's walls incites inflammation and the growth of plaque, which then ruptures, causing a clot that blocks the bloodflow to the heart. Steven E. Nissen, MD, director of the department of cardiovascular medicine at the Cleveland Clinic, provides the play-by-play:

1. LDL cholesterol particles are absorbed into the artery wall, prompting cells in the wall to summon the immune system.

2. White blood cells of the immune system squeeze into the artery wall. The white blood cells emit chemical signals that cause inflammation, specifically tiny spikes on the artery called adhesion molecules, which snare more floating immune-system cells.

3. The white blood cells evolve into macrophages, which grow and ingest LDL cholesterol particles. This is the start of plaque.

4. Some of the white blood cells die and release toxins. The plaque enlarges, and the body covers it with a cap of fibrous scar tissue and muscle cells.

5. The cap ruptures, either because of a spike in blood pressure or chronic inflammation, no one knows for sure. The plaque—a mix of fat molecules, cholesterol, and dead white blood cells—seeps out of the wound into the artery. This attracts red blood cells, which form a clot, blocking the artery and triggering a heart attack.

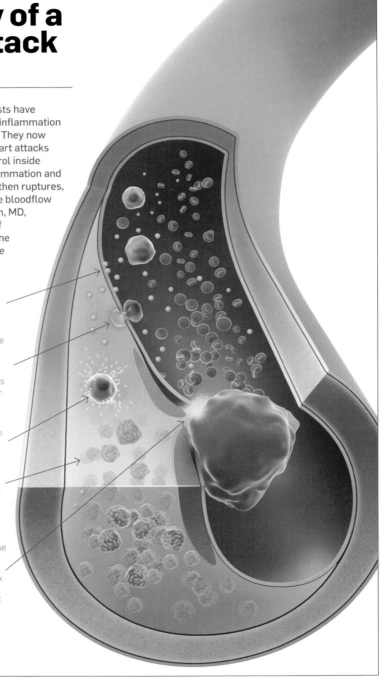

4. Blood Can Become "Sticky"

High blood sugar is like a soda spill on a counter-top—it permits plaque-forming material to fasten more easily to artery walls. It's also a symptom of diabetes, which doubles your risk of heart disease or stroke.

5. Waist Size Expands

Slowing metabolism leads to weight gain, which contributes to diabetes, high blood pressure, and high cholesterol. "Large waist size is the most important risk factor—it compounds all the others," says Annabelle Volgman, MD, medical director of the Heart Center for Women at Rush University Medical Center in Chicago.

Your Stay-Young Plan
Keep Moving

"Physical activity reduces every controllable risk factor," says Dr. Volgman. Just 10 minutes of cardiovascular exercise on most days can cut a sedentary person's heart attack risk in half.

Do Intervals

By boosting aerobic fitness and metabolism, twice-a-week interval training (short bursts of high-intensity exercise) for just 2 weeks can reduce heart risks by 20 percent, according to studies. Get started: Simply vary the pace of your daily walk for 2 minutes of every 10. (See page 280 for a full interval-training routine.)

Monitor Your Markers

Keep a copy of the blood work that's done during your annual physical and track changes over time. Make sure your numbers are always within these ranges:

Cholesterol: LDL under 100 milligrams per deciliter (mg/dl); HDL above 50 mg/dl
Blood pressure: Below 120/80 milligrams per deciliter (mg/dl)
Fasting blood sugar: Less than 100 mg/dl
Triglycerides: Less than 150 mg/dl

Get "Subclass" Cholesterol Tests

If you have heart disease or are at risk for it, ask for a test that measures your lipoprotein subfractions, the size of your cholesterol particles. If your LDL particles are very small, they are better able to burrow into artery walls; even with normal or low cholesterol readings, you may need more aggressive monitoring and treatment.

Test for Inflammation

Doctors now know that when LDL cholesterol damages the arterial wall, the artery becomes chronically inflamed, starting a cascade of events that may culminate in a heart attack. As part of this inflammatory response, your body produces a substance called C-reactive protein (CRP), which can be measured in a blood test. If you have normal cholesterol but a high level of CRP, you may need a more aggressive preventive plan (more intense monitoring of lipids). Make sure to ask for the high-sensitivity test, which rules out other causes of inflammation, such as infection, injury, and arthritis. (See the next section for more on CRP.)

2
Weeks of interval training needed to reduce heart risks by 20 percent

Brush Your Teeth, Clean Your Arteries

Cutting your risk of heart disease may be as easy as regularly flossing and brushing. Columbia University doctors have found that people whose mouths contain a high number of the bacteria that cause gum disease are more likely to have plaque-clogged arteries.

Stop Inflammation

Keep an eye on your gums—especially when you're pregnant. Research suggests women with gum disease are up to seven times more likely to deliver prematurely and that their infants often have low birth weights.

Get a Baseline Heart Scan

Prominent cardiologists recommend that women over age 50 who are postmenopausal and have any risk factors for coronary disease get a heart scan—several different technologies are available—to measure coronary artery calcium, which directly correlates to the total amount of plaque in your arteries. Getting an early baseline measurement lets your doctor monitor for signs of heart disease. Read more on this in Part Two.

8 Steps to a Healthy Heart

TAKE ACTION TO FIGHT AGAINST THE NO. 1 KILLER OF WOMEN.

By Roxanne Patel Shepelavy

FACT: Cardiovascular disease kills more women over 25 than all cancers combined.

FACT: Young women who have heart attacks are twice as likely to die from them as men are.

FACT: You can protect yourself—and you should start right now.

Erica Sharp* was the last person you'd expect to have heart problems. The 35-year-old Indianapolis bank vice president and mother of a toddler was a slight 5 foot 1 and 118 pounds. She ran marathons and competed in triathlons. She was never sick and went to the doctor only for annual physicals. So when she felt a painful pressure in the middle of her chest one February afternoon in 2004, she chalked it up to indigestion. She popped some aspirin and a couple of antacids and proceeded to conduct a 20-minute conference call in her office. Only then did she call her doctor. He said she was having an anxiety attack and referred her for a cardiac stress test just to ease her mind. Problem solved, right?

Name changed to protect identity.

Wrong. Before Sharp could even step onto the treadmill in her doctor's office 9 days later, pictures of her heart revealed something shocking: She'd had a heart attack. The tip of one of her arteries was partially blocked, the result of a congenital heart defect aggravated by high blood pressure—possibly dating back to her pregnancy, when she'd had the hypertensive disorder preeclampsia. But then her cardiologist gave her the really terrifying news: She could be headed for another attack, this one much worse than the first. "I couldn't believe it," Sharp says. "I thought I was going for my morning workout and then would be back at the office as usual. Instead, I ended up in the hospital that night and in surgery the next day with four stents in my artery."

As Sharp learned the hard way, you don't have to be old or male for cardiovascular disease to strike. In fact, it's the No. 1 cause of death for American women over 25, killing nearly 500,000 every year, and 44,000 more women than men. The American Heart Association estimates that almost a third of women have some form of heart disease. Still, most of them—cue that scary music

The Vein Event

WHAT YOUR BLOOD PRESSURE NUMBERS MEAN

When that cuff tightens and releases on your arm, it is measuring the pressure exerted by your blood on blood vessels as it travels around the body. The systolic pressure (top number) tells you how hard the blood is pushing against the artery walls when the heart contracts. The diastolic pressure (bottom number) is the pressure on the walls when the heart relaxes between beats. Ongoing elevated force damages artery walls, hardening and thickening them and interfering with bloodflow. Here's what the numbers mean for you.

SYSTOLIC PRESSURE	DIASTOLIC PRESSURE	WHAT IT MEANS	WHAT TO DO
Below 120 and . . .	Below 80	Normal	Maintain your healthy lifestyle
120 to 139 or . . .	80 to 89	Prehypertension	Reduce stress, make dietary changes, stop smoking, lose weight, exercise more, and consult your doctor
140 to 159 or . . .	90 to 99	Stage 1 hypertension	If normal blood pressure isn't achieved through lifestyle changes, your doctor may consider medication
160 or more or . . .	100 or more	Stage 2 hypertension	Adopt a heathier lifestyle, employing the changes above. Your doctor might suggest more than one medication

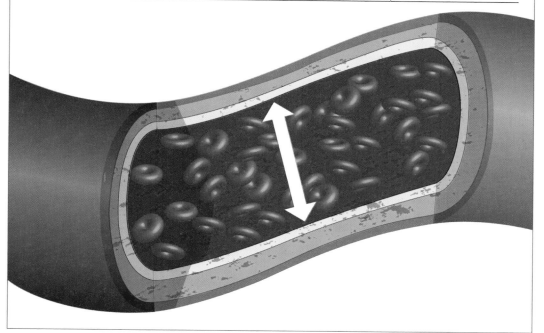

again—don't even know it. And while research shows that women under 50 have fewer heart attacks than men their age, they're twice as likely to die from them. Why? It could be because women who suffer attacks are either sicker or seeking less aggressive treatment for their symptoms.

If all this has your heart beating a little faster, well, a little worry might not be such a bad thing—assuming that it makes you start taking steps to prevent heart disease. And you can do just that, since many heart attacks in women are caused by factors like hypertension and high cholesterol that could have been treated or prevented altogether. "It's important to take care of your heart even before you have any symptoms," says Arthur Agatston, MD, a Miami cardiologist and author of *The South Beach Heart Program*. "Quite simply, the earlier you start, the easier it is to prevent heart disease."

Luckily, the latest research shows that the road to a healthy heart isn't so rough. Here, eight steps to make sure your beat goes on for a long, long time.

Step 1:
So, How's Your Mom?

Researchers have long believed that having a close family member (mom, dad, sister, or brother) with cardiovascular disease was one of the clearest predictors of heart trouble in your own future. But according to a 2006 Swedish study, it's really Mom you need to worry about. Your risk increases by 17 percent if your father has heart disease, but it shoots up by a whopping 43 percent if your mother is afflicted. This may be more environment than genetics, since children typically spend more time with their mothers and tend to learn lifestyle habits from them. But even if you don't smoke and do exercise, it's possible that your risk could still be up as much as 82 percent if both of your parents had heart disease.

Which doesn't mean you're doomed, of course. But it does mean you shouldn't waste any time. If you have a family history, Dr. Agatston recommends having in-depth tests that go beyond the normal blood workup every few years, starting in

your midforties. First, talk to your doctor about having a computed tomography (CT) scan of your heart, which can detect attack-causing plaque buildup in your arteries—even years in advance. Dr. Agatston calls these scans "mammograms for the heart." The first one establishes a baseline; subsequent images assess potential deterioration of the arteries. Opt for the 64-slice

> *Quite simply, the earlier you start, the easier it is to prevent heart disease.*

CT scanner, which measures calcium and the amount of dangerous soft plaque in the arteries. Filled primarily with cholesterol, soft plaque is prone to rupture, resulting in a blood clot that can cause a heart attack. "These are tests that really can make a difference in people's lives," Dr. Agatston says.

Dr. Agatston also suggests that all women request more detailed blood tests that measure not only the level of cholesterol but its type and size—factors that he says affect the heart in ways that scientists are only now beginning to understand. Talk to your doctor about having a standard lipid profile. A blood test can also detect the presence of CRP in the bloodstream, which may contribute to plaque formation. More prevalent in people who are overweight, sedentary, hypertensive, or smokers, CRP's presence accurately predicts the likelihood of heart attacks in women with relatively low cholesterol, and researchers speculate that it could signal heart disease before symptoms develop. Ask your doctor to check your numbers the next time you get blood work done.

Step 2:
Sorry, You're Gonna Have to Do a Little Math

The connection between cholesterol—a waxy substance made in your liver and found in blood cells—and heart disease has been known for decades, but your total cholesterol number is only

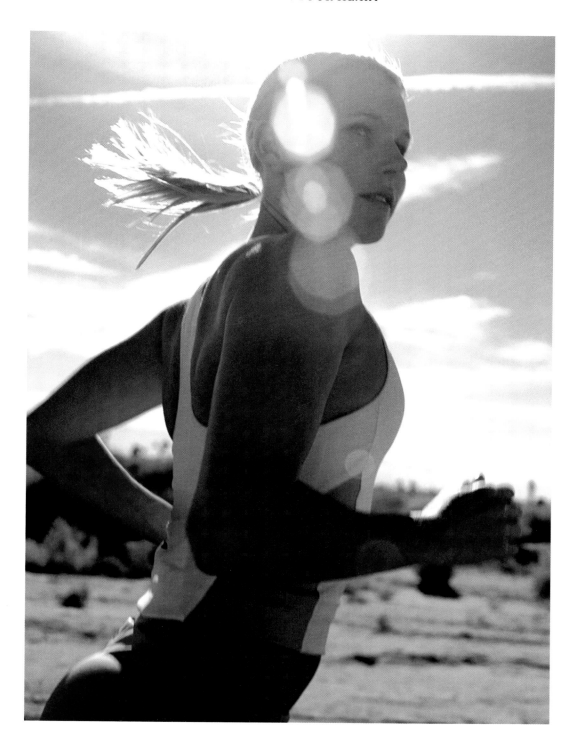

part of the equation. The real key is how much of it is LDL, the so-called "bad" cholesterol, and how much is HDL, the "good" kind.

LDL cholesterol can build up in your arterial walls, causing plaque, which can rupture in the arteries and result in blood clots and possibly heart attacks. A recent study from the University of Texas Southwestern Medical Center in Dallas indicates that keeping LDL levels low (the longer the better) can protect even people with other risk factors like smoking. Meanwhile, HDL plays the role of crime-fighting superhero to LDL's nasty villain, transporting the bad stuff through the blood to the liver, where it's metabolized and then eliminated. One Mayo Clinic newsletter even indicated that increasing HDL by even 1 mg/dl can reduce heart attack risk by 3 percent. "Basically, you want more of the good stuff, less of the bad stuff," says Sharonne N. Hayes, MD, of the Mayo Clinic Women's Heart Clinic.

For most women, total cholesterol should be under 200 mg/dl, with LDL levels no higher than 100 and HDL no lower than 50. If your numbers are in line, doctors recommend retesting your blood at least every 5 years in your twenties and thirties.

Step 3:
Don't Be Afraid to Do Drugs

If blood tests show your cholesterol is high, a

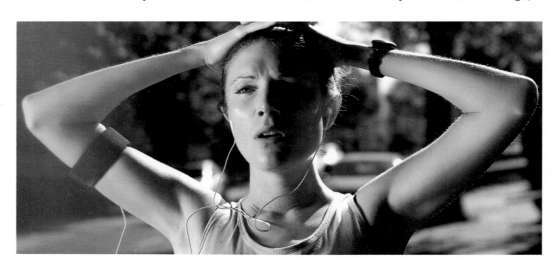

Test It Now, Trust It Later

Detecting cardiovascular disease depends on getting tested regularly—not just looking for symptoms. In addition to lipid tests, CRP, and 64-slice CTs, here are other tests to ask your doctor about.

Homocysteine blood test
What it measures:
Levels of this amino acid should be less than 13 micromoles per liter.
When to have it:
If you have unexplained hardening of the arteries or blood clots, or a family history of cardiovascular disease

Exercise stress test
What it measures:
By monitoring heart rate and blood pressure while you exercise on a treadmill or cycle, a doctor can identify the presence of a blockage.
When to have it:
If you're experiencing symptoms of heart disease, such as chest pain, shortness of breath, or lightheadedness

Thallium stress test
What it measures:
A radioactive substance is injected into your bloodstream following an exercise stress test, and a series of x-rays is taken to spot the location of blockages.
When to have it:
If you already show signs of a blockage

Angiogram
What it measures:
A catheter is inserted into the heart, dye is injected, and then a series of x-rays provides a clear look at artery blockages. It's still the diagnostic gold standard for clogged arteries.
When to have it:
After a positive stress test, in order to determine how effective surgery will be

change in diet and exercise might help (see steps 4 and 5 for some suggestions). But in many cases, it's too late or your numbers are too high for these basic steps to help. That's when your doctor may give you a cholesterol-lowering medication known as a statin, which keeps the liver from producing too much cholesterol. Some doctors have questioned the wisdom of prescribing these drugs, especially for patients who might lower their cholesterol through lifestyle changes. But recent studies show that statins can diminish LDL by as much as 40 percent, slightly raise the level of HDL, and reduce the risk of heart attacks by about 35 percent. This is why many experts say these medications are actually underprescribed. "Statins are incredible tools in lowering cholesterol and can keep many people from suffering heart attacks," Dr. Agatston says. "But there's no question: They're meant to work together with proper diet and exercise." Women taking statins may experience muscle fatigue as a side effect, though, and should get regular blood tests to check liver function.

Step 4:
Ask Yourself, "What Kind of Fruit Am I?"

Carrying extra weight around isn't just a drag during swimsuit season. It can also be dangerous, especially if those excess pounds find their way to your belly and not, say, your hips. Recent studies indicate that abdominal fat is metabolically different from the other fat in your body: As you gain padding around your middle, the individual cells swell, and their size is linked to higher triglyceride levels and lower good cholesterol.

The best treatment for belly fat? Signing up for Weight Watchers isn't enough; you're going to have to pry yourself off the couch, too. New research from Wake Forest University Baptist Medical Center in Winston-Salem, North Carolina, shows that diet and exercise together reduce the size of abdominal fat cells, which doesn't happen if you lose weight through dieting alone. Working out regularly also has a ripple effect on the body: Not only do dangerous pounds come off, but your

muscles also become more efficient at using blood; your heart gets stronger; and your blood vessels become more limber, so blood flows more easily. "A lot of things don't make you feel better in the short term," Dr. Hayes says. "Exercise is the one thing that does."

And you don't have to run a marathon every week to get these benefits. Cardiologists recommend performing an average of 30 minutes of moderate aerobic exercise a day, which has been shown to increase life expectancy by 3½ years. Whether walking, running, or swimming, you should aim to work your heart to about 50 to 70 percent of its maximum rate. Even this amount of exercise is powerful enough to combat other high-risk factors: A study out of the Cooper Institute in Dallas found that even moderately fit people had half the death rates of those who were sedentary.

While doctors used to think that weight training was bad for the heart because it increased blood pressure, research now shows it can actually lower blood pressure when transforming fat into muscle, which burns calories and keeps them from landing on your belly. This is why Nieca Goldberg, MD, a New York City cardiologist and author of *The Women's Healthy Heart Program*, recommends strengthening exercises two or three times a week for all the major muscle groups—arms, legs, shoulders, chest, back, hips, and trunk. Dr. Agatston suggests doing a Pilates- or yoga-based regimen that zeroes in on the core muscles of your abdomen and lower back. Either way, consistency is key, as is starting young: Dr. Goldberg says regular strengthening can not only help prevent age-related loss of bone and muscle mass, but also help reduce body fat and improve endurance, both of which can decrease your risk of heart disease. (See Part Two for more help.)

3.5
Years that 30 minutes of daily aerobic exercise can add to your life

Step 5:
Hey, Are Those Your Arteries Closing Up?

Exercise without diet gets you only halfway to where you need to be. But changing the way you eat doesn't mean starving yourself or signing up for a fad diet. "There's no single food that's going to kill you or save your life," Dr. Hayes says. "Proper diet is about [eating] a wide variety of healthy foods." That means, most importantly, avoiding trans and saturated fats: In a 2006 Australian study, researchers found that giving healthy subjects just one fatty meal affected bloodflow and diminished HDL's protective qualities.

The American Heart Association suggests that no more than 7 percent of your daily calories should come from saturated fats—butter, full-fat dairy products like whole milk or cheese, and meat. Meanwhile, only 1 percent of your daily diet should consist of trans fats, which are found mostly in processed foods like cookies, crackers, and chips.

This is why Dr. Goldberg encourages sticking to a "Mediterranean" diet: a moderate amount of foods high in unsaturated fats like olive oil and fish; lean meats, such as beef fillet, flank, or sirloin and pork tenderloin, and low-fat dairy; whole grains (think brown rice and barley); and at least five daily servings of colorful fruits and vegetables, which provide antioxidants that help keep blood vessels flexible. In particular, Dr. Goldberg and others tout the benefits of omega-3 fatty acids because they may help lower blood pressure and the risk of abnormal heart rhythms. Dr. Agatston also recommends incorporating foods that lower bad cholesterol, like apples, which research suggests may help prevent plaque buildup; oolong tea, which has strong antioxidant properties that can make LDL particles bigger and less likely to enter the bloodstream; and legumes, such as beans, peas, and lentils, which decrease the risk of cardiovascular disease. And he suggests partaking of foods such as almonds and walnuts and up to two glasses a day of red wine, which help reduce LDL cholesterol and protect the lining of the arteries.

Step 6:
Stop Kidding Yourself That an Occasional Cigarette Won't Hurt

Yes, you already heard the antismoking rant a few pages back. But there's a reason for it. Quitting smoking should top your list of things to do to avoid heart disease, Dr. Hayes says. And that's true even if the only time you light up is over mojitos with friends. Recent research shows that smoking between one and five cigarettes a day triples your chance of dying from a heart attack, and that it's even worse for women than for men. Smoking narrows arteries, raises blood pressure, thickens blood, and makes it more likely to clot—the classic recipe for a heart attack. This is especially true if you have other risk factors, like high blood pressure and high cholesterol, which together with smoking make you much more likely to get heart disease, according to Dr. Agatston.

Developing diabetes makes you up to seven times more prone to heart disease.

You take birth control and smoke? You've just put another bullet in the gun. That combo raises blood pressure and can lead to blood clots, further increasing your risk.

Step 7:
Get Prenatal Care

Around 135,000 women every year get gestational diabetes, high blood sugar that's likely a result of pregnancy hormones blocking adequate insulin production. Doctors used to think it came and went with pregnancy. But research now shows that having gestational diabetes gives you a 50 percent chance of developing diabetes later in life, which in turn makes you three to seven times more prone to heart disease. That puts you in line with the more than 54 million other Americans who have prediabetes. Diabetes, especially type 2, is often attributed to obesity, though many cases result from genetics and/or environment. Cardiologists consider diabetics heart patients as well: Even if they've never had an attack, they tend to have high blood pressure and high cholesterol. "Having diabetes is equivalent to having heart disease," says Paula Johnson, MD, chief of the division of women's health at Brigham and Women's Hospital in Boston. She treats diabetics and heart patients with the same regimen of aspirin and statins. "The best thing is to protect yourself with diet, weight control, and exercise so you never develop diabetes, even if you had it when pregnant."

Step 8:
Understand How Women Differ from Men

While some women do experience chest-clutching pain, many others have subtler symptoms—nausea, dizziness, and even upper back pain. In fact, a survey of women recovering from heart attacks found that many had worsening symptoms for weeks leading up to an episode, but mistook them for indigestion, fatigue, or muscle strain. Dr. Goldberg says two-thirds of women who die of heart attacks never even make it to the hospital—by the time they recognize what's happening, it's already too late.

Symptoms aren't the only way men and women differ when it comes to heart problems. Only in the last decade have scientists started to explore how heart disease manifests in each sex, and they still don't have a lot of answers. They do know that it's about more than the size of our hearts.

Research from the National Institutes of Health (NIH) shows that doctors may have missed heart disease in some 3 million women who have diffuse plaque, where plaque spreads evenly through the arteries instead of building up to create a major blockage. On angiograms (x-rays of the blood vessels) these arteries look clear. The NIH research also looked at women with microvascular disease, in which small vessels don't dilate properly during exertion. Their angiograms were often clear too. While they're not headed for immediate heart attacks, women with diffuse plaque and microvascular disease do need to be treated with either lifestyle changes or medication or both. "Doctors should diagnose intuitively," Dr. Johnson says. "If a woman comes in with symptoms"—shortness of breath, positive cardiac stress test, high cholesterol—"we can assume she needs to be treated even if her angiogram is clear. We can't just send her home and do nothing."

Indigestion or a Heart Attack?

FOR WOMEN, IT'S NOT ALWAYS EASY TO TELL.

In a study published in the journal *Circulation*, only 30 percent of women who'd had heart attacks said they had experienced any chest pain. Worrisome symptoms in women are often much subtler than they are in men. So pay attention to these possible signs.

Dizziness: It's a sign that your heart isn't pumping enough blood to your brain.

Fatigue: A weakened heart muscle can't pump enough oxygen for the body to function efficiently, so you feel tired.

Nausea: It could indicate that your blood pressure has plummeted and be accompanied by clamminess and sweating.

Pain in the upper back, upper abdomen, or lower chest: That's another sign that your heart can't pump blood where you need it.

Shortness of breath during normal activities: The heart's pumping action weakens as bloodflow to the heart diminishes.

But we all feel tired, dizzy, or short of breath sometimes. When should you worry? "If you have shortness of breath walking up stairs on one day, it's probably not a problem," says Nieca Goldberg, MD, a cardiologist in New York City. "But if it starts out once a week, then goes to three times a week, and on, you should get checked out." If you start to experience any or all of these symptoms while at rest, you may be having a heart attack or be on the verge. In that case, it's time to head for the nearest emergency room or call 911.

As many female heart attack survivors have learned, you may need to be your own strongest advocate where your heart's concerned. After all, you know your body best and can tell when something's wrong. If you need help, ask for it—and then insist that your doctor determine the cause.

Keep Your Clock Clean

CARING FOR YOUR HEART IS SERIOUS STUFF, BUT RESEARCH SUGGESTS SOMETIMES IT'S AS EASY AS CALLING A CLOSE FRIEND.

A study from the University of Maryland School of Medicine in Baltimore recently showed that laughter promotes healthy blood vessel function. Fourteen of 20 volunteers who watched a 15-minute segment of the drama *Saving Private Ryan* had artery bloodflow reduced by an average of 35 percent. In contrast, when they watched a comedy bloodflow increased by 20 percent. "The magnitude of change . . . was similar to what we might see with aerobic activity, but without the aches, pain, and muscle tension associated with exercise," says lead researcher Michael Miller, MD. He prescribes at least one good belly laugh daily, and more is even better. Have a laugh, and then try the rest of the heart-healthy tips in this list.

Break a Sweat in the PM, If Possible
As we've established, exercising for 30 minutes daily, at any time of day, strengthens your heart. But working out after noon, when the mercury peaks, may help your heart even more. In the afternoon, your muscles are warmer and more flexible, so it's easier to work out. If it feels better, you'll be more likely to exercise more vigorously and frequently, two of the keys to a healthy heart. If you can only do a morning walk, warm up by starting out slowly for 10 minutes.

Call Your Gal Pals
Stress, says Mehmet Oz, MD, a professor of surgery at Columbia University College of Physicians and Surgeons in New York City, is the greatest preventable cause of heart disease. And a landmark UCLA study found that women can counteract stress by hanging with their girlfriends. The research shows that when women face tough times, they have a self-protective response: Their bodies produce oxytocin, a hormone that compels them to nurture their loved ones and be with their friends. Called the "tend-and-befriend response," it not only relieves stress, but it's also a powerful antidote to the better-known fight-or-flight response, which is marked by the production of the heart-damaging stress hormone cortisol.

"The question I always ask my patients is 'Do you have a reason for your heart to keep beating?'" says Dr. Oz. So after a particularly stressful day, remember who makes your heart happy: Call your girlfriends and hug your kids.

Just Say No to Joe
A study published in the *American Journal of Clinical Nutrition* found that coffee drinkers who down more than about a cup a day have significantly higher levels of inflammatory markers in their bloodstream than non-java drinkers do. Chronic inflammation is thought to be an underlying factor in the development of heart disease.

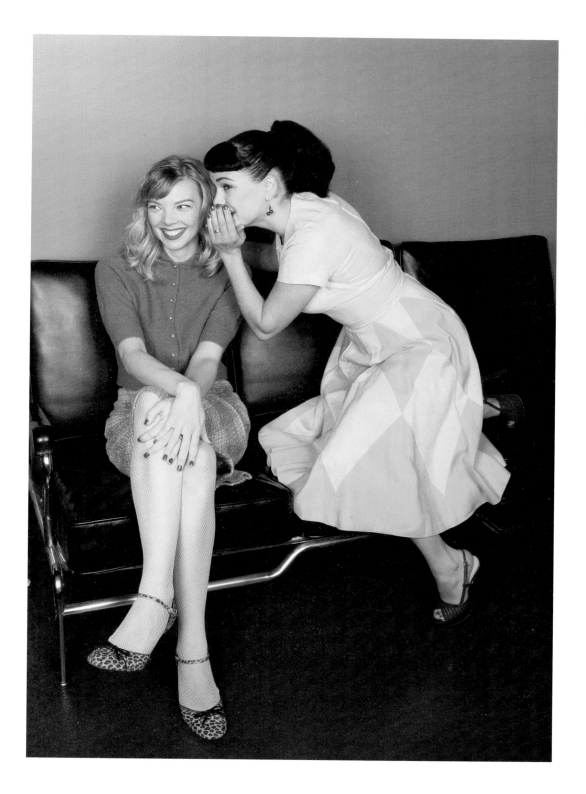

Part Two

Exercise for a Strong Ticker

The Fitness Formula

YOUR ULTIMATE EXERCISE PLAN FOR KEEPING YOUR HEART HEALTHY.

By Caroline Bollinger

There really is a fountain of youth: It's called exercise. How? Let us count the ways: In study after study, regular workouts have been proven to lower blood pressure, reduce body fat, raise "good" cholesterol, lower "bad" cholesterol, improve bloodflow, and regulate key hormones.

To ensure that you reap all these benefits, leading experts on aging and exercise agreed that your ultimate training plan should include the four cornerstones of age prevention: consistent cardio, intense intervals, yoga, and weight training. Start now and you can turn back the clock . . . for life.

1. Do: Consistent Cardio

The verdict is in: People who exercise almost daily really do keep ticking longer. When scientists pored over data from the famous Framingham Heart Study of more than 5,000 women and men, they discovered that active folks lived nearly 4 years longer than their inactive peers, largely because they sidestep heart disease—the nation's leading killer. Aerobic exercise such as walking, cycling, jogging, and swimming protects your heart by lowering blood pressure, reducing "bad" cholesterol, and keeping arteries flexible to improve bloodflow.

Age Eraser: 30 minutes, 5 days a week of moderate-intensity aerobic exercise. Work at a pace that allows you to talk freely; if you can sing, you're not exercising hard enough.

To get started, choose an activity you enjoy and do 10 minutes, 5 days a week. Then increase by 5 minutes each week until you're doing 30 minutes at a time. Dividing your exercise into three 10-minute bouts throughout the day works, too.

2. Do: Intense Intervals

Exercise keeps your mind fit by bringing more blood and oxygen to the noggin, rejuvenating your brain in the process. "The hippocampus, the main area of the brain where memory resides, is particularly susceptible to damage from low bloodflow or lack of oxygen—both of which become more likely as we age," says brain researcher Eric B. Larson, MD, of the Group Health Cooperative in Seattle. Doing bursts of higher-intensity activity will increase bloodflow and oxygen even more.

Age Eraser: 45 minutes, twice a week (moderate-paced cardio exercise interspersed with 1-minute speed bursts every 2 minutes). Based on a 1-to-10 scale, you should feel like you're working at an intensity of 7 or 8 (brisk enough that you can talk, but you'd rather not) during the speed bursts

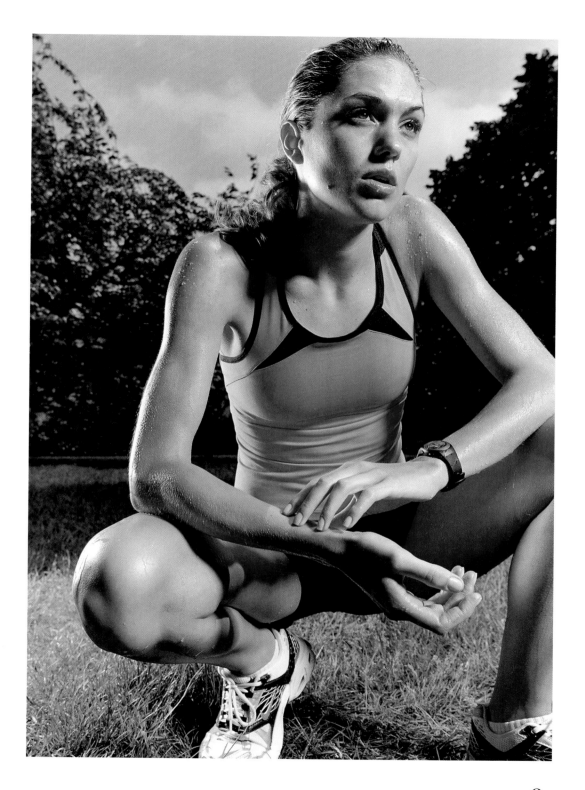

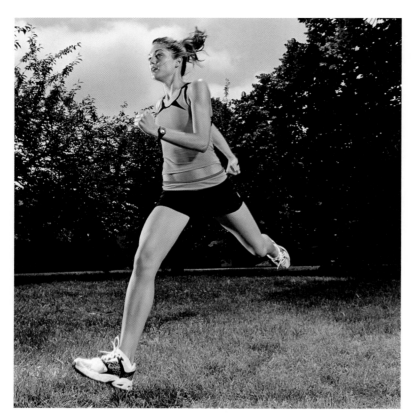

YOUR ULTIMATE 7-DAY PLAN
30 Minutes, Four Times a Week
This routine combines everything into one easy-to-follow schedule.

Day 1
30 minutes of cardio
30 minutes of yoga

Day 2
45 minutes of intervals/cardio
(Try the routine on the opposite page.)

Day 3
20 minutes of weight training
30 minutes of yoga

Day 4
30 minutes of cardio
30 minutes of yoga

Day 5
45 minutes of intervals/cardio
20 minutes of weight training

Day 6
30 minutes of cardio
30 minutes of yoga

Day 7
Rest

and an intensity of 5 or 6 (moderate enough that you can talk freely) the rest of the time.

If you're just starting out, do 15-second intervals, slowly building up to 1 minute as your endurance increases. Because this is cardio exercise, you don't have to do these workouts on top of the steady-paced cardio session above (though you can if you have the time, and you'll shape up even faster). Just extend two of those workouts and make them intervals. (See "A Better Way to Train" for another interval workout.)

3. Do: Weight Training

A healthy heart is key, but unless you have strong bones and muscles, getting up off the couch and walking out the door to enjoy life won't be so easy. Lifting weights is one of the best ways to keep these body systems in tip-top shape, says Wendy Kohrt, PhD, a professor in the division of geriatric medicine at the University of Colorado Health

Sciences Center in Denver. And it can help you stand tall—a quick way to look younger.

Age Eraser: 20 minutes, twice a week. Pick up two sets of dumbbells (3 and 5 pounds for beginners; 5 and 10 or 10 and 20 if you need an even bigger challenge), and do simple strength-building workouts, such as the ones on page 223.

4. Do: Yoga

The less tense you are, the fewer lines and wrinkles you'll develop. One of the best workouts to fight stress? Yoga. In a German study, 3 hours of practice a week lowered the anxiety levels of 16 women ages 26 to 51 by a whopping 30 percent. "As your mouth, jaw, and brows relax, you can literally see the creases soften," says Larry Payne, PhD, director of the Yoga Therapy Rx program at Loyola Marymount University in Los Angeles. It may also protect against free radicals, compounds that break down skin's elasticity.

A Better Way to Train

TEACH YOUR HEART TO PUMP MORE BLOOD WITH THIS REGIMEN.

As we've said, interval training is best for building heart strength. "In order to increase the strength of any muscle, you have to stress it," says Paul Robbins, a metabolic specialist with Athletes' Performance in Arizona. Interval training works better than other exercise because the rest periods make it possible to complete short workouts at higher intensities. We asked Robbins and exercise physiologist Ulrik Wisløff, PhD, to design the ultimate heart-strengthening regimen. Do the 42-minute program (which requires a heart rate monitor) twice a week, alternating it with your strength sessions. In addition to running, you can also use this same structure for any cardio activity that involves the large muscle groups, such as cycling, rowing, or swimming.

Warmup: Jog for 5 minutes at a pace at which you can easily hold a conversation.

Five-Minute Intervals: Complete a full cycle of 5-minute intervals and active recovery four times.

Minute 1:
Run at 90 to 95 percent of your maximum heart rate.

Minute 2:
Run at 75 to 80 percent of your maximum heart rate.

Minute 3:
Run at 90 to 95 percent of your maximum heart rate.

Minute 4:
Run at 75 to 80 percent of your maximum heart rate.

Minute 5:
Run at 90 to 95 percent of your maximum heart rate.

Active Recovery:
Walk or jog for 3 minutes during this "rest" period.

Cooldown: Walk or jog for 5 minutes at a pace at which you can hold a conversation.

Bonus: Bump up your heart fitness another notch by alternating intervals between the treadmill and other equipment. "The more large-muscle groups you use, and the more you vary the equipment, the better it is for cardiovascular fitness," says Robbins.

Tip 1: There are 12 1-minute sprints in the workout. Maintain consistency from the first sprint to the last sprint, and if possible, finish stronger than you start.

Tip 2: Initially, take more rest between sprints, if need be, to make sure that your form stays good throughout the exercise. If your heart rate is not dropping by 20-plus beats between intervals, then take more rest and skip an interval.

Feel the Burn without the Run

You don't have to hit the pavement or the elliptical machine to get a decent cardio workout. Strength training in a circuit—going rapidly from one move to the next—will keep your heart rate up, blasting calories while building muscle. Plus, you don't need any gear, you can do them anywhere, and you'll reduce your risk of overuse injuries—a common side effect of traditional cardio.
Note: If you're not used to vigorous activity, ask a doctor to evaluate you before starting any exercise program.

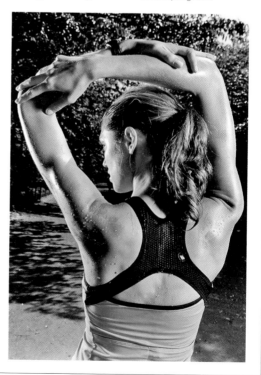

How to Lower Your Heart Rate

QUIT MAKING YOUR TICKER WORK SO HARD
AND YOU'LL PROLONG ITS LIFE—AND YOUR OWN.

*B*efore rising from bed in the morning, take your pulse. (Place the tips of your index and middle fingers on your wrist and count the beats for a minute.) Do this for 3 days and figure the average. An average person's rate is around 70 beats per minute (bpm), but in athletes it's lower. If an exercise program refers to maximum heart rate, find yours by subtracting your age from 220. Italian researchers found that having a resting heart rate above 70 bpm increases your risk of dying of heart disease by at least 78 percent. Follow the tips below to help drop your bpm and improve your odds.

1. Run Hard, Don't Just Jog

"Exercise increases your heart's efficiency, reducing the number of heartbeats you need to achieve bloodflow," says John Eleftheriades, MD, the chief of cardiothoracic surgery at Yale University. Interval training increases the amount of blood pumped with each heartbeat by about 10 percent, but slower, sustained running has no effect on it, according to an American College of Sports Medicine study.

2. Trade Massages with Him

Regular massages may soothe a rapid heartbeat. Relaxation techniques reduce your body's production of adrenaline, norepinephrine, and epinephrine, stress hormones that rev up your heart in the face of danger, says Atman P. Shah, MD, an assistant professor of medicine at UCLA. A 2007 British study found that people who received an hour of reflexology treatment (a type of foot or hand massage) had rates that averaged almost 8 bpm lower than when they went without.

3. Sleep More Soundly

The neighbor's barking dog can wreak havoc on your heart rate. Plus, "fewer than 7 hours of sleep a night increases arterial aging and your risk of a heart attack," says Mehmet Oz, MD, author of *Healing from the Heart*. In a 2007 study, Australian researchers used sound to wake people multiple times. After each noise-induced arousal, heart rates spiked an average of 13 bpm. Try Hearos Xtreme Protection Series earplugs—they can reduce noise by 33 decibels and are available at most drugstores.

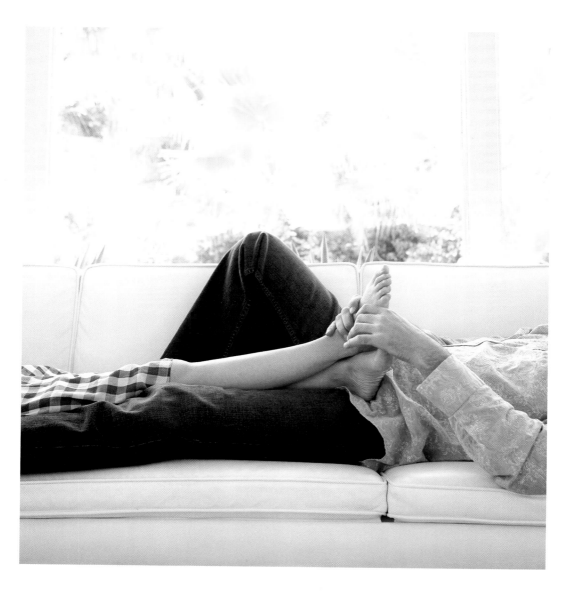

4. Don't Try to Hold It

If you gotta go, you really should go. Taiwanese researchers who studied forty people with early heart disease found that the stress of having a full bladder steps up the heart rate by an average of 9 bpm. When your bladder expands, it increases activity in your sympathetic nervous system. This may cause your coronary vessels to constrict, forcing your heart to beat more often—all of which might boost your heart attack risk.

5. Get Fishy

In a UCLA study, people who took a 1-gram fish-oil capsule every day reduced their resting heart rates by an average of 6 bpm after 2 weeks. Fish oil may help your heart respond better to your vagus nerve, which controls the heart rate. The result is a slower resting heart rate and better heart-rate responsiveness, says Dariush Mozaffarian, MD, DrPH, a cardiologist at Harvard Medical School. Try Ocean Nutrition (www.ocean-nutrition.com).

Part Three:
Your Healthy-Heart Diet

The 10 Best Foods for Your Heart

YOUR MOUTH CAN HELP YOU SERIOUSLY REDUCE
YOUR RISK OF A HEART ATTACK.
HERE'S HOW.

By Nicole Collins

You know what you should be eating by now, but if you're just paying lip service to the need for a diet rich in whole grains, fruit, vegetables, and fish, your lack of commitment could be fatal. A heart-healthy diet can reduce your LDL ("bad") cholesterol by 30 percent—a drop similar to what you can get from statin drugs. These foods are dietary magic bullets: They lower LDL cholesterol, raise "good" HDL cholesterol, and, best of all, don't require a prescription.

1. Nuts
People who eat 1½ ounces of nuts—pistachios, almonds, and walnuts are

best—more than four times a week have a 37 percent lower risk of coronary heart disease than those who seldom eat nuts, according to a study in the *British Journal of Nutrition*.

2. Fish
We'll say it again: Two servings a week of omega-3-rich fish is all it takes to significantly reduce the risk of heart disease, according to the American Heart Association. Docosahexaenoic acid (DHA) and eicosapentaenoic acid (EPA) are the omega-3 fatty acids in fish that do the coronary dark work. (See "Go Fish" on page 290 for details on getting more seafood—safely—into your diet.)

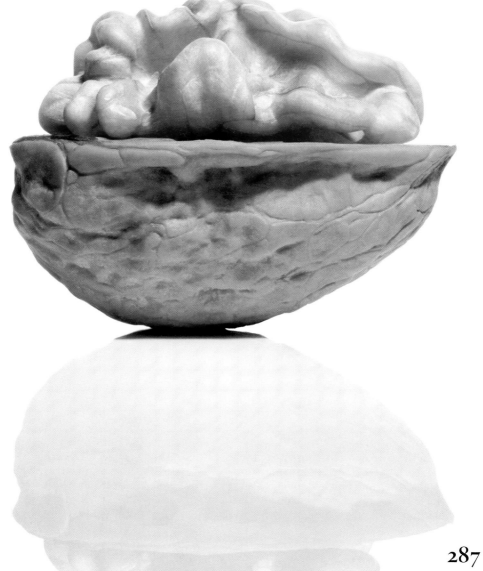

3. Oats

Eating an average of two and a half servings of whole grains a day (e.g., oats, brown rice, barley) reduces your risk of cardiovascular disease by 21 percent, according to a study in the journal *Nutrition, Metabolism and Cardiovascular Diseases*.

4. Avocados

Chock-full of monounsaturated fat and beta-sitosterol, avocados give a double-barreled blast to LDL cholesterol. They are also rich in folate, a water-soluble B vitamin that helps lower the levels of homocysteine, an amino acid that can hinder blood flow.

5. Black Beans

People who eat one 3-ounce serving of black beans a day decrease their risk of heart attack by 38 percent, according to a recent study in the *Journal of Nutrition*. Black beans are packed with superstar nutrients, including protein, healthy fats, folate, magnesium, B vitamins, potassium, and fiber.

6. Ground Flaxseed

A recent study of people with high cholesterol (greater than 240 mg/dl) compared statin treatment with eating 20 grams (about 2 Tbsp) of flaxseed a day. After 60 days, those eating flaxseed were doing just as well as those on statins. Sprinkle it on oatmeal, yogurt, and salads.

7. Green Tea

Epigallocatechin gallate (EGCG), an antioxidant that helps fight heart disease, is plentiful in green tea. Drink it like water: 5 cups of green tea daily can boost your cardiovascular health, according to several recent studies. But don't add milk—it eliminates the benefits.

8. Watermelon

High in blood pressure-lowering potassium, a good source of inflammation-reducing vitamin C, and rich in lycopene, a slice of watermelon or a glass of watermelon juice is a smart addition to your daily diet.

9. Spinach

Spinach is packed with the essential minerals potassium and magnesium, and it's one of the top sources of lutein, an antioxidant that may help prevent clogged arteries. Eat 1 cup a day of fresh or ½ cup cooked.

10. Red Wine

Swimming in resveratrol—a natural compound that lowers LDL, raises HDL, and prevents blood clots—red wine can truly be a lifesaver. Vin rouge is also a rich source of flavonoids, antioxidants that help protect the lining of blood vessels in your heart. Limit yourself to two glasses a day. Not a drinker? Nibble dark chocolate. It contains the same flavonoids as red wine.

4 New Heart Attack Fighters

THE AMERICAN HEART ASSOCIATION RECENTLY RELEASED NEW PREVENTION GUIDELINES FOR WOMEN.

1. Take aspirin with a doctor's okay. Low doses prevent clots that cause heart attacks, but regular use can cause stomach bleeding and increase stroke risk. "Whether you should take it depends on your age and family history," says Columbia University's Lori Mosca, MD, PhD.

2. Cut saturated fat even further. Artery-damaging fat should account for less than 10 percent of daily calories. Ideally, you should keep it below 7 percent. Be vigilant about reading food labels to avoid eating partially hydrogenated (trans) fats.

3. Trim 200 calories a day after menopause. After 50, your metabolism slows about 5 percent a decade, so your body burns less energy even if you're moderately active.

4. Limit antioxidant supplements. And don't expect them to prevent cardiovascular disease, either. Recent research suggests that high doses of beta-carotene, vitamin A, and vitamin E actually may increase the risk of premature death, and too much vitamin C may boost the risk of dying for women over age 50 with diabetes. Up your vegetable intake instead.

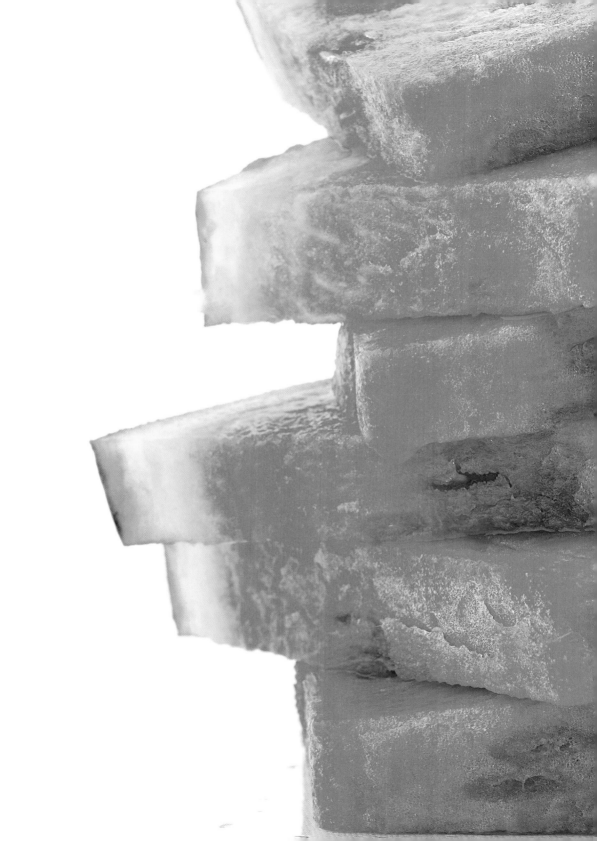

Go Fish

PUT SEAFOOD ON YOUR PLATE—AND HEART DISEASE ON ICE.

By Suzanne Schlosberg

If the only fish to cross your lips on a regular basis is the crunchy Cheddar cheese kind, it's time to find Nemo—and eat him. Not only is seafood a nutrient-packed source of protein, it's one of the richest sources of omega-3 fatty acids, the super-healthy polyunsaturated fat linked to fewer cases of heart disease, depression, stroke, and possibly even Alzheimer's disease and nonmelanoma skin cancer. On top of all that, seafood is slim on calories and artery-clogging saturated fat, and can be easier to prepare than a cheeseburger.

Despite the finer points of fish, we still don't devour enough of it. Just one in four women eats two 4-ounce servings a week, the absolute minimum the American Heart Association recommends. Why isn't seafood on the menu more often? Aside from its often hefty price tag (which you can beat by buying the good stuff frozen), recent news reports about "toxic seafood" are enough to make tuna sound like a swimming bullet.

But don't believe the scary headlines. Many respected health experts agree that seafood is one of the best things you can put down your gullet. "The benefits of fish are well established, while the risks are overblown," says Dariush Mozaffarian, MD, assistant professor of medicine and epidemiology at Harvard Medical School and lead author of a 2006 article in the *Journal of the American Medical Association* that weighed the pros and cons of eating seafood. One positive finding: Adding just 3 to 6 ounces of fish to your diet every week, especially those high in omega-3 fatty acids reduces the risk of death from a heart attack by a staggering 36 percent.

According to Dr. Mozaffarian and his crew, omega-3s seep into the cell membranes of the heart and blood vessels and help protect them against irregular heartbeats, blood clotting, and other disturbances that can cause heart attacks. The *JAMA* study concluded that we should all be getting an average of 250 milligrams of omega-3s daily to safeguard our tickers. And since fatty acids from fish are also crucial to a fetus's developing brain—including vision, memory, and language comprehension—women considering having kids should eat no less than four 3-ounce servings of seafood a week.

On the flip side, many types of seafood do contain mercury—and at very high levels, mercury kills brain cells. We know this from studies of industrial accidents like the one in Japan in the '50s, when a petrochemical company discharged heavy-metal waste into the ocean, poisoned the fish supply, and caused pregnant women who ate contaminated fish to bear children with damaged nervous systems. Megadoses of mercury can remain in your bloodstream for more than a year. Still, getting mercury poisoning isn't easy—your body removes most of it

36
Percentage that adding fish to your diet reduces your risk of death by heart attack

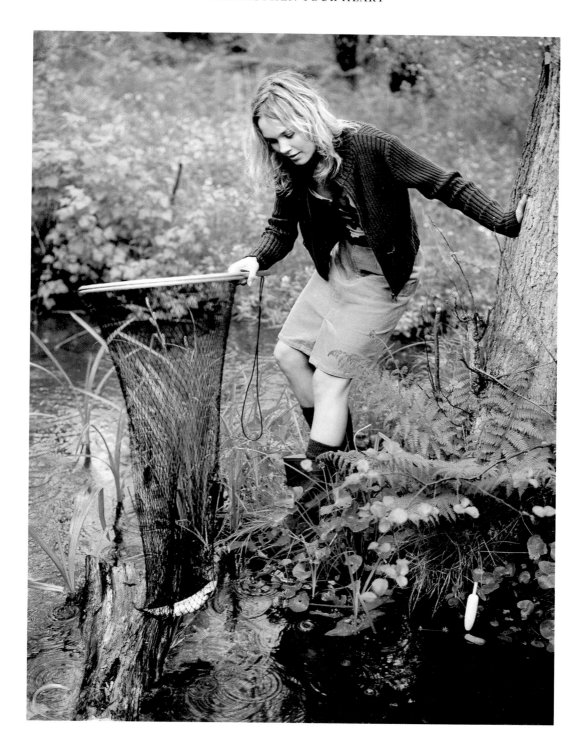

naturally via the filtering action of your kidneys and other metabolic pathways. In order to rack up a dangerous amount of the toxin, you'd have to consume the most mercury-laden fish several times a month. Which fish are in that same sorry boat? Since large bodies soak up more chemicals than small ones, the victims include king mackerel, sharks, swordfish, tilefish, and whales.

When a society does down tainted fish at the same ungodly rate that Americans scarf junk food, the results seem to vary. One study of kids living in the Seychelles, a group of islands in the Indian Ocean where pregnant women eat an average of 12 fish meals per week, was reassuring. "We've examined 700 children on six occasions over 16 years and haven't found adverse effects that are consistent with mercury consumption," says Gary Myers, MD, a professor of neurology and pediatrics at the University of Rochester in New York. He notes that seafood in the Seychelles has mercury levels similar to those of commercial fish eaten in New York. But an equally comprehensive study of children in the Faroe Islands, located between Norway and Iceland, produced worrisome results. Researchers found brain impairment due to high prenatal mercury exposure. One theory: In the Faroes, most mercury comes from whale meat eaten in large quantities during hunting season, which possibly causes a rush of mercury that the body takes much longer to flush.

The other dark spot on seafood's shining reputation comes from polychlorinated biphenyls (PCBs). These industrial chemicals were banned 30 years ago but hang around in the environment for decades. While animal studies have linked PCBs to cancer, it's unclear whether they cause the disease in humans. But Dr. Mozaffarian and colleagues hold firm that PCB levels in fish—which are considerably lower than in poultry or beef—are so minuscule that the cardiovascular benefits of seafood surpass the potential cancer risks several hundred times over.

All that said, since brain damage and cancer are at stake here, it's still better to err on the side of caution. Luckily, the simple solution is to score your 250-milligram minimum of omega-3 fats from fish with as few toxins as possible. What follows ranks the most commonly eaten seafoods

according to how much of the good and the bad they deliver. To access the most comprehensive list with definitive information about sustainability, visit www.montereybayaquarium.org/seafoodwatch.

Ocean's Twenty: The Health Rewards of Your Favorite Seafood

There are plenty of fish in the sea, but finding the best takes thorough analysis. The list below started with a list of the 20 most popular types of seafood in the US (which explains why hairy anchovies are missing). The omega-3 (DHA and EPA) content of each fish was calculated using Food and Drug Administration data and a serving size of 3 ounces. Other nutritional perks were factored in, like selenium, a mineral that bolsters cancer-fighting antioxidants, and B_{12} vitamins, which are crucial to nerve health. The average levels of toxins in each fish, like mercury and PCBs, was also added. (See "Mercury Meter" on page 294 to learn your limit.) Use this list to navigate the fish counter like Captain Ahab.

1. **Salmon** (the wild kind) wins by a waterslide. Most varieties, including coho and sockeye, provide more than three times the 250-milligram recommended minimum daily dose of omega-3s. Wild Atlantic salmon is king of the sea with a mighty 1.6 grams of the good stuff and a mini mercury count of 0.01 parts per million (ppm). A serving also gets you 72 percent of your 55-microgram daily dietary reference intake (DRI) of selenium. Avoid farmed salmon, which may contain PCBs from polluted water.

2. **Rainbow trout** (the farmed kind) gets the silver medal for a full gram of omega-3s. Tests on mixed varieties of trout show only 0.07 ppm of mercury, and farmed may contain even less. It also boasts more than twice the 2-microgram DRI for B_{12} and half the 15-milligram DRI for niacin, which lowers bad cholesterol and plays a key role in metabolism.

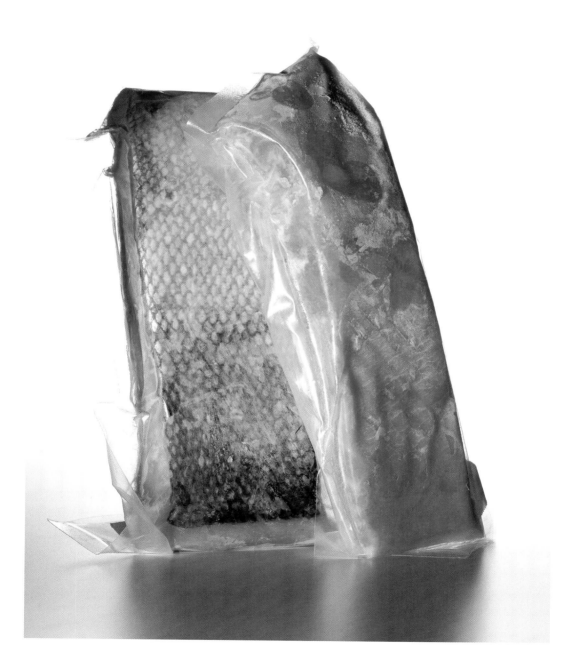

3. **Oysters** (from the Pacific) are almost devoid of mercury (0.01 ppm) and pack 1.2 grams of omega-3s per 3 ounces. Each slippery serving also delivers more than twice the 12-milligram DRI of immunity- and libido-boosting zinc. Kumamotos, a smaller variety, is particularly tasty and a good choice for newcomers. Avoid wild Eastern oysters as they may contain PCBs.

4. **Striped bass** (if farmed) is not known to contain mercury in any measurable quantity and packs 0.8 gram of omega-3s, more than twice the suggested minimum. Bonus nutrients include about double the DRI of B_{12} and 72 percent of your daily selenium. Avoid mercury-laden wild striped bass (0.22 ppm).

5. **Pollock** (from the Atlantic)—often used to make fillet of fish, fish sticks, and imitation crab (aka surimi)—is rich in B_{12} (3 micrograms) and selenium (40 micrograms) and extremely low in mercury (0.04 ppm). And its 0.5 gram of omega-3s is nothing to shake a fin at. Avoid Pacific pollock—it's more likely to contain PCBs.

6. **Flounder and sole** are nutritional twins and contain a healthy 0.4 gram of omega-3s and just 0.04 ppm of mercury. A single serving has nearly 100 percent of your daily DRI of selenium and B_{12}. Avoid "blackback" and summer varieties—they can pack PCBs.

7. **Alaskan king crab** deserves its crown as the crustacean with the biggest omega-3 bang (0.4 gram) and a piddling 0.06 ppm of mercury. It's low cal (82 calories per 3 ounces), and it contains 50 percent of your zinc DRI and—check it out—five times your B_{12} DRI. Avoid blue crab, which has higher levels of PCBs and mercury.

8. **Perch** (freshwater). One serving provides more than 100 percent of your omega-3 minimum, almost all of your selenium (47 micrograms), and half of your B_{12}, with no measurable mercury. So eat up!

Also on the Menu

MORE FISH THAT SINK OR SWIM BY HEALTH AND ENVIRONMENTAL STANDARDS

Order This . . .

Arctic char: It looks and tastes a lot like superstar salmon and has similar nutritional properties.

Herring: Ask for this fatty acid–packed cold-water fish grilled or boiled (1.7 grams omega-3s). The pickled stuff is sky-high in sodium.

Mussels: These are yummy little protein bombs with 0.7 gram of omega-3s.

Sablefish: Also known as black cod, butterfish, or pompano, sablefish is chock-full of healthy fats (1.5 grams omega-3s).

Squid: Request this heart-friendly critter grilled, not fried (0.5 gram omega-3s).

Not That . . .

Chilean sea bass: It's high in mercury (0.39 ppm) and often caught with lines that kill seabirds.

Grouper: This fish fails on the mercury front (0.47 ppm) and has been overfished.

Swordfish: Jammed with 0.98 ppm of mercury, it's best avoided.

Wahoo: Related to toxic king mackerel, it's not worthy of your plate, either.

Mercury Meter

MERCURY (IN PPM)	EAT IT
Less than 0.08	In unlimited quantities
0.08–0.12	No more than 8 times a month
0.13–0.23	No more than 4 times a month
0.24–0.31	No more than 3 times a month
0.32–0.47	No more than twice a month
0.48–0.94	No more than once a month

Source: Environmental Defense Fund Seafood Selector (www.edf.org)

9. **Clams** score you 0.2 gram of omega-3s (some tests reveal that they can contain as much as 0.5 gram). A single serving also has 350 percent of the 15-milligram DRI for iron and a colossal 84 micrograms of B_{12}. All that with a mere 0.02 ppm of mercury.

10. **Scallops** have a meaty texture even steak lovers can appreciate. Both the bay and sea varieties are heart friendly, with 0.3 gram of omega-3s, more than half your B_{12} DRI, and only a hint of mercury (0.05 ppm).

11. **Shrimp** are a dieter's dream at only 84 calories per serving, with 0.3 gram of omega-3s and a supersafe mercury level of 0.05 ppm. The drawback: A serving of shrimp has 166 milligrams of cholesterol (almost as much as an egg), so if you're watching your cholesterol, don't eat the pink critters more than once a week.

12. **Catfish** (if farmed) has 0.2 gram of healthy fats, more than 100 percent of your B_{12} DRI, and only 0.05 ppm of mercury. But the whiskered fish's biggest claim to fame is 14.3 micrograms of muscle- and bone-building vitamin D—almost three times your DRI.

13. **Haddock** gives up a good bit of omega-3s (0.2 gram), 63 percent of your selenium, and over half of your B_{12} DRI. And barely-there mercury (0.03 ppm) makes it an anytime entrée.

14. **Tilapia** is a freshwater dweller similar to catfish. Though it has only 0.1 gram of omega-3s, tilapia is nearly free of mercury (0.01 ppm) and contains 84 percent of your daily selenium and 79 percent of your B_{12}. So you can eat it till the sharks come home.

15. **Spiny Lobster** doesn't have claws like the monsters from Maine, but its tail has tons more omega-3s (0.4 gram versus 0.07 gram) and a lot less mercury (0.09 ppm versus 0.3 ppm). Other highlights include 50 percent of your zinc DRI, 91 percent of your selenium DRI, and nearly twice your DRI of B_{12}.

16. **Canned tuna** (packed in water). It's saddled with more mercury (0.12 ppm) than most fish on this list, but it has the least of all other types of tuna and still provides 0.2 gram of omega-3s. Eat it no more than eight times a month and feel good about getting 75 percent of your niacin DRI and more than 100 percent of your selenium and B_{12}.

17. **Cod** (from the Pacific) supplies almost twice the omega-3s of Atlantic cod (0.2 gram versus 0.1 gram) and racks up 72 percent of your selenium for just 89 calories a serving. But don't dine on it more than twice a week, because its mercury count is on the high side (0.1 ppm).

18. **Halibut** is a very good source of omega-3s (0.4 gram) and provides more than 40 percent of your DRI of niacin, 72 percent of your selenium, and 58 percent of B_{12}, so eating it every once in a while is a healthy option. Just keep it to no more than four meals per month, because its 0.2-ppm mercury count is twice as high as cod's.

19. **Skipjack tuna** is smaller than bluefin or yellowfin and therefore soaks up fewer toxins. It delivers an impressive 0.3 gram of omega-3s, 72 percent of your selenium DRI, and 93 percent of the B_{12} DRI. Still, it has 0.2 ppm of mercury, so limit it to four meals a month.

20. **Orange roughy** has two strikes against it: minimal omega-3s (0.02 gram) and way more mercury (0.6 ppm) than any other fish listed here. But it's low in calories and high in protein and selenium (75 micrograms). So if you're craving it, go ahead—just not more than once a month.

10 Foods Your Heart Doc Won't Eat

THESE RESTAURANT MEALS ARE SO SALTY YOU COULD
THROW THEM OVER YOUR SHOULDER FOR
GOOD LUCK. IF YOU CARE ABOUT YOUR BLOOD PRESSURE,
DON'T LET THEM PAST YOUR LIPS.

By David Zinczenko with Matt Goulding

Few things in world history have done as much good, and caused as much damage, as the simple mineral salt.

On the upside, salt made modern civilization possible, allowing ancient man to preserve food so he could concentrate on more important things, like curing ulcers with leeches and creating the subprime mortgage crisis. But while salt has long been used to make food more easily available, it can also be used to cause starvation—"salting the land" meant poisoning crops with salt so your enemies couldn't grow grains and produce. In fact, salt was once so precious and powerful that some scholars believe the word "salary" comes from the Latin *salarium,* which was how Roman soldiers were paid. (I believe it means "Thanks for killing the natives, here's some money, go buy salt.")

Today, salt is cheaper than dirt. (Literally—just go to a gardening store and you'll see.) But salt isn't done causing its damage. When you eat out at most restaurants, from the highest of the high-end to the cheapest and fastest of the drive-thrus, you're all but guaranteed to take in more than your recommended daily amount of sodium—

about 2,300 milligrams (mg) of sodium, max. But salt is so cheap and, let's face it, makes so many foods taste delicious, that it's in nearly everything. In fact, the average American takes in about 3,300 milligrams of sodium every single day!

And it's not because of what comes out of our saltshakers. According to researchers at the Monell Chemical Senses Center in Philadelphia, 77 percent of that sodium intake originates from processed-food purveyors. Their motivation: Pile on the salt so we don't miss natural flavors and fresh ingredients.

Why is that a problem? With ever-expanding portion sizes, supersalty foods are displacing fresh fruits and vegetables, which are rich in potassium. And a one-to-one ratio of dietary salt to potassium is critical for your health (even better if it's closer to one-to-two). Studies show that a high-sodium, low-potassium diet is linked to a host of maladies, including high blood pressure, stroke, osteoporosis, and exercise-induced asthma.

To protect your heart, your bones, your muscles, and your taste buds, we scoured takeout menus and supermarket shelves to expose the 10 saltiest foods in America. No need to take the information with a grain of salt. These dishes provide plenty.

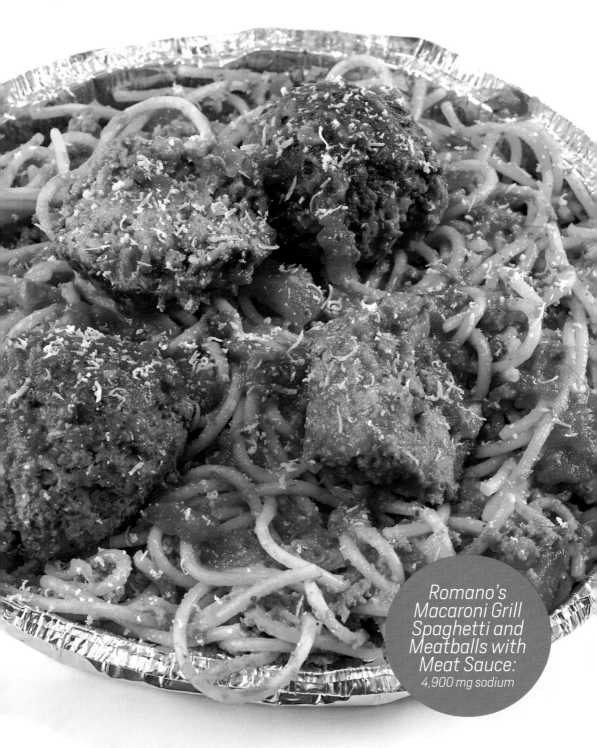

Romano's Macaroni Grill Spaghetti and Meatballs with Meat Sauce:
4,900 mg sodium

10. Saltiest Side

Dairy Queen Chili Cheese Fries

*2,550 mg sodium, 1,240 calories, 71 g fat
(28 g saturated, 0.5 g trans)*

Sodium equivalent: *15 strips of bacon*

This one's a no-brainer: chili, cheese, fried potatoes. But even a savvy eater couldn't possibly anticipate how bad these three ingredients could be when combined by one heavy-handed fast-food company. Stick with classic ketchup and recapture nearly a day's worth of sodium and 930 calories.

Eat This Instead!

French Fries (regular)

640 mg sodium, 310 calories, 13 g fat (2 g saturated)

9. Saltiest "Healthy" Meal

Olive Garden Grilled Shrimp Caprese

*3,490 mg sodium, 900 calories, 41 g fat
(17 g saturated), 82 g carbohydrates*

Sodium equivalent: *20 individual canisters
of Pringles Originals*

Grilled shrimp on its own makes for one of the healthiest sources of protein on the planet, but when corrupted by the imaginations of the corporate cooks at Olive Garden, the result is considerably bleaker. The melted mozzarella and the garlic butter sauce are to blame for the high sodium numbers. Stick with the sea, but choose grilled salmon instead of a platter that's soaked in salty sauce.

Eat This Instead!

Herb-Grilled Salmon

*760 mg sodium, 510 calories, 26 g fat (6 g saturated)
5 g carbohydrates*

8. Saltiest Burger

**Chili's Southern Smokehouse Bacon
Big Mouth Burger**

*4,200 mg sodium, 1,650 calories, 108 g fat
(36 g saturated)*

Sodium equivalent: *A pound of salted peanuts*

Where there's smoke, there's salt, at least when left in the hands of the restaurant industry. Here, smoky, thick-cut bacon combines with smoked Cheddar cheese and an ancho chile barbecue

sauce to smother this huge patty and buttered bun with nearly 2 days' worth of salt. We can't argue that any of the burgers at Chili's are actually "good" for you, but switching to the Oldtimer will cut nearly three-quarters of the sodium and 64 grams of fat.

Eat This Instead!

Oldtimer

1,310 mg sodium, 821 calories, 44 g fat (12 g saturated)

7. Saltiest Seafood Dish

Red Lobster Admiral's Feast

*4,662 mg sodium, 1,506 calories, 93 g fat
(9 g saturated)*

Sodium equivalent: *7 medium orders of Burger King
Onion Rings*

The admiral is piloting a sinking ship if this is the vessel he's steering. It's a sea of dreaded beige, with 4 different varieties of deep-fried seafood filling out the plate. Add on the Caesar salad and the fries that come with the meal and you're looking at more than 6,000 milligrams of sodium before you. Red Lobster is filled with low-calorie options, but sodium's definitely an enduring issue here, so choose wisely. Grilled fish and vegetables is a great place to start.

Eat This Instead!

Wood Grilled Sole with Fresh Asparagus

590 mg sodium, 305 calories, 7.5 g fat (2.5 g saturated)

6. Saltiest Breakfast

Arby's Sausage Gravy Biscuit

*4,699 mg sodium, 1,040 calories, 60 g fat
(22 g saturated, 2 g trans)*

Sodium equivalent: *13 large orders of McDonald's
French Fries*

This is absolutely one of the worst ways you could start your day. Make a date with this and you'll have consumed 2 full days' worth of sodium before noon. The key to maintaining a reasonable blood pressure level for most folks is to take in an equivalent amount of sodium and potassium throughout your day. The problem with this biscuit is that you're consuming a heart-stopping level of sodium and almost no potassium. Throw in the abundance of calories and trans fats and you may have been better off sleeping in.

Eat This Instead!
Bacon and Egg Croissant
651 mg sodium, 337 calories, 22 g fat (10 g saturated)

---

5. Saltiest Pasta
Romano's Macaroni Grill Spaghetti and Meatballs with Meat Sauce (dinner)
4,900 mg sodium, 1,810 calories, 118 g fat (54 g saturated)
Sodium equivalent: *8 ½ cups of Original Chex Party Mix*
The only thing more unappetizing than the sky-high sodium level here is the fact that a single bowl of pasta can pack as much saturated fat as 54 strips of bacon. Unfortunately, when ordering pasta out, options that contain any kind of meat or seafood usually come with an unnaturally large dose of calories, fat, and sodium. Save those dish-

es for the stove at home and stick to the tomato-based capellini next time you find yourself at Macaroni Grill.

Eat This Instead!
Capellini Tre Pomodoro
990 mg sodium, 640 calories, 25 g fat (3 g saturated)

---

4. Saltiest Sandwich
Blimpie 12-Inch Super Stacked Turkey and Bacon
5,244 mg sodium, 1,165 calories, 48 g fat (21 g saturated)
Sodium equivalent: *28 strips of bacon*
Deli meats are typically injected with salt solutions to lend them more moisture and flavor, but in the case of this turkey terror, it lends the consumer nearly 2 ½ days' worth of sodium intake. A word to the wise: If you're watching your salt intake, processed meats, processed cheeses, and bacon will never serve you well. This is one of

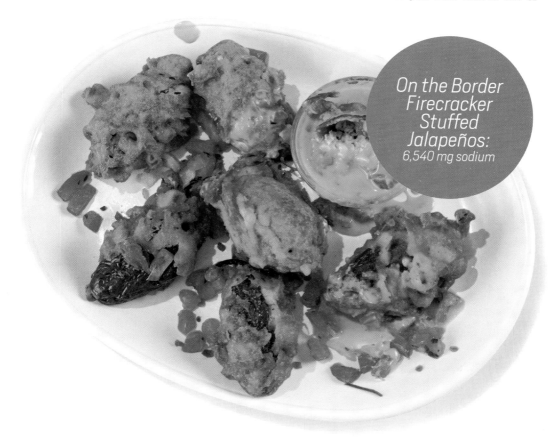

On the Border Firecracker Stuffed Jalapeños: 6,540 mg sodium

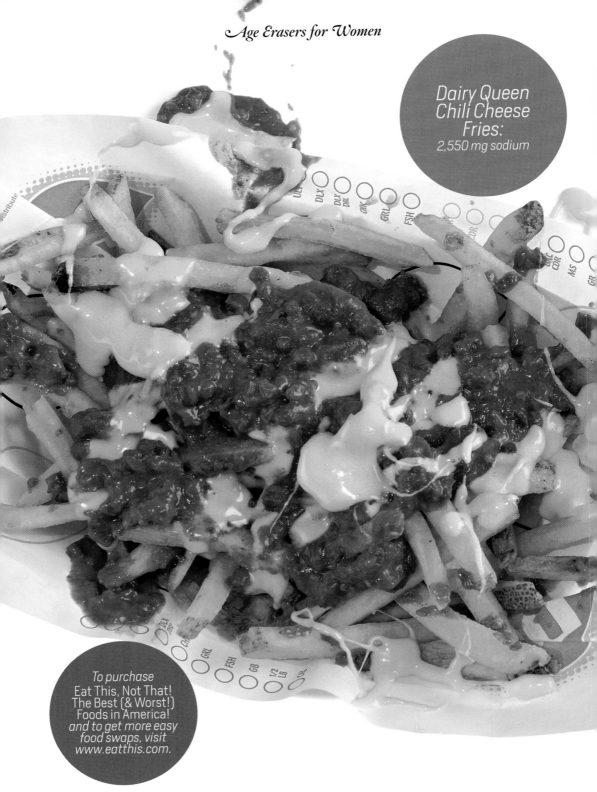

Dairy Queen
Chili Cheese
Fries:
2,550 mg sodium

To purchase
Eat This, Not That!
The Best (& Worst!)
Foods in America!
and to get more easy
food swaps, visit
www.eatthis.com.

the few times that tuna is actually the smart sandwich selection.

Eat This Instead!
Six-Inch Tuna Regular

776 mg sodium, 483 calories, 21 g fat (3 g saturated)

3. Saltiest Appetizer
On the Border Firecracker Stuffed Jalapeños with Chili con Queso

6,540 mg sodium, 1950 calories, 134 g fat (36 g saturated)
Sodium equivalent: *1,453 Pepperidge Farms Cheddar Goldfish*

Appetizers are the most problematic area on most chain-restaurant menus. That's because they're disproportionately reliant on the type of cheesy, greasy ingredients that catch hungry diners' eyes when they're most vulnerable—right when they sit down. Seek out lean protein options like grilled shrimp skewers or ahi tuna when available; if not, simple is best—like chips and salsa.

Eat This Instead!
Chips and Salsa

440 mg sodium, 430 calories, 22 g fat (3.5 g saturated)

2. Saltiest Entrée
Chili's Buffalo Chicken Fajitas with condiments and four flour tortillas

6,846 mg sodium, 1,782 calories, 108 g fat (29 g saturated)
Sodium equivalent: *68 cups of Pop Secret Homestyle Popcorn*

After Chinese food, Tex-Mex may be the saltiest cuisine on the planet, dedicated as it is to shredded cheese, refried beans, and massive tortillas. Even if you split this dish three ways, you'd still consume an entire day's allotment of sodium. Your best bet at Chili's is to avoid the Tex-Mex treatment and opt for more basic fare, like their Classic Sirloin.

Eat This Instead!
Chili's Classic Sirloin

990 mg sodium, 540 calories, 50 g fat (18 g saturated)

The Sodium Spectrum

Studies show the average woman significantly underestimates her sodium intake at every meal. Use this scale to see how much you know about the salt content of America's favorite foods.

150 mg:	*1 strip bacon*
300 mg:	*1 cup cornflakes with nonfat milk*
360 mg:	*2 handfuls potato chips*
500 mg:	*2 tablespoons Italian dressing*
600 mg:	*Large french fries*
700 mg:	*2 pickle spears*
775 mg:	*1 cup chicken noodle soup*
850 mg:	*10 tablespoons shredded parmesan*
1,100 mg:	*18 pretzel twists*
1,200 mg:	*¼-pound cheeseburger*
1,300 mg:	*Large glass tomato juice*
1,400 mg:	*4 Buffalo wings*
1,550 mg:	*3 ounces blue cheese*
1,800 mg:	*8 slices salami*
1,916 mg:	*3 tablespoons teriyaki sauce*
2,818 mg:	*3 tablespoons soy sauce*

1. The Saltiest Food in America
P.F. Chang's Hot and Sour Soup Bowl

6,878 mg sodium, 534 calories, 20 g fat (4 g saturated)
Sodium equivalent: *208 saltine crackers*

P.F. Chang's has published its nutrition facts for years sans sodium counts, which was cause for concern and—as it turns out—justified suspicion. Chinese food runs high on the sodium spectrum because of its reliance on viscous stir-fry sauces and salt-laden condiments like soy sauce. But this is an unfathomable amount of salt to pack into one 534-calorie bowl of soup. Unless you stick to vegetable sides and small servings of a select few entrées (Orange Peel Beef, Chang's Lemon Scallops), you're all but guaranteed to absorb 1 or more day's worth of sodium in a single sitting at P.F. Chang's.

Eat This Instead!
Sichuan-Style Asparagus Side

263 mg sodium, 213 calories, 11 g fat (2 g saturated)

Chapter Eleven

Bring Out Your Beautiful Best

FAST AND EASY WAYS TO LOOK YOUNGER, SEXIER, AND HEALTHIER IN MINUTES

> INVESTMENT: 1 WEEK
> AGE ERASED: 3 YEARS

Introduction

Part One:
Get (Even More) Gorgeous!
• Your Custom Beauty Guide
• Look Great Anytime, Anyplace
• Become Sexier in Seconds
• Secret Steps to Softer Lips

Part Two:
Lustrous Hair Starts Here
• Your Hair's Most Important Ally
• Guarantee a Good Cut
• Banish Bad Hair Days
• Be Your Own Colorist
• The Gorgeous Way to Go Gray

Part Three:
Dress Your Best
• How Shopping Can Save Your Life
• 10 Style Mistakes That Instantly Age You
• Find Your Perfect Swimsuit
• A Woman's Guide to Denim

Introduction

Birthdays may be inevitable, but looking older than you feel doesn't have to be. The first step is to recognize your own natural beauty. The question is, are you ready to set it free? Nobody knows your body—assets, liabilities, and everything in between—more intimately than you do. But with each passing year, it gets easier and easier to fixate on the so-called flaws. That's why it's time to clean the mirror and move in for a whole new look.

Start here: Picture your perfect outfit. Ten options probably just fluttered through your brain, but it's the one that fits your body. In fact, it fits your body so well that your eyes will seek out every shiny surface just to catch a glimpse of your fabulous reflection as you walk by. Can you see it yet? Now imagine if every piece of clothing you own made you feel the same way.

As long as you're checking yourself out, take a look at your makeup and your hair. Since before you hit your teen years, you've been experimenting with both—enhancing what you have, covering up what you dislike . . . and maybe making some mistakes along the way. Do you like how they're making you look now? Because ultimately they're tools, and by changing how you use them you can make yourself look better than you've ever imagined. If you have a few lines, for example, start by throwing your face powder away—it lingers in them and immediately adds years to your face.

The age-defying solutions in this chapter will help you discover a younger-looking version of your current self, and soon you'll replace your critical inner eye with sunnier thoughts. And those flaws? Completely forgotten. Now that's something to look forward to.

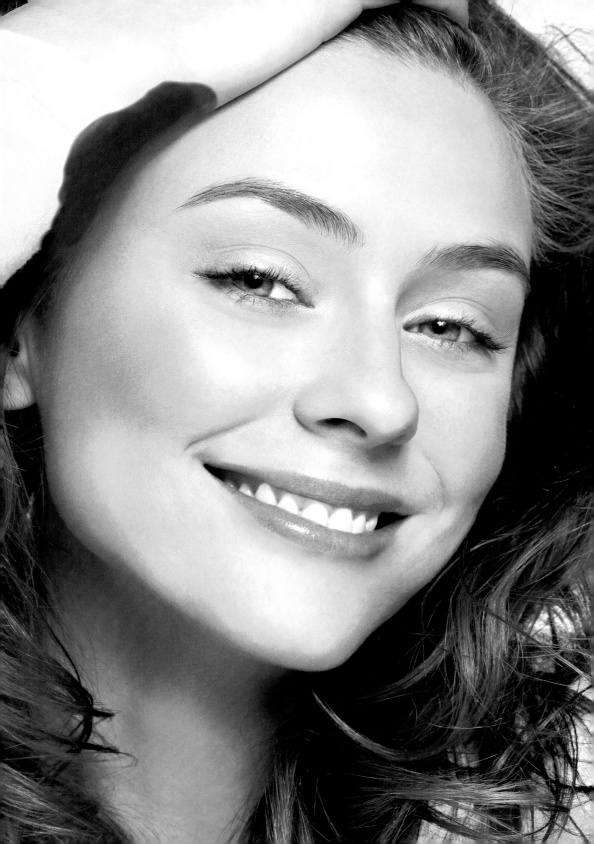

Part One

Get (Even More) Gorgeous!

Your Custom Beauty Guide

THREE TOP MAKEUP ARTISTS SHOW YOU HOW TO LOOK
JUST LIKE YOURSELF—ONLY BETTER.

Porcelain Skin
Erase Imperfections
Use a small synthetic brush to dot on yellow-toned concealer and blend over red and dark areas. "Yellow/orange is great to camouflage any red/blue discoloration," says makeup artist and Stila Cosmetics founder Jeanine Lobell. Next, smooth tinted moisturizer over your entire face "like you would a regular moisturizer. It's less detectable than foundation."

Create a Sunny Glow
Whisk a hint of shimmering bronzer up cheekbones, then over temples and forehead. Brighten the apples with a hint of peachy-pink blush (bright red-pinks make cheeks look ruddy).

Wake Up Eyes
Sweep a sheer white-gold shadow over the entire lid, blending at the inner corners to make eyes look brighter. Smudge a bronzy gold shadow across the upper and lower lash lines. For the smoothest application, "load up your brush with powder, then press it on the back of your hand to secure the shadow onto the brush," Lobell says. Curl lashes and apply mascara "to lift eyes even further." Try clear eyebrow gel for a polished look.

Add Lip Shine
Use a lip-liner that's close to your natural lip color, and then top with gloss. "Since gloss is transparent, it lets the natural lip pigment come through," says Lobell.

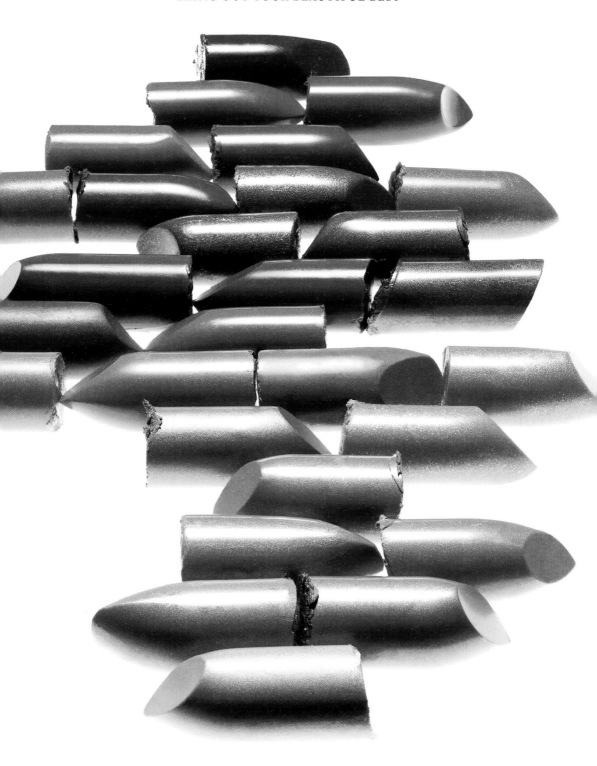

Line the lower inside rims of your eyes with a flesh-toned pencil to erase redness and open up the eye.

Olive Skin

Warm Up Skin
For the most natural look, choose products with yellow undertones; they work best because they match your skin. Apply a sheer, tinted moisturizer with your fingertips (don't forget your neck). "Go one shade darker than your natural skin tone to warm the complexion," Roncal suggests.

Pop On Some Pink
Brush a bright (but sheer!) pink blush on the apples of cheeks and the tip of the nose, "where the sun would naturally make your skin a little rosier," says makeup artist Mally Roncal, founder of Mally Beauty. "A flush of pink makes cheekbones pop and prevents a bronze face from looking like flat, brown wallpaper."

Brighten Eyes
Sweep bronzer instead of shadow over eyelids, then add the merest touch of shimmer at the very center of the lid from lash line to crease. Smudge a pale gold shadow in a V-shape at the inner corners to open and widen eyes. Define lashes with black mascara.

Play Up Your Pout
A pink-berry hue accentuates the natural color in your lips. For a soft, stained look, apply sheer lipstick with a fingertip. Dab a pearly beige gloss on the center of the lower lip, then press lips together to blend.

Freckled Skin

Even Out the Complexion
The winning concealer here is—yup—yellow-based: It's best at camouflaging redness, darkness, or broken capillaries. Alexandra Kwiatkowski, a New York–based Nouba makeup artist, likes liquid or cream formulations that are undetectable and blend easily. Following concealer with tinted moisturizer "provides natural color and coverage without looking too heavy," she says.

Get Sun-Kissed (Without the Sun)
Lightly apply a medium-toned bronzer over your cheeks, then swipe some on the bridge of the nose and top of the forehead to balance the face (bronzed cheeks alone scream "fake tan"). "Never go too dark," Kwiatkowski warns. "Bronzer can appear dirty and ruddy on freckled skin. Pick one with a slight shimmer that reflects light and makes the whole face glow."

Boost Radiance
Apply a pink blush to the apples of your cheeks for a pop of healthy color. Tap it onto skin with fingers to blend. Next, pat a tiny bit of liquid shimmer to cheek and brow bones to highlight and brighten them. To keep skin looking fresh, touch up with blotting papers instead of powder.

Wash Lids with Emerald Green
"This warm, golden green gives your skin a boost and draws attention to blue eyes," Kwiatkowski says. Dust shadow on lids, then make it sheerer by blending with a finger from lash line to crease. Use a small, dampened brush to smudge a sable-brown shadow across the upper and lower lash lines to define them softly. Lining the lower inside rims of the eyes with a flesh-toned pencil will erase redness and open up the eye. You can also make pale lashes look lusher with black mascara.

Stain Lips
Dab lips with a berry lipstick. "Gently press in the color to create a soft, kissable lip," Kwiatkowski says. For extra staying power, use the same trick with a soft lip pencil in a rosy hue, then top it off with clear lip balm.

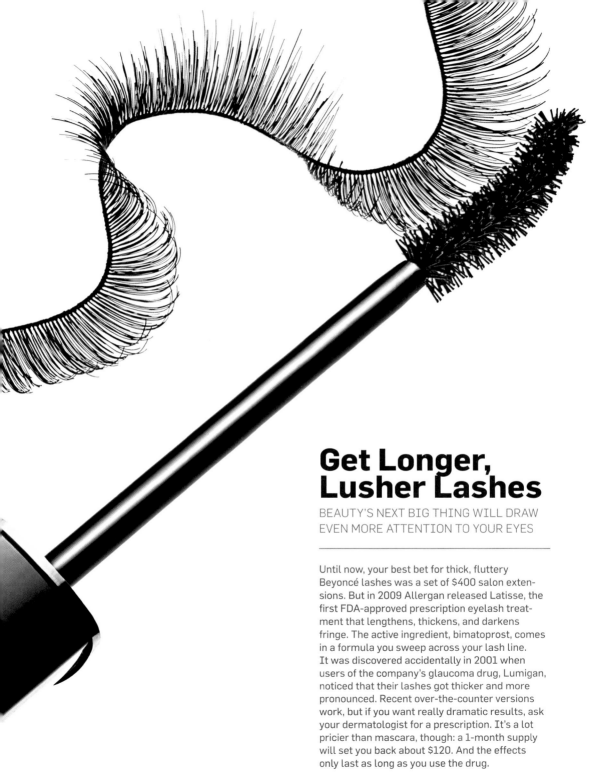

Get Longer, Lusher Lashes

BEAUTY'S NEXT BIG THING WILL DRAW EVEN MORE ATTENTION TO YOUR EYES

Until now, your best bet for thick, fluttery Beyoncé lashes was a set of $400 salon extensions. But in 2009 Allergan released Latisse, the first FDA-approved prescription eyelash treatment that lengthens, thickens, and darkens fringe. The active ingredient, bimatoprost, comes in a formula you sweep across your lash line. It was discovered accidentally in 2001 when users of the company's glaucoma drug, Lumigan, noticed that their lashes got thicker and more pronounced. Recent over-the-counter versions work, but if you want really dramatic results, ask your dermatologist for a prescription. It's a lot pricier than mascara, though: a 1-month supply will set you back about $120. And the effects only last as long as you use the drug.

Look Great Anytime, Anyplace

A SEASON–BY–SEASON CALENDAR OF THE EXPERTS'
BEST GET–GORGEOUS HAIR, SKIN, AND MAKEUP TRICKS.

Summer Is Prime Time to . . .

Lay Off the Bottle (and Brush and Tube)

When the weather warms up, cut back on cosmetics. A study in the *Journal of the European Academy of Dermatology and Venereology* found that reports of sensitive skin rise during the summer months, especially in women. So it's time to simplify your regimen. "Look for out products with a short ingredient list," says study author Laurent Misery, MD, PhD. "The fewer ingredients a product has, the less likely it is to irritate the skin."

Wear It Short

Have you been thinking about getting cropped Katie Holmes-style? Schedule an appointment with your hair stylist so that she can do her magic now. Hair grows faster when the weather is warm, so if you don't like the results, you won't be stuck with a less-than-desirable 'do for long.

Let the Waxing Wane

Yes, it gets rid of that annoying fuzz, but waxing also removes a thin layer of skin—unfortunately, just enough to make you a lot more vulnerable to the sun's rays. If you'll be spending a lot of time outdoors, consider shaving, depilatories, or bleaching instead.

Switch to the Bright Side

The more intense your nail polish color, the better your pedicure will look, says Donna Perillo, owner of Sweet Lily Natural Nail Spa in New York City. That's because brighter shades hide the yellowing effect the sun has on pigments.

Go Faux

Skin cancer rates continue to rise. Satisfy your baking needs by hitting the bottle behind closed doors. Apply self-tanner about 2 hours before bed so it has enough time to absorb (otherwise, you'll end up with streaks).

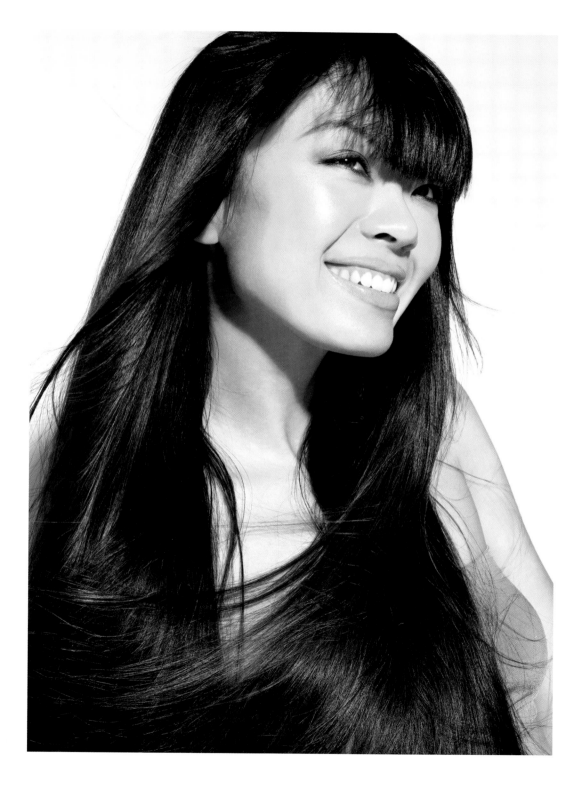

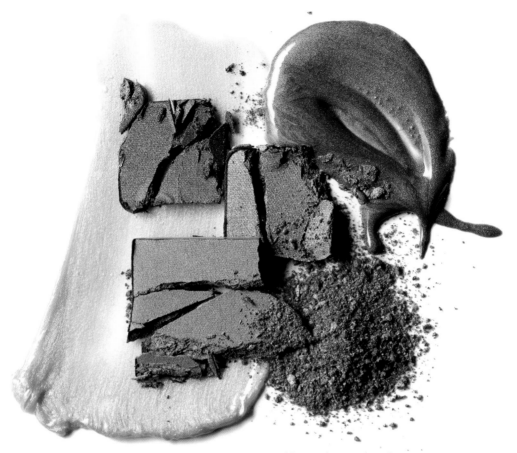

Try Acid

Salicylic acid, that is. Sweat trapped against your skin can clog pores and cause acne-producing bacteria to grow. Prevent backne and buttne with a quick mist of a salicylic acid spray to keep pores clear and kill bacteria.

Take It Easy

Don't be so hard on your nails. "People spend more time in the water when the weather turns hot, and that's where bacteria and yeast can breed," says dermatologist and nail specialist Dana Stern, MD. Your cuticles act as a natural barrier, preventing the bad stuff from entering the nail bed, so make sure your manicurist doesn't cut your cuticles and isn't otherwise overly aggressive when she works her magic on your poor hands.

Fall Is the Ideal Season to . . .

Scan Your Skin

"Now's the time to go in for your yearly checkup with your dermatologist," Francesca Fusco, MD, assistant clinical professor of dermatology at Mount Sinai School of Medicine in New York City, says. "Have your doctor do a skin scan so she can catch any sun damage that may have occurred during the summer."

Schedule Spa Time

If you get only one facial this year, do it in the fall. "After a summer in the sun, ask for alpha hydroxy acid (AHA) and retinol treatments to get rid of dead skin cells and firm up your skin," says Christine Chin, owner of Christine Chin Spa in New York City. Need another reason to be pampered? After enduring months of sweat and sunscreen, your skin may be feeling rebellious, and a facial can help head off any breakouts.

Turn Down the Lights

Take sun-bleached strands a shade or two darker and they'll look healthier and more natural. "Plus the richer hue will make your skin look warmer and better," says celebrity colorist Rita Hazan, owner of Rita Hazan Salon in New York City.

Mask Skin Flaws

Sure, it's Halloween season, but your skin doesn't have to be scary. Prep your complexion for harsh winter weather by applying a mask—hydrating for dry skin, purifying for acne-prone, and calming for sensitive.

Winter Is the Best Time to . . .

Leave Nails Naked

A study in the *Journal of the American Academy of Dermatology* found that brittle nails were three times more common in women who used nail polish remover at least twice a month (acetone is the likely culprit). Dry, cold weather can also wreak havoc on your digits. So take some time off from polish, and moisturize your hands and nails every day.

Skip Shampoo

Minerals in tap water and detergents in shampoo can cause your winter-stressed scalp to itch and flake. One solution: Before bed, rub a dry shampoo into your roots to absorb the excess oil, then comb it out in the morning (bypassing the blow-dryer also means you'll get to hit snooze a few extra times).

Experiment with Fragrance

"Winter is the best time of year to find a deal on perfume," says Tania Sanchez, coauthor of *Perfumes: The Guide*. That's because cosmetics counters are crammed full of gift sets for the holidays, and the leftovers go on sale after the fat guy sings. Grab a marked-down fragrance and get a whiff of something you've been meaning to test-drive.

Stop Flaking

Your skin needs extra moisture during the cold, dry months. But the hydrators in lotions and creams can't do their job if there's a coat of dead, rough skin blocking your pores, explains Dr. Fusco. Send your flaky winter layers down the drain with a gentle body wash containing exfoliants like AHA or urea.

Drown Your Skin's Sorrows

Once you've exfoliated, follow these steps to keep your skin happy: Layer on a moisturizer with sunscreen in the morning, apply a thick night cream before hitting the sheets, and make a humidifier part of your bedroom decor.

Fight Fuzz

If you've been considering laser hair removal, now's the best time to do it. "The devices are designed to target the darker pigments in your hair," Dr. Fusco says. Now that your summer glow is gone, there's more contrast between your hair and skin, so the treatment will work better.

Forget Foundation

The heavier pigments and thick consistency of foundation tend to make it settle into dry areas on

If you get only one facial a year, do it in the fall—after a long summer in the sun.

your skin and give your complexion a patchy look that only brings attention to imperfections. Save time—and your skin—by using a tinted moisturizer instead. It will quench thirsty skin, and the hint of pigment will brighten your complexion.

Check Your Conditioner's Contents

Is your hair dry and static-y? Protein could be the guilty party. To find out for sure, check the label on your favorite conditioner; if the P-word is high on the ingredient list, alternate between it and a conditioner that contains lubricants such as panthenol, glycerine, or shea butter to keep your strands smooth. (Learn more about shampoo and conditioner on page 318.)

Go for the Bronze

Hey, pasty face, a quick swipe of a peachy bronzer will wake up your skin. When brushing on color, make a "3" shape on the right side of your face (a backwards "3" on the left), so the bronzer hits all the right places: your forehead, cheekbones, and jawline.

In Spring You Should . . .

Think about Wrinkles

Retinoids, which we introduced you to earlier in Chapter 4, are the gold standard of antiaging ingredients, but dry air or lots of sun exposure can make it difficult for your skin to tolerate these high-powered creams, says Ranella Hirsch, MD, past president of the American Society of Cosmetic Dermatology and Aesthetic Surgery. Translation: This is the perfect season to introduce them into your skin-care arsenal.

Get Rubbed the Right Way

After winter hibernation, your muscles are likely to be a bit creaky, says Holly Miller, concierge of Willow Stream Spa in Scottsdale, Arizona. "A sports massage will help work out the kinks that come from taking your body out of cold storage," Miller says. If you don't have the time—or the funds—for an hour, don't stress it: One study found that even a 15-minute rubdown brings physical benefits.

Play with New Products

Milder temps mean your skin is less likely to be sensitive—and it's not hot enough yet to sweat off anything new you try. So go ahead—this is the safest time to experiment with new moisturizers and foundations to see which suit your skin best.

Ditch Your Hair Dryer

Don't wait for tropical heat to hit to unplug your dryer or flat iron. Give your hair as much R&R as possible by letting it air-dry before the serious humidity settles in. You'll save your strands from damage and give your hair time to adapt to a new styling routine.

Up the Ante

Nicer weather and more daylight mean more sun exposure: Even if you try to protect your skin, it's still soaking up the ultraviolet (UV) rays. So increase your daily dose now.

Shed Some Skin

The increased humidity makes spring the ideal season for sloughing off dead layers of dry winter skin, Dr. Fusco says. Since you're less likely to be irritated, try a mild enzyme or AHA peel to reveal skin that's softer than a downy chick.

Become Sexier in Seconds

GO FROM FRAZZLED TO FABULOUS IN LESS THAN A MINUTE WITH THESE EXPERT TIME-SAVING TIPS

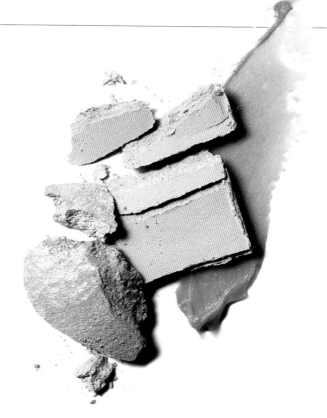

Ditch Under-Eye Bags

Surgery to lift your lids? Absolutely not! Just brush on a rich, satiny shade like topaz or amethyst, then blend into the crease. Dark colors create depth, distracting from bags (light, sparkly colors exaggerate the problem).

Play Up Your Lashes (without Looking Made-Up)

Use a skinny pencil to smudge between lashes. If you're going to use mascara, wrap a paper towel around the wand and give it a squeeze before swiping it over your lashes.

Take 10 Pounds Off Your Face

A sweep of a bronzer just below your cheekbones creates slimming definition.

Wake Up Your Eyes

Apply a dab of white shadow at the inner corners of your eyes.

Lash Out like a Pro

Bend the brush end of your mascara wand to a 45-degree angle. Using a tissue to keep your hand from getting inky, gently bend it toward the cap (it will still slide in and out of the tube). This will allow you to hit every lash without smearing your lids. Just don't apply mascara in the car. One of the most common eye injuries: corneal abrasions caused by mascara wands.

Amp Up Your Smile

No need to soak in peroxide: Just wear a coral lipstick with a pink tint. It flatters everyone.

Painlessly Plump Your Lips

Outline your mouth with a little concealer, and your lips will look full and defined. Or add a burst of dramatic color to make your lips look plumper. Lightly tap the color on with your finger and smooth out any unevenness with a clear gloss.

Polish Your Brows

All you need to look pulled together is to brush a bit of powder a shade lighter than your hair color through your brows. Another idea: Draw a thin line under your brows with a highlighting pencil to fake a brow grooming—your arches will look defined and lifted.

De-Puff a Party Face

To calm cranky skin, hold a bag of frozen peas to your face for 30 seconds. Make sure the peas are loose, so they conform to the shape of your face. They'll reduce swelling and redness all over.

Downplay Dark Circles

Play up something else instead—your mouth or your cheeks, for instance.

Secret Steps to Softer Lips

A 5–STEP GUIDE TO A KISSER
THAT FEELS FULLER AND LOOKS YOUNGER

You could have the skin of a goddess, the hair of an actress, and the looks of a supermodel. But when your lips start getting as dry and as cracked as the Mojave Desert, it's hard not to notice them. Use these simple shortcuts to keep them healthy and inviting.

Step 1: Prep

"The skin on your lips is very thin and contains less natural pigment, so it's more susceptible to sun damage and dryness," says Erin Welch, MD, a dermatologist at Denver Dermatology Consultants. Keep that smacker supple by locking in moisture as soon as you step out of the shower. Take a warm, moist washcloth and press it against your mouth for a full minute to saturate lips before the next step, exfoliation.

Step 2: Gently Exfoliate

Once a week, squeeze a pea-size amount of lip balm into your hand and combine it with an equal amount of granulated sugar. With a clean finger, scrub the mix onto your lips, using a circular motion, for 1 minute. "The sugar is therapeutic and removes dry skin, while the ointment protects and relieves pain associated with cracking," says Charles Zugerman, MD, associate professor of dermatology at Northwestern University's Feinberg School of Medicine in Chicago.

Step 3: Boost Moisture

To amp up hydration and lock in moisture at night, apply a lip salve containing shea butter or petroleum jelly. "These heavy emollients create a watertight seal on the lips' surface, protecting against moisture loss," Dr. Welch says.

Step 4: Apply Protection

The sun can fry your lips, especially if you wear light-attracting glosses. Experts suggest swiping on a balm with an SPF of 15 or higher every day. "Wearing adequate sun protection guards against cancer-causing ultraviolet B rays," Dr. Zugerman says. It also slows collagen loss and the development of vertical wrinkles and prevents scaliness.

Step 5: Smooth on Color

Since you're already wearing a barrier balm, you can use any lipstick you like. If your lipstick has a sunscreen, Dr. Zugerman says, you can skip Step 4 if you want. To make your color last, follow up by pressing a tissue over your lips and patting on translucent powder. A tiny amount of powder will filter through the tissue, sealing in the color.

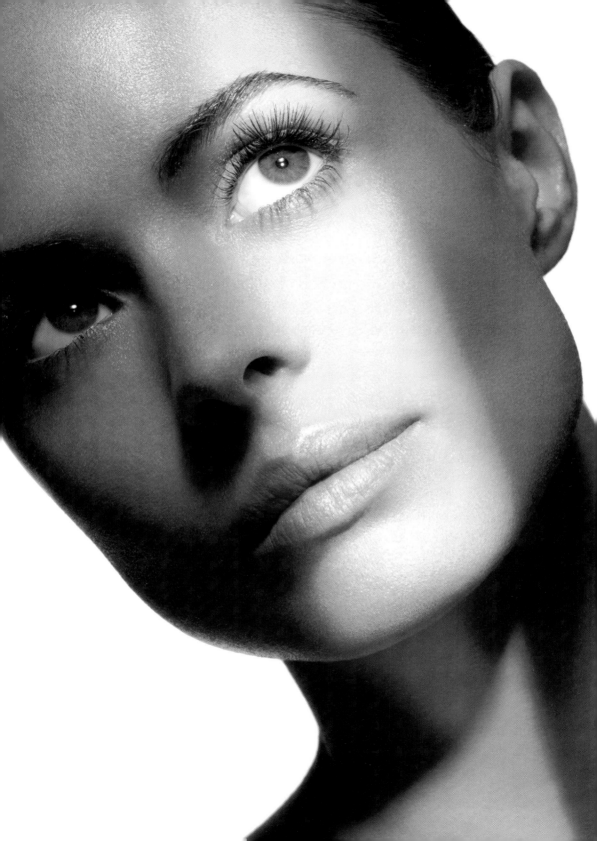

Part Two:
Lustrous Hair Starts Here

Your Hair's Most Important Ally

HOW OFTEN TO SHAMPOO? WHAT'S REALLY BEST FOR YOUR HAIR?
GET THE FACTS ON THIS AGE–OLD DEBATE.

At first glance, it looks like an unassuming three-story office building. But inside, there's some seriously cool stuff going on. Teams of chemists in white lab coats are hunched over electron microscopes, analyzing slides, and mixing mysterious cobalt-blue potions in Pyrex containers. No, they're not coming up with a cure for some exotic disease. All of this scientific activity, worthy of a Michael Crichton thriller, is about . . . clean hair.

Here at the Procter and Gamble (P&G) Sharon Woods Innovation Center, just outside Cincinnati, experts with degrees in microbiology, chemistry, and mechanical engineering create shampoos that'll rock your world. Want a mini-tour? There's the sensory department, where testers evaluate products in simulated bathrooms complete with sinks and mirrors; a testing lab where thousands of swatches of hair are washed, rinsed, dried, and stretched; hot and cold rooms, where technicians keep hair samples at precise temperatures and humidity levels to evaluate how they react; and a hair styling studio, where real women test products. And that's just one floor.

At P&G, one of the world's largest hair-care-product manufacturers and the maker of Aussie, Herbal Essences, Head and Shoulders, and Pantene, shampoo is serious business. It can take more than 2 years to develop a shampoo—worth it, considering that Americans spend more than $4 billion a year on the stuff. "There's more surface area to clean on your hair than on your skin," says Teca Gillespie, a beauty scientist at P&G. "The average woman has about 100,000 hairs on her head. That surface area can be as big as that of a queen-size bedsheet." So finding the right cleanser matters. A lot. "Shampoo is the most important factor in how good your hair looks," Gillespie says. "It's the foundation for everything else." Translation: You can slather on a shea-butter deep conditioner and shell out $250 for an ionic blow dryer, but if you're not using the right shampoo, you're screwed.

The good news is that shampoos are better than ever. The ones your mom used got hair clean, period. Composed of surfactants (soaps) made from animal fats and plant compounds, they left a residue, didn't lather well, and tended to be harsh. Today, women typically shampoo three times a week, and 63 percent have recently colored their hair. So today's formulas contain

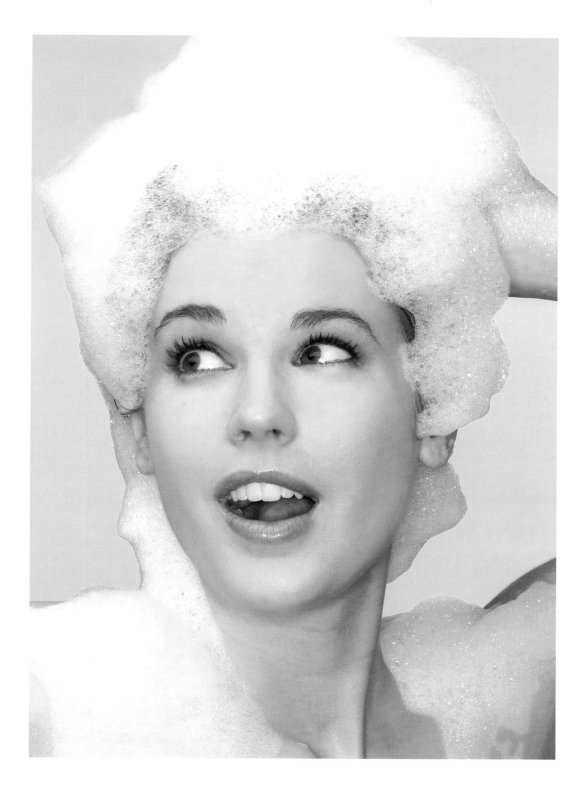

gentler synthetic surfactants, conditioning ingredients, and more. "Now it's all about a shampoo's perceived benefits—the fragrance, the lather, how it feels on your hair, the way it pours from the bottle," says Julia Youssef, vice president of L'Oréal USA's Technical Center. "It's a little like Starbucks. It's not just about coffee—it's the total experience."

But before you buy your next bottle, know this, says Mort Westman, a cosmetics chemist and president of Westman Associates in Oak Brook, Illinois: "There's a presumption that the more expensive a shampoo is, the better it is. Wrong. There's good and bad at all prices, so don't be impressed with labels—be impressed with what it does for your hair."

Myth versus Fact

Experts spill the dirty little secrets behind the most common shampoo "truths"

"You need lather to know it's really working."

MYTH. The more foam a shampoo produces, the cleaner your hair's getting, right? Not exactly. You may love working up a good head on your head, but those suds are mostly created for psychological effect (oooh, it's cleaning!). Foaming occurs when surfactant molecules in the shampoo mix with air and create tons of tiny bubbles. Ideally, your head should have only enough lather to lubricate the hair and scalp, so a quarter-size blob of shampoo will usually do the trick.

"You should use a clarifying formula to get rid of buildup."

PARTLY FACT. Unless you're using heavy-duty styling products, like pomade, mousse, or gel, regular shampooing prevents styling-product residue from collecting on your hair. If you do need a clarifier, don't use it more than once a week. These detergent-heavy cleansers, which do such a great job of removing buildup, will also do a great job of damaging the hair cuticle.

"Washing every day can be bad for your hair."

MOSTLY MYTH. "Daily washing is safe and healthy," says Mort Westman, the cosmetics chemist. If you have oily hair, it's fine to suds up every day—but even oily types should use a gentle formula (translation: one with moisturizing ingredients, like silicones, shea butter, or panthenol). People with coarse or dry hair might want to be more conservative and wash every other day, says L'Oréal's Youssef. No matter what kind of hair you have, as long as you stay away from harsh formulas that strip natural oils and treat your strands with conditioner, regular shampooing won't do any harm.

"For best results, follow with a conditioner."

FACT. No, this isn't a scam to sell you two products. Chemists can pack only so many ingredients into each bottle. And a shampoo can't clean properly and deposit enough conditioner to moisturize your locks. Using a separate conditioner will coat strands with ingredients that hydrate and protect. By the way, if your hair's super-oily, apply the thick stuff only from the ears to the ends.

"After a while, your hair gets used to your shampoo. That's why you need to switch to a new brand occasionally."

MYTH. "Hair is dead, period," says Westman, the cosmetics chemist. "So it can't 'get used to' anything. It's just your perception of how your hair responds to a new formula." So if you love your brand, there's no reason to switch.

Turn Up the Volume

A THICKER MANE WITH MINERALS

In the past few years, the popularity of mineral makeup has gone through the roof. Now hair-care companies are covering the same territory. In January 2009, L'Oréal launched its Professionnel Série Expert Volume Expand line. These shampoos and styling products use calcium to strengthen hair and silica to smooth cuticles. The result: volume and shine. "Depositing these minerals on hair increases each strand's diameter and 'adds space' between hair fibers," says Ni'Kita Wilson, a cosmetic chemist in Fairfield, New Jersey.

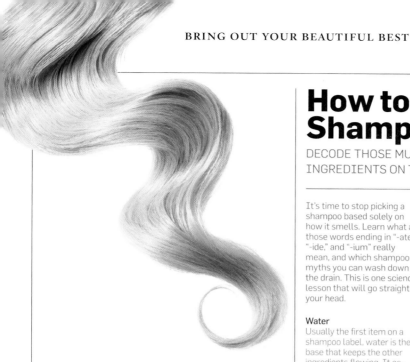

How to Speak Shampoo-ese

DECODE THOSE MULTISYLLABIC INGREDIENTS ON THE LABEL

It's time to stop picking a shampoo based solely on how it smells. Learn what all those words ending in "-ate," "-ide," and "-ium" really mean, and which shampoo myths you can wash down the drain. This is one science lesson that will go straight to your head.

Water
Usually the first item on a shampoo label, water is the base that keeps the other ingredients flowing. It accounts for up to 80 percent of what's in the bottle.

Ammonium Lauryl Sulfate/ Ammonium Laureth Sulfate/ Sodium Lauryl Sulfate
Surfactants is basically, a fancy word for detergents. These are the muscles that do all the cleaning.

Cocamide DEA, MEA, or TEA/ Cocamidopropyl Betaine
These milder foaming detergents are added to create suds. But they also moisturize and thicken the formula so the shampoo is easier to pour.

Sodium Citrate
Buffering agent that keeps the shampoo at the proper pH level (slightly acidic) as you wash, allowing dirt and oil to wash off and helping cuticles (the overlapping scales on each strand) lie flat so hair looks smooth and shiny.

Glycol Distearate/Stearate
These waxes are kind of like hunky Swedish masseurs: primarily there for look and feel. They're what give the formula a pearly sheen and allow it to flow easily from the bottle.

Polyquaternium/Quaternium
These softening compounds—also found in some fabric softeners—thicken shampoos and condition hair.

Dimethicone/Cyclomethicone
These silicone oils coat and smooth down the cuticles to add thickness, reduce static, and provide shine. They also make comb-outs easier. If you have coarse, curly, or damaged hair, make sure your shampoo contains one of these conditioning ingredients.

Panthenol
A form of vitamin B, this hardworking humectant (that's a substance that helps hair attract and retain moisture) works inside and out: It penetrates the hair cuticle to plump it up and coats it for added shine.

Cetyl/Oleyl/Stearyl Alcohol
Seeing the word "alcohol" may set off an alarm (drying = bad!). But these are hydrating alcohols that attach themselves to the outsides of the hair shafts and act as lubricants. Result: Combs effortlessly glide through hair.

Nut Oils/Shea Butter
These super-rich natural moisturizers, found in hydrating shampoos, coat cuticles so water stays locked inside.

Ascorbic Acid/Citric Acid
Natural acids derived from vitamin C, they smooth cuticles and add shine.

Octyl Salicylate/PABA
These sunscreens are added to protect your scalp and hair from chaos-causing UV rays—so your color lasts longer.

Head Games

WHY A SALON SHAMPOO FEELS SO FREAKIN' GOOD

As anyone who's ever experienced a thorough salon scrubbing knows, getting your hair shampooed can be an almost orgasmic experience. No big surprise there. After all, your scalp is an erogenous zone—a place supersensitive to touch—and just like your nipples or the nape of your neck, it's rarely handled by other people. "Hands-on scalp stimulation works the same way it does during a massage: by increasing bloodflow and releasing tension," says Amy Wechsler, MD, a New York dermatologist and psychiatrist.

But there's a scientific reason for the overwhelming pleasure response: As you're being rubbed the right way, the nerve endings in your scalp send information to the sensory cortex (the brain's "Goody!" center, which registers comfort and relaxation). In response, the sensory cortex lights up like a switchboard during an *American Idol* voting night and releases such feel-good hormones dopamine and serotonin, says neurosurgeon Larry McCleary, MD, author of *The Brain Trust Program*. Add to that the soothing stimulus of the hot water, and you've got one toe-curling experience.

Guarantee a Good Cut

FOLLOW THESE PRO TIPS AND WALK OUT OF THE SALON SMILING.

Find Mr. or Ms. Right

Step number one (no big surprise here) is finding a stylist. When you see a hairstyle you like—whether a friend's blunt cut or a layered 'do on a total stranger—ask who created it. Or do some detective work. Check out a salon's Web site to see samples of the handiwork. When you call for an appointment, ask if a stylist on staff specializes in your hair type. Some cutters are pros with curls, others at turning thin, baby-fine strands into lions' manes.

Case the Joint

Before you lock down an appointment, visit the salon to check out the vibe. Is it too chaotic (or low-key) for your taste? Are women leaving with Victoria Beckham cuts? Winehouse beehives? Overly shellacked beauty-pageant hair? If you don't like what you see, walk out. Quickly.

Schedule Smart

An early appointment is always best. Sure, a good stylist should always be on top of her game, but wouldn't you be less fresh if you'd just spent 7 hours on your feet? And ask how far apart appointments are spaced, says stylist Kevin Mancuso, creative director of Nexxus Salon Hair Care. Look for a salon that schedules clients at least 30 minutes apart—rather than stacked up like a clipping assembly line every 15 minutes.

Have "the Talk"

Any stylist worth her weight in mousse will do a consult to find out your styling routine and vision for the style before picking up the shears. And by all means, bring a photo of a hairstyle you like. Even if you don't love everything about the cut, a snap can offer insight on what you're after. Is it the layering around the face? Blunt bangs? "A picture is easy to translate," says Antonio Prieto, owner of New York's Antonio Prieto Salon. "Your vision of layers may be different from mine. A picture can clear that up."

Stare and Share

Sure, Brad and Angelina's kids are cute, but if your eyes are glued to that glossy instead of what's going on in the mirror, you could be in for a nasty surprise. Watch the cut as it progresses, and if you're unhappy at any point—even the first snip—speak up! Also, pay close attention to how your hair is being styled and what products are being used so you can achieve the look on your own.

Ask for a Re-Do

"There's nothing wrong with going back to your stylist if you decide after a few days that you hate the cut," says stylist George Ortiz. "In fact, most salons will fix the problem for free." Just be prepared to articulate exactly what you don't like.

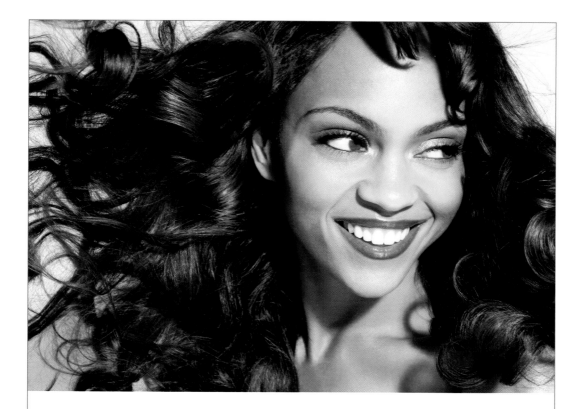

Banish Bad Hair Days

TRAUMATIZED TRESSES AREN'T PRETTY. HERE'S HOW TO NURSE EVEN THE MOST MANGLED MANES BACK TO HEALTH.

The Damage: Overprocessing
The Cause: Bleaching and dyeing strip natural pigments and create tears that make hair porous and weak.
The Remedy: Once a week, use a deep-conditioning protein treatment to coat the cuticle and fill in those hollow areas. Apply it evenly all over freshly shampooed hair, then twist your hair into a bun and sleep with a towel on your pillow. Then rinse your hair out in the morning.

The Damage: Fried Strands
The Cause: If your styling tools top 212°F, the water inside each hair will start to boil. As the moisture tries to escape, hair blisters and eventually breaks. (Read: Not good.)
The Remedy: Set styling tools to low, and use shampoo and conditioner that will hydrate your hair's most fragile spots (like the ends). Follow with stylers containing protective oils like glycerin. Spritz a bit on the top layers of your hair before using high-temp tools.

The Damage: Breakage
The Cause: The friction of brush bristles rubbing against the cuticle—the overlapping cells along the outer layer of your hair—tears the surface.
The Remedy: Keep the cuticle smooth and intact by coating damp or dry hair from the midshaft to the ends with a pea-size dab of serum that contains silicone (or search the ingredient list for words ending in "ethicone").

The Damage: Split Ends
The Cause: When the protective cuticle at the end of the hair shaft wears away, the tip frays; that crack then travels up the hair shaft.
The Remedy: The only way to cure split ends is with a trim every 6 to 8 weeks. For a temporary fix, apply a styling product to just the tips. Find one that has glycerin or hyaluronic acid—both bond the ends together.

The Damage: Chemical Chaos
The Cause: Perming and straightening change the structure of hair, making it weak, coarse, and brittle. The parched strands soak up moisture from the air, causing frizz.
The Remedy: Look for styling products that contain stearyl alcohol, a fatty alcohol that strengthens and softens hair. Run a quarter-size blob through damp hair, then blow-dry, or use it on dry hair to tame and style.

Be Your Own Colorist

USE THIS STEP-BY-STEP, MISTAKE-PROOF GUIDE TO PICK THE PERFECT SHADE AND APPLY IT LIKE A PRO.

By Jessica Matlin

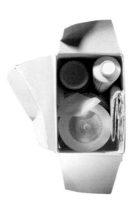

*T*here's nothing like a great dye job to turn back the clock. Hair color not only covers gray—it also boosts volume and shine, makes fine lines less noticeable, and brightens a dull complexion. But your technique should change over time. "What worked then might be aging you now," says colorist Kim Vo of the Mirage Las Vegas. To the rescue: new, definitive rules for do-it-yourself dyeing that can make you look and feel a decade younger—no salon required.

Think Inside the Box

Before you hit the hair-color aisle of your local drugstore, ask yourself: How much of a commit-

ment am I willing to make? Then, pick a formula based on your comfort level. Semipermanent dye is like a fling from your youth: It rinses away after about 10 shampoos, so you won't be left with any of those nasty telltale roots. Since semiperms don't use peroxide or ammonia, they can't lighten your hair or give you a drastic color transformation. They only deposit pigment, enhancing or adding depth to your current shade.

Want something a bit more serious? Go with demipermanent. It contains low levels of ammonia, so it will stay in your hair longer and fade out over about 25 washes. A demi can take you, at most, one shade lighter or two shades darker; it can also change your hair's tone—from, say, a

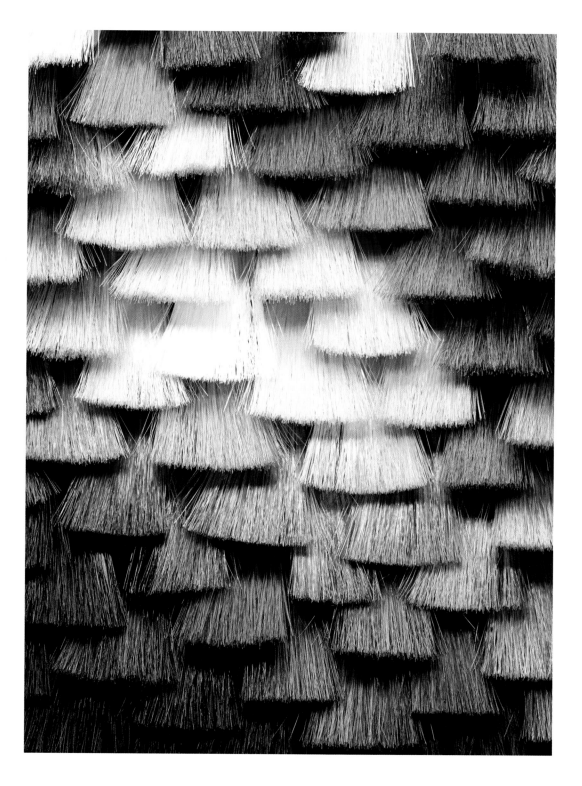

325

medium brown to a medium auburn.

If you're ready to commit to a serious color change, you want a permanent option. These dyes alter your shade with peroxide and ammonia, so the color will last until it gets cut or grows out. These formulas give you the most versatility in altering your color, letting you achieve more dramatic results.

Consider Your Undertones

Just like your skin, your hair's got them (they're either warm or cool), and the peroxide in hair color will expose them. "Brunettes tend to have warm undertones, which is why they're often surprised by how red their hair turns after coloring—especially when going lighter," says Lisa Evans, a colorist at Salon Mario Russo in Boston. If you're worried about your hair looking brassy, choose a cooler, ashier tone. Another trick for forecasting how your hair will react to hair color, according to Eva Scrivo, owner of Eva Scrivo Salon in New York City: Take a look at your grade-school pictures. If your hair was a warm, honey blonde in second grade, there's a good chance it'll go warmer when you color it now. And if you were a cooler, ash blonde or brunette, dying or bleaching will probably reveal those undertones. It's important to keep that in mind before you try out a new shade on your own.

Find the Right Hue

For the most youthful effect, lighten hair about two shades from your current natural color (for instance, from medium brown to light brown or dark blonde; dark blonde to medium or light blonde). "When in doubt, start lighter," says Rita Hazan, owner of Rita Hazan Salon in New York City. "If the shade isn't right, it's easier to go darker than lighter."

"Going lighter softens your face, so fine lines and age spots look less noticeable," adds Gary Howse, creative director of Seattle's Gary Manuel Salon. Besides being more flattering, it also minimizes the possibility of mistakes and avoids noticeable roots.

Choose a Multitonal Shade

The vibrancy of youthful hair comes from the subtle contrast of colors— a mix of highlights and lowlights against your base color. "Nothing is more aging and looks more unnatural than hair that's flat and all one color," says Brad Johns, Clairol's global color director.

To recreate this radiant effect, first use a multitonal dye. Both demi and permanent formulas of this type feature a combination of dye molecules that mimics the nuances of younger hair—dark strands will be deepened and grays washed into lighter glints. A tip-off that a dye delivers multidimensional color: The product name or description contains words such as "shimmering," "blended," or "tone-on-tone." To hide a smattering of silver, choose a demipermanent dye; if you're more than 40 percent gray, opt for a permanent color.

Next, add highlights. If you want more visible contrast than a multitonal dye delivers, frame your face with a few strategically placed highlights. Bonus: These winning streaks make eyes look brighter and give skin a healthy glow. "Go two to three shades lighter than the rest of your hair," says Mary Button, a colorist at Philadelphia's Adolf Biecker Salon. Opt for a warm shade to compensate for skin sallowness—look for words such as "golden," "honey," or "amber" in the product's name or description. Stick with hues that are close to your hair color; for example, brunettes, use light brown, not blonde, and redheads, use copper. Remember, less is more: Aim for about 10 quarter-inch streaks on each side, beginning about $1/8$ inch back from your face and spaced $1/2$ inch apart until just past your ears. Perfect your technique by "sketching" your pattern beforehand with conditioner, which has a consistency that's similar to that of hair color.

Go Deep, with Conditioner

You'd never slap a coat of paint on a cracked wall, so don't even think about applying color without conditioning. "If your hair is damaged, the pigment won't adhere well to your strands and it will end up looking streaky," says Nicolas Cornuot, spa director of Phyto Universe in New York City. "So at least 1 week before coloring, pamper your hair with a deep-conditioning treatment." Think of it as spackling holes before painting—you're creating an even surface for the color to attach to. Giving your strands a dose of intense hydration also helps protect them from the harsh chemicals used in coloring so you can avoid fried, crispy ends.

And don't shampoo for a day or two before you color. "Your hair's natural oils will protect your scalp and prevent irritation," says Nathaniel Hawkins, a hair stylist for Tresemmé. Don't worry about any styling products that are left in your hair—they won't affect the coloring process. If you do wash the day of, lather up with a gentle formula; strong detergents can irritate your scalp. Mix that with the chemicals in dye and you could end up with itching and burning.

Do Your Prep Work

Coloring your hair is kind of like baking a soufflé: If you don't pay careful attention to every step, you'll likely end up with a big, hot mess. "I often hear about women who dye their hair when they're exhausted, in a hurry, or have had a couple glasses of wine," Scrivo says. "That's when mistakes happen. Always, always concentrate and take your time."

Before you even rip open the box, "apply a thin layer of Vaseline along your hairline—from earlobe

The Right Makeup for Your Hair Color

YOU'VE TRIED ON MORE MAKEUP SHADES THAN SHOES BUT CAN NEVER SEEM TO FIND THAT PERFECT COLOR. THE TRICK: USE YOUR HAIR'S HUE AS A GUIDE TO PICKING YOUR PRETTIEST PALETTE.

"*Dark brown hair frames the face, creating a gorgeous canvas for bolder colors.*" —Petra Strand, makeup artist; creator, Pixi by Petra

Make it work for you: Those with lighter complexions can carry off shimmery oyster white shadow and strawberry-red lipstick.

"*Play up the mysterious, sexy vibe of black hair by accentuating just one feature with sultry color.*" —Jerrod Blandino, founder and creative director, Too Faced Cosmetics

Make it work for you: If you're raven-haired and have a darker complexion, keep a neutral palette: sand, honey, and caramel.

"*Since blonde hair surrounds your face with light, play up that golden glow with a touch of iridescence.*" —Brett Freedman, Los Angeles makeup artist; founder, Vanitymark Cosmetics

Make it work for you: If you're not a fair-skinned blonde, but medium- to olive-toned in complexion, then try sheer, rosy pinks on your eyes, cheeks, and lips.

"*Red hair naturally adds warmth to the complexion; colors that have a hint of brown or apricot enhance that without looking too bright.*" —Bobbi Brown, author of *Bobbi Brown Makeup Manual*

Make it work for you: A sheer coral lip color and a bronze eye shadow and blush will flatter redheads with warmer skin tones.

"*Soft shades of brown—from caramel to chestnut—are the furthest thing from severe; just about any color of makeup complements them.*" —Troy Surratt, New York City makeup artist

Make it work for you: If you're a brunette with a lighter complexion, golden apricots and rosy pinks will work better.

to earlobe and along your neckline—to prevent the dye from staining your skin," advises Harry Josh, celebrity colorist and a creative consultant for the John Frieda Collection.

Next, mist the ends of your hair with water. "Since the tips of your hair tend to be dry and damaged, they can soak up too much color," says Jason Backe, the color director for Clairol. "Some extra moisture will help color go on more evenly and prevent the ends from turning out darker than the roots."

Ready, Set, Color!

Pull out a comb and divide your hair into quadrants: Make one part down the middle and another from ear to ear, then clip each section securely in place. Apply the color one section at a time. "This is an organized approach to working with color that prevents any section of your hair from 'taking a holiday,' which is colorist-speak for 'you missed a spot,'" says Chuck Hezekiah, a color expert for Garnier Nutrisse. Apply color from the roots to the ends, working it through with gloved hands. As soon as you've applied color to the last strand, start the timer—most color takes about 20 minutes to develop.

If you're applying a shade close to your natural color to hide grays, deviate from your kit's instructions and instead concentrate on your roots. Younger hair is naturally lightest at the ends. To recreate this effect, apply dye to your roots, but not your ends. Then during the last 3 minutes of processing, splash water onto the crown of your head and then comb color through from top to bottom. "That shot of water dilutes the dye, creating a more natural-looking hue," says James Corbett, owner of James Corbett Studio in New York City. Rinse hair until the water runs clear. Then apply the kit's conditioning treatment, and rinse well.

Another tip: Because heat opens the hair's cuticle, warming an old towel in the dryer and wrapping it around your head after applying the dye allows the formula to soak into the hair shaft.

After dying, hold off on shampooing for 3 days. "This will give the cuticles—which open during the coloring process—time to close and seal in the color molecules," Scrivo says. And watch the water temperature when you wash: "Hot water can cause cuticles to expand and open, allowing some of the color to escape. The cooler the rinse, the better," says David Stanko, a color consultant for Redken.

Keep Your Color Longer

For extra shine, try a gloss. There's now a host of at-home glosses (once available only at salons), including tinted formulas that help intensify a fading shade. "They contain silicones that coat and smooth the cuticle, allowing light to reflect evenly," says Vo. Use monthly to maintain shine and vibrancy.

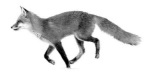

The Gorgeous Way to Go Gray

Wash that gray out of your hair? More and more women are saying "No way!" According to L'Oréal, nearly half of women over age 40 are no longer hitting the bottle. Besides being profoundly liberating (no more pesky roots!), going gray makes a statement of supreme confidence: *This is who I am, and I'm proud of my natural beauty*. It can also look pretty darn fabulous: Think Meryl Streep's chic silver cut in *The Devil Wears Prada*, Jamie Lee Curtis's stylish silver pixie, or Emmylou Harris's stunning silver mane. Still, if you want to give gray a try, you'll need to know how to avoid the awkward growing-in stage that occurs when you stop dyeing your hair. The mere thought of clashing incoming and outgoing tones keeps many women from returning to their roots. Follow these steps to look terrific every minute of the way to gray.

Step 1:
Go Gradually

Wait until your roots are at least 60 percent silver before giving up your dye job, so your new hue will look symmetrical and natural as it grows in, suggests colorist Jennifer Jahanbigloo, owner of Juan Juan Salons in Beverly Hills, California. But don't give up color altogether just yet. "The contrast in texture and tone as your hair grows can look unkempt," she notes. During this phase, which can last up to a year, get a do-it-yourself highlighting kit or ask your colorist to weave in a few fine highlights or lowlights (darker streaks) to add dimension and blend in roots.

Step 2:
Consider a New Cut

Cropping your hair above your collarbone during the in-between period will lessen the contrast between silver and pigmented strands. Layers can also help camouflage multiple hues. "A choppy cut looks youthful and helps hide your roots," says Jonathan Gale, a colorist at the John Frieda Salon in Los Angeles. When your gray has grown out, don't regress to a matronly 'do. "For gray to look glamorous and chic, your cut should be contemporary," says Mark DeVincenzo, creative director at the Frédéric Fekkai Salon in New York City. Silver strands absorb light, making your mane look dull, so style your hair straight (use a flatiron or a dryer and a round brush) to promote shine. Once your hair is completely white, talk to your stylist about adopting an above-the-shoulder, layered style that provides movement and softly frames your face.

Step 3:
Pick Silver-Specific Products

When hair turns gray, the protective cuticle thins out, which can make strands coarse and prone to breakage. Keep tresses soft and healthy by doing the following:

• Choose a moisturizing shampoo to soften and smooth hair and make it appear more lustrous.

• Wash hair with a formula geared for gray once a week to counteract yellowing caused by sun, pollutants, hard water, and smoke. But don't overdo it: Many of these products contain a blue tint that can cause a purplish cast.

• Apply a clear gloss or glaze monthly to coat the cuticle and boost shine.

• Opt for gels and mousses that are clear: The dyes in colored stylers can tarnish gray hair.

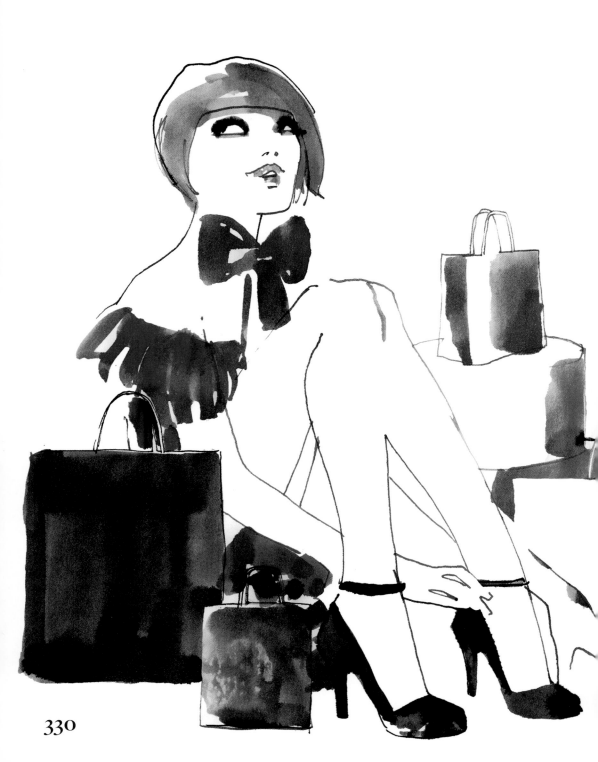

Part Three:
Dress Your Best

How Shopping Can Save Your Life

A QUICK TRIP TO THE MALL COULD GIVE YOUR BRAIN,
YOUR HEALTH, AND EVEN YOUR RELATIONSHIPS A BOOST.
YOU DON'T EVEN HAVE TO BUY ANYTHING!

By Dan Tynan

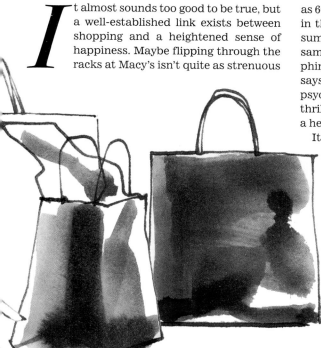

It almost sounds too good to be true, but a well-established link exists between shopping and a heightened sense of happiness. Maybe flipping through the racks at Macy's isn't quite as strenuous as 60 minutes on the treadmill or as fun as a romp in the sack with your significant other, but assuming you enjoy it, shopping will give you the same kind of high by releasing a flood of endorphins—the feel-good chemicals in your brain, says Nancy Irwin, PsyD, a Los Angeles–based psychotherapist. "Shopping can be extremely thrilling," she says. "It's a peak experience to get a hell of a deal."

It may not sound like news to you, but at last, there's scientific proof: In a paper published in 2007, researchers at West London's Brunel University noted that shopping is associated with increased activity in the left prefrontal cortex, a part of the brain that has been linked to pleasure and positive thinking. In fact, levels of dopamine, a neurotransmitter released during pleasurable experiences like sex, can rise sharply even when you're merely window-shopping. In another study, published in the journal *Neuron*, researchers at MIT, Carnegie Mellon, and Stanford strapped volunteers to a

331

If ever there were welcome news, experts think that shopping may even help us maintain our mental acuity in old age.

functional magnetic resonance imaging (fMRI) machine and showed them photos of products. When shoppers saw something they wanted to buy, a flood of dopamine to the nucleus accumbens—the brain's reward center—lit up their fMRI images like a dashboard. (The downside: When the charge for those Frye boots shows up on your credit-card statement, that dopamine is nowhere to be found. Sneaky.)

Luckily—for your brain, not your bank account—science has discovered a way to sidestep buyer's remorse: Imagine yourself enjoying your purchase a decade from now. Anat Keinan, PhD, an assistant professor at the Harvard Business School, and Ran Kivetz, PhD, a professor of marketing at Columbia Business School, gave 57 shoppers a hypothetical scenario: Choose between an expensive article of clothing they loved and a cheaper, less desirable version of the same thing. Then the researchers randomly divided the shoppers into two groups and asked one group to guess how much they thought they would regret their choice the next day and the other group how much they thought they would regret their choice in 10 years. Shoppers in the 10-year group were much more likely to be disappointed that they'd chosen a cost-cutting option; when they were later turned loose in an actual mall, they were more likely to purchase expensive, nonessential items. In their findings, published in the December 2008 issue of the *Journal of Marketing Research*, Dr. Keinan and Dr. Kivetz concluded that thinking about short-term regret drives consumers to be virtuous, while thinking about long-term regret leads them to be extravagant.

Whether that information makes you fear for your financial ruin or lunge for your American

32.1
Percentage that using self-checkout lines lowers impulse buys among women

Express Gold card, Paul Zak, PhD, director of the Center for Neuroeconomics Studies at Claremont Graduate University in California, is sure about one thing: Shopping is good for all humanity. Take a typical exchange between sales-person and customer: When you buy a dress, you're psyched because you have a new outfit. But the saleswoman is psyched too, because she just scored a commission. You help her, and she helps you. The positive effects continue to pile up, often unintentionally, even after your purchase. Thanks to your newly elevated mood, you might smile at a stranger on the bus or offer to make dinner for your guy when you get home, passing along residual happiness. Everybody wins.

And it's not only about pleasure. Shopping may even help women maintain their mental acuity in old age, says Guy McKhann, MD, a professor of neurology at Johns Hopkins University in Baltimore and a coauthor of *Keep Your Brain Young*. "People who are doing really well as they get older tend to be mentally engaged, physically active, and socially involved," he says. "And women are all of those things when they shop." Meanwhile, if he's back on the couch, Grandpa scores none of the above.

Coed Browsing

So if shopping is so good for you, why do most men in a store look like they want to curl up next to the checkout counter and die? Not surprisingly, shopping can affect men and women differently, say S. Christian Wheeler, PhD, of Stanford University, and Jonah Berger, PhD, of the University of Pennsylvania in Philadelphia. In a study published in the *Journal of Consumer Research*, the two marketing professors asked men and women to think about

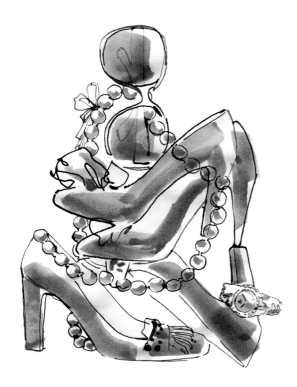

store and he can shop for hours while his wife slowly slips into a coma.

The solution for couples who dread shopping together isn't very complicated, Dr. Lefton says. Just ditch the idea that you have to stay side by side as you browse. "I've been married for 39 years. When my wife and I go to the mall, we split up. I don't have to go shoe shopping, and she doesn't have to come to the Apple store. We meet up for lunch." As long as you're both looking for stuff you love, coed shopping excursions will help keep you—and your relationship—going strong.

Less Is More

Why can shopping sometimes feel so stressful? It's not just the relentless crowds, sparse parking, and cheesy music. If you ask psychologist Barry Schwartz, PhD, author of *The Paradox of Choice: Why More Is Less*, it's all about options: We have too many.

Being Picky Doesn't Pay
"When people have too much to choose from, some will be less satisfied with their choices," Dr. Schwartz says. "It's easy to think about the opportunities they rejected." Researchers have dubbed those people "maximizers." They've found that it's really the "satisfiers"—those who aim for just good enough—who are happiest with their purchases.

Save Your Brain Waves
Indecisiveness strains the brain, says economist Paul Zak, PhD, of Claremont Graduate University in California: "You have a limited amount of mental energy, and your brain wants to conserve it." For every pair of boots you try on, your gray matter works hard to picture your owning them (and strutting by a catty co-worker in them). Now multiply that fantasy process by 12.

The Fewer, the Better
The secret to Zen shopping, then, is to limit yourself from the get-go. Consider skipping the gargantuan stores and head to smaller ones instead. Take only a few items into the dressing room. And meditate on the fact that "good enough" really is.

clothes shopping and then plot a trip on a map. Men tended to map the most direct driving route possible (as in "Get me the hell out of here, pronto"). Women were more likely to take the scenic route. The scientists' explanation: Many men tend to shop for specific items and only when they are needed, whereas women generally browse to see what's out there. (Interestingly, when subjects weren't asked to think about shopping beforehand, the researchers found the opposite trend: Women went direct, while men meandered.)

That doesn't mean that shopping is any less beneficial for men, says Lester Lefton, PhD, formerly a professor of experimental psychology at Kent State University in Ohio. It's not shopping per se that men dislike—it's shopping for things that hold no interest for them, says Dr. Lefton, who admits that he has been buying the same shoes (size 12EEE Byrons from Allen Edmonds) for more than 30 years. But bring him into a nicely stocked hardware or electronics

10 Style Mistakes That Instantly Age You

HERE'S A CHEAT SHEET OF WHAT YOU SHOULD NEVER WEAR— AS WELL AS A FEW INGENIOUS AGE–ERASING FASHION SECRETS.

It happens to the best of us: Somewhere in our thirties or forties we let our sense of style slip, even if ever so slightly. The pressures of work and family, the time crunch, the changes to our bodies— they all conspire against us, and sometimes we take the easy way out, stop updating our look, and just reach for the same old stuff. But just because you're getting older, you don't have to look the part. Here's a collection of decisions that will instantly add years to your appearance. Avoid them at all costs.

Instant Ager #1: A Kitchen-Sink Purse
No matter how much you love your giant piece of arm candy, eventually you're going to feel the effects of the relationship in your neck and shoulders. That's because the trapezius (the muscle that connects the shoulder to the neck) and levator scapulae (which elevates the shoulder blade) fatigue in the effort to support your bag. The muscles begin to tear, and headaches may even develop. "Heavy purses pull the muscles that go up to the base of your skull," says Karen Erickson, DC, a New York City chiropractor. Fast-forward 5 to 10 years and you've got shoulder numbness and tingling from pinched nerves, back pain, and arthritis of the neck— and then you're forced to wear a fanny pack, the

worst fashion sin of all. Sort through your mess, separate the essentials from the junk, and keep your bag as light as possible.

Instant Ager #2: Bad Sunglasses
Large "wraparound" lenses, while popular with the younger crowd, probably won't help you fit in with them. Always keep your sunglasses in proportion to your face by selecting frames that complement your face's shape (see page 74 for examples). A smaller face with small features, for instance, will appear overwhelmed when paired with enormous sunglasses. But don't go for beady Yoko Ono lenses, either; lenses that cover the corners of your eyes can help prevent crow's feet. If in doubt, stick with one of the three traditional frames: cat-eyes, aviators, or wayfarers, which were popularized by Audrey Hepburn in *Breakfast at Tiffany's*. Other eyewear taboos: wearing either transition lenses or clip-ons. Do yourself a favor and invest in prescription sunglasses instead.

Instant Ager #3: An Ill-Fitting Bra
It's a statistic you've no doubt heard before: Some 80 percent of women are wearing the wrong bra size. Your tried and true bra of your twenties most certainly will not be the go-to of your thirties and forties—your breasts will change and

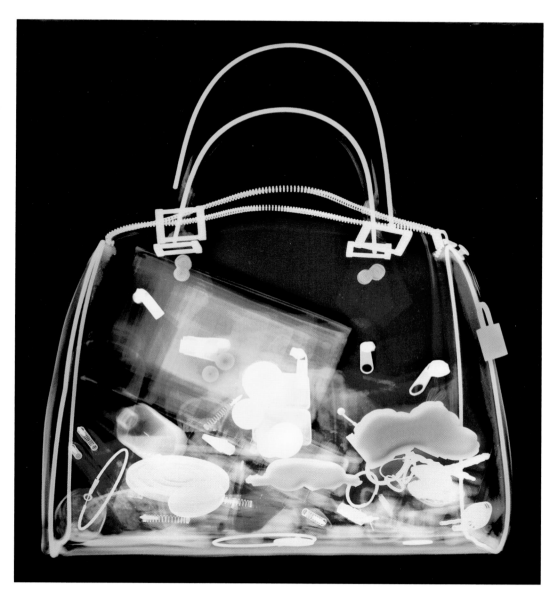

you'll likely need something larger with more underwire support. Schedule a professional bra fitting at least once a decade. When you find a model that lifts and separates to your liking, double (or triple) down. It's great to feel perky.

Instant Ager #4: A Bulge in Front

Be aware of changes in your body. If you have a bit of a stomach, whether from having a baby—congratulations!—or just being away from the gym too long—and, hey, it happens to the best of us—never stretch denim over it. The ensuing bulge this fashion sin creates is probably popular at your local Applebee's, and therein lies the problem. Don't go there. Simply opt for a midrise cut instead.

335

Instant Ager #5: A Bulge in Back

If someday you discover that you've developed a large pear-shaped bottom, look for jeans with pockets that are as far apart as possible—the closer they are, the larger your butt will look. You'll also need to say no to the no-pocket look, which makes your butt look much larger than it actually is. Same rule applies for the slip pocket, a pouch without any external stitching. Denim gives your behind shape, but you need to "break up" the fabric's monotony in order to make your butt look less daunting.

Instant Ager #6: Crop Tops

These are sexy, right? Wrong! Unless you're wearing a swimsuit at the beach, nobody but your lover should see your tummy. Fortunately most designers are cutting their tees at longer lengths. The style to look for is called "tunic," which extends all the way through your torso and helps elongate your body. Plus you can tuck it in and layer with it, something you simply can't do when you're showing the world your belly button.

Instant Ager #7: Shapeless Garments

Muumuus flatter no one, not even the Hawaiians who invented them. But if your goal is to cover up, rein in all that material with a belt. Or opt for empire dresses—with waistlines that hit directly below the bust—which have a slimming effect and help your legs look longer.

Instant Ager #8: Visors

Wearing a visor automatically makes you look like an AARP member and spend the majority of the day on an Arizona golf course. These "half hats" do not serve any fashion purpose whatsoever.

Instant Ager #9: Over-Accessorizing

Having a nice jewelry collection is great . . . so long as you don't wear it all at once. Wearing a chunky ring, an eye-catching necklace, long earrings, and oversized bangles simultaneously will overpower the eye. Pick a focal point and let it flatter. The best way to do that is to take a look in the mirror on your way out the door and remove one accessory.

Instant Ager #10: Sweats

Wear them at home, just not in public.

10 Instant Age Erasers

1. Lightweight, oversize scarves can conceal your décolletage, hiding sun damage and chest wrinkles.

2. Leather jackets, especially bombers, lend a flirty, adventurous air.

3. Cinching belts add shape and help carve out a waist.

4. If you wear shoes that match your skin color when you're dressed in a skirt, you'll create the illusion of having longer legs, which slims your entire body.

5. Bangs hide trouble areas like your forehead, where fine lines will begin appearing as early as your thirties. Similarly, layered bangs (meaning they're longer on the sides) disguise eye wrinkles.

6. Ballet flats, with their low-profile soles, round toe boxes, and little bows, provide a girlish quality. The inspiration for most designs is Capezio, maker of the original ballet slipper.

7. Skinny jeans hug your hips and ankles, but not everyone can pull them off. Boot-cut and slim-fitting jeans are the most flattering styles.

8. Lip gloss creates an illusion of fuller, smoother puckers.

9. Cream-based blushes and eye shadows as well as tinted moisturizers give your skin a youthful, dewy glow, as opposed to a powder foundation, which gets into your creases and leaves you looking caked and stale.

10. Heels add immediate sex appeal, as will harnessing a swing. "Here's a trick Marilyn Monroe used," says Camilla Morton, author of *A Year in High Heels*. "She had a half inch cut off of just one of her heels. The slight imbalance gave her hips a natural wiggle." No need to be so extreme—just have a cobbler shave a few millimeters off the tip of one heel to give your inner goddess a kick start.

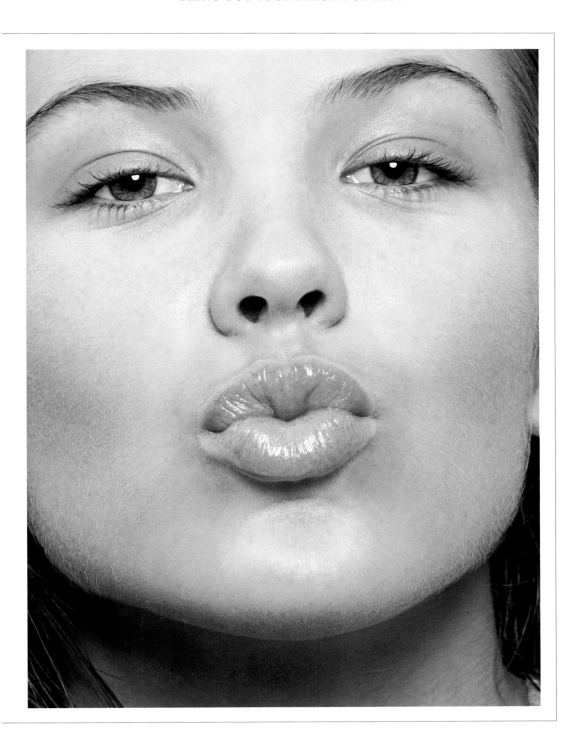

Find Your Perfect Swimsuit

THE LAST THING YOU WANT ON YOUR MIND
AT THE BEACH IS YOUR BODY. SURE, WE ALL HAVE A "PROBLEM
AREA" OR TWO—BUT THESE SOLUTIONS
WILL HELP YOU WORK WITH WHAT YOU'VE GOT.

L et's get real. You don't hate your figure, but balancing a top-heavy build with a slender waist and wide hips can still be a challenge. So match your body type with our advice on how to hide the bumps and complement the curves. You'll be a show-off in no time.

Big Tops

Balance out a top-heavy body by drawing attention away from the twins. Forget the myth that a thick-strapped, racerback tank is the only solution for keeping them in line. But unless your generous chest is also unnaturally perky, support is your first priority. Find it with wide straps and underwire construction, both of which come in bikini and one-piece styles. High tank-style necklines are the ultimate minimizers, but you can also pull off a strapless or bandeau top if it has wide side stays. (Try this test: Wiggle! The top shouldn't scrunch or slide down at all.) Low-slung bikini bottoms pull the eye down and look great with a full-coverage tankini (hooray for mix-and-match separates). All-over patterns play down your busty proportions, while halter tops not only distract by making shoulders appear sexy, but provide gravity-defying support with their upward pull. Embrace your inner Marilyn with a sexy, '40s-style halter—or try a cinched sweetheart neckline that highlights cleavage without neglecting support.

Booty Bounties

Minimize your oversized load with suits that slim your backside and hips, and highlight what's on top. To bring a bottom-heavy body

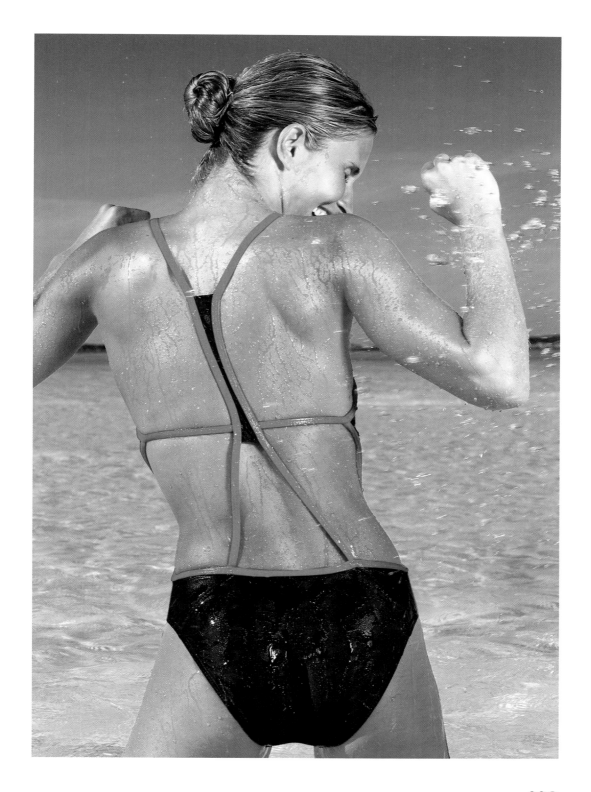

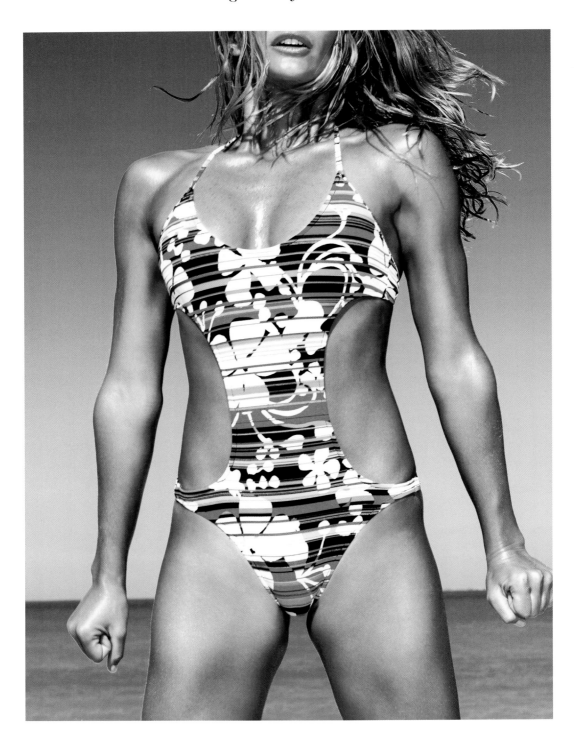

into proportion, choose a top with an interesting neckline or unusual bust detailing—beading, fringe, a bright flower appliqué—to keep eyes front and center. (One peek at you in a deep, plunging V-neck, and no one will even notice what lies beneath.) Save the bold prints and crazy colors for up top and stick with dark solids down south. Avoid hip-huggers and string bikinis, both of which hit at—and therefore highlight—your widest part. And please: Don't be fooled by skirted bottoms, which can leave you looking like an overstuffed couch slip covered in yards of fabric from behind. Instead, choose a cut that covers most—but not all—of your backside for the most flattering profile. High-cut legs elongate your gams and call attention to a trim waist, especially in a revealing bikini.

Middle Management

Create the illusion of a magnificent middle in styles that strike the perfect balance between conceal and reveal. For the 98 percent of us with not-so-fab abs, there's the tankini—strapless or halter styles play up an amazing upper half while covering trouble spots.

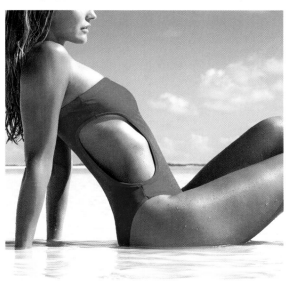

Pair either one with boy-style briefs for a combo that gives you maximum coverage and still allows a sexy sliver of skin to peek through (perfect for moms-to-be too). One-piece suits with shirring at the waist or princess seams work like corsets to create an hourglass shape; diagonal stripes or detailing do the same trick visually. Patterns and horizontal stripes are a notice-me no-no. Ruching, however, conceals and slenderizes your midriff to help you cover up that postbrunch bulge. Another can't-miss: a sexy, solid number in rich, dark chocolate, navy, or black. It's timeless, durable, and hides all evidence of the last time you satisfied your cravings.

Hourglass Honeys

Move the focus above your hips with a plunging neckline. This visually distributes the rest of your weight. The goal here is to create a sense of balance between your top and bottom, so stay away from belts and sporadic patterns. If anyone can sport an allover print, it's you.

Boyish Builds and Bitty Boobies

Reshape a boyish silhouette in suits that play up (and add inches to) your assets. If you're shaped like the wrong timepiece—grandfather clock instead of hourglass—first rejoice that you're not a sundial, then choose a one-piece with side cutouts. They visually nip in your waist and give you a look that's not so straight-up-and-down. Pair them with V-cut bottoms to create even more curvy illusions. Up top, horizontal stripes are an A-cup's best friend—they create the illusion of width. Underwire bikinis lift and separate. Likewise, a little padding can take your cleavage from boylike to bouncy in an instant. (For extra va-va-voom, gel inserts slide into padding pockets to replace, not supplement, the fabric freebies already in the suit. If padding makes you nervous, strategically placed ruffles work the same magic.) Light colors amplify, as do suits with a metallic sheen, so find separates in these fabrics to make your desired body parts pop. And since bikinis cause visual breaks, choose tube tops with molded cups and low-rise bottoms to maximize the distance between color blocks.

341

A Woman's Guide to Denim

AVOID DRESSING ROOM DRAMA BY TAKING THESE FACTORS INTO CONSIDERATION BEFORE YOU HEAD IN TO TRY ON.

*T*he right pair of jeans feels just like an old friend. Comfortable and comforting, they bring out your greatest assets and forgive the occasional flaw (no, your legs do not look too short; no, you do not have a gut; and no, your butt absolutely does not look big). And with a wide range of styles and lengths that flatter all different kinds of figures, "jeans aren't one-size-fits-all anymore," says Danielle de Marne of the boutique Scoop NYC. All of these options, she says, assure you a better fit becuase "the overall package is better." In the interest of making your overall package look better, consider this a denim directory. It'll cut through the confusion and help you find the jeans that work best for your butt, belly, legs, and height. After all, what are friends for?

Pockets

We all know back pockets have a practical purpose (stashing cash and your grocery list). But they can also create an illusion of lift, form, or fullness that flatters your shape. For better or worse, pockets can virtually rebuild your butt, so here's how to choose wisely.

Pleated

"Angled pockets make your tush look smaller and higher," says Scoop NYC's de Marne. The stitching gives slight shape to the jeans even when they're off, so it adds that much more dimension to a flat butt when they're on you.

Drop Yoke

Back pockets don't need to be on your backside—flat ones are most flattering sewn lower. "When the top hits in the middle of your bum, it makes your butt look lifted and fit," de Marne says. The pocket hugs your butt's underside for a perkier-looking back porch.

Embellished

"If your butt is flat, a pocket with embroidery is a good choice," says Paige Adams-Geller, longtime denim-fit model and founder of Paige Premium Denim. By adding a focal point and decorative texture, the stitching gives the illusion of shape.

Flap Patch

There's a reason flap pockets are so closely associated with Eva Longoria: "They look good

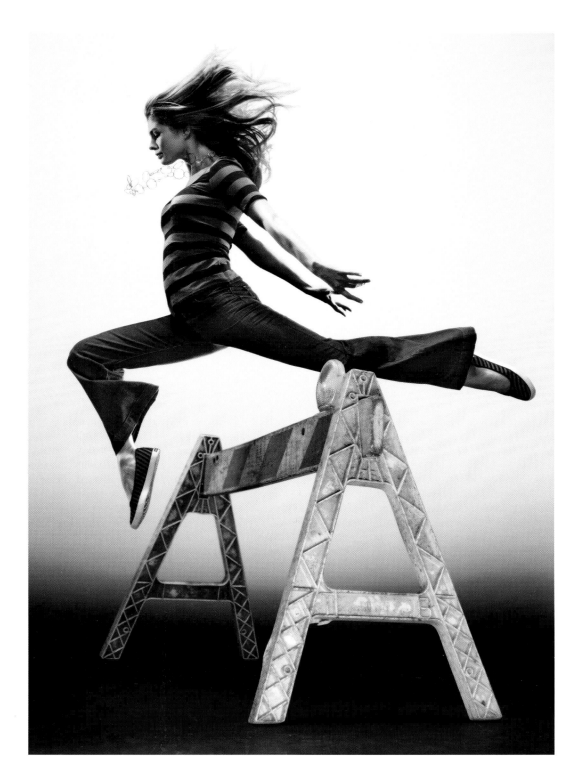

343

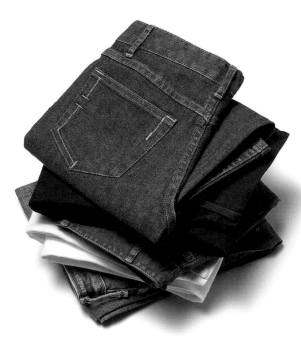

if you have a perfect butt," says Adams-Geller. And if you're not a member of that camp? Since they're bulkier than patch pockets, flaps give shape to a less-round derriere.

Rise

Sometimes a bikini wax isn't just for bikinis. That's how low some rises, or the distance from crotch to waistline, have become. Don't want to go that low? Then there's a higher rise for you. It all depends on your butt, your belly—and your comfort level.

Super Low

Flat abs get full attention here. Adams-Geller recommends this rise for petites, because the short zipper looks appropriate. Super-lows also help on bloated-belly days (with a long, loose top)—the waistline hits below your pooch.

Low

Jodi McMillen, owner of the online boutique Blaec.com, says this split-the-difference rise is "easiest to wear, most comfortable, and good for bigger behinds." Why? The waist hits low in the back, making the butt appear compact.

Classic Waist

Women, sick of peekaboo thongs, are returning to higher rises. The classic waist is good for obscuring a belly, McMillen says, and the longer zipper is appropriate for taller women.

Cut

In the same way that pockets can improve the look of your butt, the cut and hem of your jeans make the most of your height and the length of your legs—even if you come up a little short in either category. Not that there's anything wrong with that.

Cropped

"[Almost] anyone can get away with the crop, unless you're short. Then they can look like floods," Adams-Geller says. (If you're petite, you can rehem your pants so they hit in the middle of the calf.) They're fun with flip-flops and sexy with boots or high-heeled sandals, McMillen says, but they look too childish when worn with sneakers.

Straight Leg

After years of boot-cut domination, this cut is again a denim designer's favorite. Adams-Geller recommends it for women with boyish figures. She also likes it for women with a bit of a belly and thin legs, since it draws attention downward. Straight legs look best with the lift of high-heeled boots or stilettos, which make your legs look even longer.

Boot Cut

Jeans with this cut give you two major things every woman wants: thinner hips and longer legs. The slight flare at the ankle offsets width at the hips, and that same flare draws attention down the leg, thereby creating the appearance of more length. "They're good for everybody, every shoe, dressed up or dressed down," McMillen says.

Flare

Flared jeans do boot-cut one better, with the extra width at the bottom offsetting wider hips up top. But the broad ankle opening and taper of the leg can look disproportional (especially when hemmed) on short or long-torsoed women, so flares work best for tall or long-legged types.

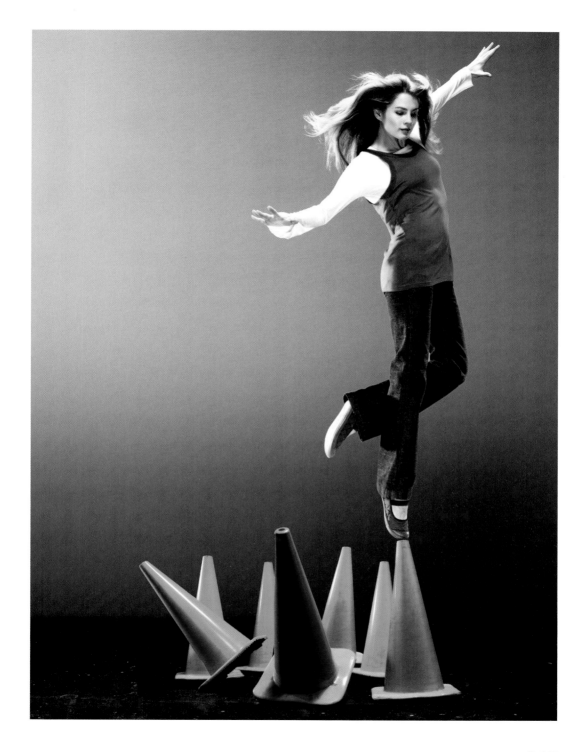

Age Erasers

Credits

Photographs

Akos: pages 311, 323
American Images Inc. / Getty
  Images: page 173
James Archer: page 268
Claire Artman/ Corbis: page 83
Ondrea Barbe: pages 59, 199, 201,
  202, 205, 213, 305, 313
Randi Berez: pages 5, 265
Beth Bischoff: pages 136, 138–139,
  247, 250–251, 252–253, 254–255
Darren Braun: pages 162, 165, 166
Greg Broom: page 119
Levi Brown: pages 260, 324, 325,
  326, 328
Bryan Christie: page 125
Jamie Chung: page 21
Craig Cutler: page 293
Bill Diodato: pages 67, 69
Emely / Veer: page 159
Darryl Estrine: pages 207, 209
Dennis Galante/ Corbis: page 108
Sally Gall: pages 145, 147–148
Steve Granitz/ Getty Images:
  page 75
Nicolai Grosell: pages 11, 17, 257
Claude Guillaumin/ Getty Images:
  page 337
Brian Hagiwara/ Getty Images:
  page 173
Philippe Halsman/ Magnum Photos
  (Marilyn Monroe): page viii
Spencer Heyfron: pages 187–188,
  193–194
Todd Huffman: page 259
D. Hurst / Alamy: page 158
Image Source Black / Alamy:
  page 175

iStock: pages 143, 171, 173, 261, 289
Matt Jones/ Trunk Archive: pages
  98–99
Christophe Jouany: page 157
Kasiam / iStock: page 63
Elizabeth Knox/ Getty Images:
  page 72
John Kuczala: page 191
David Lawrence: pages 151, 153
Pascal Le Segretain/ Getty Images:
  page 175
Robert Llewellyn/ Corbis: page 3
Nicola Majocchi: pages 131–132, 135
Mitch Mandel: pages 297, 299
Masterfile: pages 112, 160, 279
Chayo Mata: pages 231, 233–234
Josh McKible: page 223
Andrew McLeod: page 77
mgkaya / iStock: page 74
David Muir / Masterfile: page 97
Michael Muller: pages 225, 239,
  340–341
Taghi Naderzad: page 15
Nicographer / Getty Images: page 329
Nuts / Getty Images: page 319
Sonja Pacho / Corbis: page 169
Arne Pastoor / Getty Images:
  page 291
Plamen Petkov: pages 217–218
Trinette Reed / Getty Images:
  page 285
Christa Renee: page 61
Nicholas Rigg / Getty Images:
  page 36
Christopher Robbins / Getty
  Images: page 111
Rubberball Productions: page 105

Nick Ruechel: pages 177, 179, 181
Philippe Salomon: page 317
Anchles Schmitt: pages 43–45, 48–49,
  53–54, 126–129, 220–221, 226–227
Gregor Schuster / Getty Image:
  page 287
Carlos Serrao: pages 55, 245–246,
  249, 343, 345
John Shearer / Getty Images: page 75
Lisa Shin: pages 307, 309, 312–313,
  321, 344
Chris Shipman: pages 41, 46–47, 123,
  137, 222, 237
Steven Simko: pages 239, 241–242
Sara Singh: pages 330–331, 333
SMC / Getty Images: page 335
Lisa Spindler / Veer: page 87
Jordan Strauss / Getty Images:
  page 74
Kevin Summers: page 173
TMG / Getty Images: page 85
Dimitri Vervitsiotis / Getty Images:
  page 185
Vistalux: pages 267, 273
Mark Watkinson: page 224
Nathaniel Welch: pages 281–283
Ansgar Werrelmann,/ Corbis: page 91
Jesse Winter: pages 50–51
James Wojcik: pages 23–33
YOCO: page 71

Illustrations

James Archer: page 268
Bryan Christie: page 125
Josh McKible: page 223
Mark Watkinson: page 224
YOCO: page 71

Age Erasers

Index

Boldface page references indicate photographs or illustrations.
Underscored references indicate boxed text.

A

Abdominal muscles
    activities for shaping,
        244–49
    anatomy, **237**
    benefits of strong, 236
    exercises for, 250–55,
        250–55
    interval training, 248
    rules for flat, 232–36
Abdominal rotation, 45, **45**
Acne, treatment of, 64, 312
Acupressure, 184
Adenosine, 178
Adrenaline, 211
Adventure sports, 211
Age Erasers Score, 2–9
    Fitness Age, 4–5
    Heart Age, 8
    Mental Age, 9
    Skin Age, 6–7
Agent Provacateur Strip
    Poker, 119
AHA, 312
Airplane/superman
    extension, 46, **46**
Alcohol consumption, effects
    of, 149, 183, 215
All-fours kickback, 141–42
Aloe, 65
Alphagon, 73
Alpha hydroxy acid (AHA),
    312

Alpha-linolenic acid, 25
Alzheimer's disease, 170
Angiogram, 274, 277
Anterior cruciate ligament, 22
Anthocyanins, 31
Antiaging serum, 63
Antidepressants, 25
Antioxidants, 19, 32–34. *See
    also specific antioxidants*
Anxiety, effect on libido,
    100–101
Apples, 30, 172, 276
Arctic char, 18, 294
Arms, toning, **223**
Arthritis, 45
Artificial tears, 73
Asparagus, 20
Aspirin, 276, 288
Avobenzone, 62
Avocados, 216, 288

B

Back pain, 171–72, 184
Bagels, whole grain, 216
Baked potatoes, 219
Baking soda, 78
Balance
    exercises for improving,
        211
    measuring, 4
Balance pushup, 4

Balancing squat, 133
Bananas, 96, 216
Barbell back squat, 49, **49**
Barbells, vaginal, 88–89
Bar bridge, 226, **226**
Bartholin's glands, 86
Beans, 26–27
Beauty guide, 306–8
Beef
    grass-fed, 20
    as iron source, 20
    as muscle food, 22
    Tex-Mex salad, 22, 24
Belly fat, 240, 242, 275
Bent-over row, 223, **223**
Benzoyl peroxide, 65
Berries
    antioxidants in, 218
    for brain health, 31
Biological clock, 180–81
Birth control, libido loss and,
    104–6
Black beans, 288
Blackberries, 31
Bladder
    strengthening control
        with sexual activity, 88
    stress of holding full, 285
Bleaching teeth, 79
Bloat, 234
Bloodflow, increasing with
    yoga, 93